Computed Tomography of Congenital Brain Malformations

Computed Tomography of Congenital Brain Malformations

By

MOHAMMAD SARWAR, M.D.

Associate Professor of Diagnostic Radiology
Section of Neuroradiology
Yale University School of Medicine
New Haven, CT

1985
MARTINUS NIJHOFF PUBLISHING
A MEMBER OF THE KLUWER ACADEMIC PUBLISHERS GROUP
BOSTON/THE HAGUE/DORDRECHT/LANCASTER

Published by

WARREN H. GREEN, INC.
8356 Olive Blvd.
St. Louis, Missouir 63132
U.S.A.

Sole distributor outside the U.S.A. and Canada
KLUWER ACADEMIC PUBLISHERS GROUP
Distribution Centre
P.O. Box 322
3300 AH Dordrecht
The Netherlands

ISBN No. 0-8527-231-2

Printed in the United States of America

DEDICATION

I dedicate this book to the loving memory of my father and to my adorable wife, Zahida, and our three precious daughters, Huma, Sadiya and Sina.

Preface

Computed tomography (CT) interpretation of congenital malformations of the brain can be quite a difficult and an intimidating task. This book has been written to help allay that intimidation and make CT interpretation of these disorders easier. The embryologic and pathogenetic aspects of these malformations are not clearly defined in every instance; I have tried to present in this work these aspects as I understand them. I hope I have accomplished my objective.

Acknowledgments

I gratefully acknowledge the superb editorial assistance of Joan Wallace, manuscript typing by Eve VanDine and Susan Morrissey, and the preparation of the illustrations by Tom McCarthy and Ann Curley.

Last, but not least, I appreciate the understanding shown by my family during the long preparation of this work.

Contents

Computed Tomography of Congenital Brain Malformations

1

Introduction

Central nervous system (CNS) malformations constitute an important aspect of neurologic diseases; nearly 2,000 such entities are recognized at present. They occur in almost one percent of all live births (80–100/10,000 live births) and represent at least ten percent of all systemic malformations. Approximately 75 percent of fetal deaths, 40 percent of infant deaths and .05 percent of deaths in children under one year of age are caused by CNS disorders. However, clinically encountered CNS malformations are relatively mild; the more severe forms are incompatible with life and are discarded by nature as abortions. As a whole, these malformations occur in about two percent of all conceptions. Concurrent with the successful control of many diseases (e.g., infections) of infancy and childhood is an increase in the relative incidence of morbidity and mortality due to CNS malformations. Only about half of the CNS malformations are recognizable at birth or in the newborn; others become manifest as the child develops. It is well-recognized that many disorders remain silent for years to decades or until the morbid process converts the malformation into a disease. Incidence of major congenital disorders of the brain are shown in Table I.

ETIOLOGY

Basically, the development of CNS malformations is governed by genetic changes that occur before or soon after conception and by environmental factors operating between conception and birth. The main causes of congenital disorders of the brain are indicated below (6).

1. Genetic factors and chromosomal aberration
2. Irradiation
3. Infections (Torch*)
4. Environmental
5. Drugs
    - Thalidomide
    - Cortisone, ACTH
    - Methotrexate
    - Hypervitaminosis A
    - Anticonvulsants
    - Cyclophosphamide
    - Masculinizing progesterones and estrogens
    - Fetal alcohol syndrome
6. Maternal Disorders
    - Diabetes
    - Hypoxia
    - Endemic goitre and cretinism
    - Phenylketonuria
    - Vitamin A deficiency
    - Carbon monoxide, Lead and Mercury poisoning

*Torch (Toxoplasmosis, Rubella, Cytomegalic inclusion disease, and Herpes simplex encephalitis).

Absence of histologic changes (e.g., inflammatory cellular response and glial reaction) does not exclude a noxious agent (e.g., infection) as the underlying cause of CNS malformation, since the immature immune system at the embryonic and early fetal stage offers little or no defense (7,8). That is, the earlier in gestation that a noxious process occurs, the less effective the defensive cellular reaction will be as judged by the presence or absence of lipid-filled macrophages and proliferation of astrocytes. It has been shown that the immature brain reacts only one way to a necrotizing damage from whatever cause; there is almost traceless resorption (resolution) of the brain parenchyma – only glia-lined cavities and sclerotic microgyria (ulegyria) remain around the defects. Observations in animals have indicated that intrauterine viral infections can cause a variety of CNS malformations resembling those seen in humans, e.g., hydrencephaly, Arnold-Chiari malformation, myeloschisis and aqueductal stenosis.

TABLE I
INCIDENCE OF VARIOUS CNS MALFORMATIONS (After Myrianthopoulos (1))

Name	Incidence	Comment
Arnold-Chiari Malformation	If one considers that almost all patients with neural tube defects (spina bifida= Myelo-Meningocele) and hydrocephalus have Arnold-Chiari malformation as well then its incidence would be about 10/10,000 births. Incidence without associated spina bifida is less than 1/10,000 births	Prenatal detection of neural tube defects is possible in about 95% of cases by assaying amniotic fluid for A-feto-protein (AFP)
Dandy-Walker Syndrome	0.25-0.5/10,000 births	In hydrocephalus patients, its incidence is about 2-4% (2,3)
Dysgenesis of the Corpus Callosum	Less that 1/10,000 births	The reported incidence seems to be far less than actually encountered in clinical practice. As more and more children are being examined with CT scanning, this entity is being recognized more often. Unless this malformation is part of a chromosomal aberration, it is compatible with life. A great majority of these patients show no symptoms unless thoroughly examined by specialized neuropsychiatric testing.
Holoprosencephaly	Incidence varies with type. Overall incidence is less that 1/10,000 births	Somewhat more common in females. Parental consanguinity with autosomal recessive inheritance is reported in some families.
Hydrocephalus	In different countries its incidence varies. In the United States its incidence is about 15-17/10,000 births; in about 1/2 to 1/3 of these patients there is associated spina bifida. The incidence in Dublin is 35/10,000 and in Japan 2-3/10,000 births.	Associated commonly with other serious malformations of the brain. It shows considerable ethnic, geographic and sex variation.
Hydrencephaly	0.5-1/10,000 births	Rare cases of genetic origin have been described.
Neurocutaneous Syndromes (Phakomatoses)		
1. von Recklinghausen neurofibromatosis	4/10,000 births (It is difficult to diagnose in infancy).	Autosomal dominant inheritance. 58% have family history. Sporadic cases are from new mutations.
2. Tuberous Sclerosis	0.2-0.3/10,000 births or 1/300,000 to 500,000 population.	Comprises about 0.1-0.6% of inmates in mentally retarded institutions.
3. Sturge-Weber Syndrome	Less than 1/10,000 births	About 0.1% incidence in inmates of institutions for mentally retarded.
4. von Hippel-Lindau Syndrome	No known figures	Approximately 20% of cases have family history – autosomal dominant inheritance.
Encephalocele/Meningocele	2/10,000 births	Shows practically no ethnic, geographic, or sex variation. About 3/4 of cases of occipital encephalocele are females; anterior encephalocele/meningocele occurs more often in males.

Anencephaly	Overall incidence is about 6-7/10,000 births. Incidence varies in different countries and races, e.g., in USA it is 10/10,000 births, in Belfast 45-70/10,000 births and in Egypt 40/10,000 births.	Shows great variation according to geography, race and ethnic background. More common in whites than in negroes in the USA (white to negro ratio is 4 to 1). Associated spina bifida occurs in at least 10-50% of cases.
Craniosynostosis	Reported incidence varies widely; no good data available. From Cooperative Perinatal Project its incidence seems to be about 5/10,000 births.	Has male predominance (male to female ratio is 3 to 1). Genetic factors are important in its etiology.
Porencephaly	About 1/10,000 births	Associated with other CNS malformations in about 10% of cases.
Chromosomal anomalies		
1. Down Syndrome (Trisomy 21)	10-20/10,000 births	
2. Trisomy 13 Syndrome	2/10,000 births	
3. Trisomy 18 Syndrome	2/10,000 births	
Orbital Hypertelorism	About 10/10,000 births	
Iniencephaly	About 2-6/10,000 births	According to Warkarny (4) iniencephaly more common in areas where anencephaly is common. About 90% of cases are females.
Congenital tumors of the brain	Less than 1/10,000 births	
Agenesis and cavum of the septum pellucidum; cavum vergae; cavum velum interpositum	1. Agenesis of septum pellucidum. In PEG series, its incidence varies from 0.2-0.3/10,000 births 2. Cavum septum pellucidum. In formalin fixed brains, its incidence has been reported at 20% 3. Cavum vergae. In formalin fixed brains, its incidence is about 2.3%. It is hardly ever present without the concomitant presence of cavum septum pellucidum. 4. Cavum velum interpositum. Rarely found in children over two years of age; not as rare in mentally retarded children	The incidence of cavum septum pellucidum diminishes with age. It is seen on CT scan in a great majority of premature infants. Its incidence on CT scan has been reported at 10% under one year, 5-6% at 2 to 5 years, 2-7% at 6 to 9 years and 2-3% at 10 to 14 years (5).
Micrencephaly	1-5/10,000 births. True ("genetic"): 0.5/10,000 births.	Frequently associated with other CNS malformations. "Genetic" type can be free of other CNS malformations.
Aqueductal stanosis	2/10,000 births	Responsible for about 15-20% of cases of hydrocephalus. Sex-linked recessive inheritance known.

TERATOGENESIS

The vast majority of congenital malformations occur in the embryonic stage (before 8 weeks); this is the period when major organogenesis takes place. It has been suggested that injury to the neural crest may be the cause of major congenital malformations. As the process of differentiation proceeds and becomes more established, the susceptibility to teratogenesis diminishes. A very small number of genes impart "class instructions" for many different cellular interactions, and these few genes then control the detailed structure of a large number of neurons. Thus, it is not difficult to understand how genetic disorders can lead to various and complex morphologic alterations resulting in congenital malformations of the CNS and of other parts of the body.

Environmental factors also seem important in the etiology of congenital malformations. It has been shown in the chick embryo that oxygen deficiency can interfere with normal development. Also, neural defects have been induced in mammals (mice, hamsters) by hypervitaminesis A. It is well established that during the period of brain growth spurt (from mid-gestation to 2-3 years after birth) the brain is especially vulnerable to the deleterious effects of nutritional deprivation, inborn errors of metabolism, irradiation and endocrine imbalance (9). It should be noted that in addition to the effects of a teratogen at a certain developmental period, the nature and dose of the noxious agent and the genotype have a major bearing on teratogenesis.

Considering the complex processes involved in the development of the brain, it is indeed surprising that we do not encounter more errors in its morphology. It seems more likely that we are as yet incapable of recognizing many of these disorders.

METHODS OF DIAGNOSIS

The radiologic diagnosis of these CNS manformations is highly important in prognosis and genetic counseling. Non-radiologic methods have been used to diagnose CNS malformations, but their use is not yet extensive and their overall yield is low. Such techniques include fetoscopy, amniocentesis (e.g., analysis of alphfetoprotein for neural tube closure defects; this is useful in 85-95% of cases), and culture of fetal cells. CT scanning is now widely used for the investigation of neurological diseases. This modality has played an important role in the early investigation and morphologic characterization of most of the major CNS disorders. It has made air studies obsolete. However, CT scanning after introduction of a small dose of Metrizamide into the ventricular system or the subarachnoid space helps in establishing whether or not a cystic lesion communicates with either. Although angiography can add significant information in the overall morphologic analysis of these complex malformations, possible complications preclude more frequent use. It is hoped that digital subtraction angiography will be employed relatively more often in the assessment of, at least, the very bizarre and confusing malformations. Ultrasonography has a very promising future role in the investigation of these disorders (10,11). Nuclear Magnetic Resonance (NMR) is expected to provide a revolutionary insight into the morphology and chemical constitution of these disorders.

Malformations in which the role of CT scanning has been clearly established are discussed at length in the chapters to follow; those in which the CT scan provides marginal assistance are alluded to briefly.

REFERENCES

1. Myrianthopoulos NC: Epidemiology of central nervous system malformations. In: Viken PJ, Bruyn GW, eds. *Handbook of Clinical Neurology,* Vol 30, p. 139, Amsterdam, Elsevier/North-Holland Biomedical Press, 1977.
2. Raimondi J, Samuelson G, Yaszagary G, Norton T: Atresia of the foramina of Luschka and Magendie: the Dandy-Walker cyst. *J Neurosurg* 31:202-216, 1969.
3. LaTorre E, Fortuna A, Occhip E: Angiographic differentiation between Dandy-Walker cyst and arachnoid cyst of the posterior fossa in newborn infants and children. *J Neurosurg* 38:298-308, 1973.
4. Warkany J: *Congenital Malformations. Notes and Comments.* Year Book Med Publisher, Inc. 1971.
5. Nakano S, Hojo H, Kataoka K, Yamasaki S: Age related incidence of cavum septi pellucidi and cavum vergae on CT scans of pediatric patients. *J Computer Assist Tomogr* 5:348-349, 1981.
6. Melnick M: The etiologies of central nervous system malformations. In: Viken PJ, Bruyn GW, eds. *Handbook of Clinical Neurology,* Vol 30, p. 85, Amsterdam, Elsevier/North-Holland Biomedical Press, 1977.
7. Johnson RT: Effects of viral infection on the developing nervous system. *N Engl J Med* 287:599-604, 1972.
8. Thompson JA, Glasgow LA: Intrauterine viral infection and the cell-mediated immune response. *Neurology* 30:212-215, 1980.
9. Dobbing J, Sands J: Quantitative growth and development of human brain. *Arch Dis Child* 48:757-767, 1973.
10. Mack LA, Rumack CM, Johnson ML: Ultrasound evaluation of cystic intracranial lesions in the neonate. *Radiology* 137:451-455, 1980.
11. Babcock DS, Bokyung KH: *Cranial Untrasonography of Infants.* Williams and Wilkins, Baltimore/London, 1982.

2

Embryology of the Central Nervous System

A basic understanding of the embryology of the central nervous system is necessary to appreciate the dysmorphology of congenital malformations of the brain and attendant neurologic dysfunction. The number of neurons at birth is 100 billion. Since there is little increase in that number after birth, the rate of neuron production can be estimated at 250,000/min. The glial cells number about one trillion. Because the brain must pass through several critical processes during its development, its liability to morphologic alteration and physiologic dysfunction is high.

These processes are as follows:

i) Induction of the neural tube.
ii) Cell proliferation in different regions.
iii) Migration of cells to their place of normal residence.
iv) Aggregation of cells to form definite structures.
v) Neural differentiation.
vi) Interneuronal connection.
vii) Selective death of certain cells.
viii) Elimination of some and stabilization of other cell populations.

The three germ layers – ectoderm, mesoderm and entoderm – are recognizable by the second week. At this point, the mesoderm induces the midline ectoderm to transform into the **neural tube**. In the third week, the ectodermally derived neural plate, induced by the mesoderm and ectodermally derived notochord, forms a longitudinal groove that exhibits external features of the future brain, brainstem and spinal cord. The neural folds demonstrate continuing apposition. Commencing in the primordial cervical region and proceeding cephalad and caudad, these folds fuse dorsally to enclose the neural tube during the foruth week (Fig. 1). The cephalic end of the closed neural tube then **dilates into three primary vesicles – the prosencephalon** (forebrain), the **mesencephalon** (midbrain) and the **rhombencephalon** (hindbrain) (Fig. 2). These vesicles undergo further subdivisions to form all the brain structures (Fig. 3). Defective closure of the neural tube at the anterior neuropore leads to anencephaly.

(cerebral hemispheres) in man exhibits the most striking morphologic changes, growing rapidly and overlapping almost the entire brain by about the seventh month of fetal life. These cerebral hemispheres are separated by falx, which develops from a thin layer of mesoblast. Corpus striatum develops from the ventro-lateral telencephalic wall. The layered pattern of the brain is formed as early as the fourth month of gestation; regional differences begin to appear at about the fifth month of gestation. It may be pointed out that at about 50 days of gestation, the cerebral hemispheres, basal ganglia, thalamus, autonomic nervous system, eyes and cerebral blood vessels are well-differentiated.

Concomitant with changes in size and shape of the brain (Fig. 4), adaptive changes occur in the brain cavities (ventricles). Prior to 20 weeks gestation, the ventricles normally occupy more than 50 percent of the hemispheres. These cavities progressively diminish in size as the brain increases in volume (Fig. 5). The relatively wide communication between the lateral ventricles and the third ventricle narrows to form the interventricular foramen (one on either side). The outlet foramina of the fourth ventricle are formed at the third month of gestation.

The prosencephalon (forebrain) is divided into its two components – telencephalon and diencephalon – by about the 36th day of gestation. The telencephalic vesicles (which lead to the formation of recognizable cerebral hemispheres by the third gestational month) extend anterior to the cephalic end (the lamina terminalis) of the neural tube. The telencephalon

In the fourth week, the foregut entoderm elaborates to create anlage for facial structures. This process is influenced by cephalic neural tube (anlage for telencephalon) and by cephalic mesoderm (anlage for facial bones and skull). Proper development of the brain, skull and facial skeleton depends on the intricate interplay of various inductive processes among the three germ layers. Any process that impairs such induction results in facio-telencephalopathy (holoprosencephaly).

Cell proliferation occurs at the subventricular level; this cell population, called germinal matrix, is

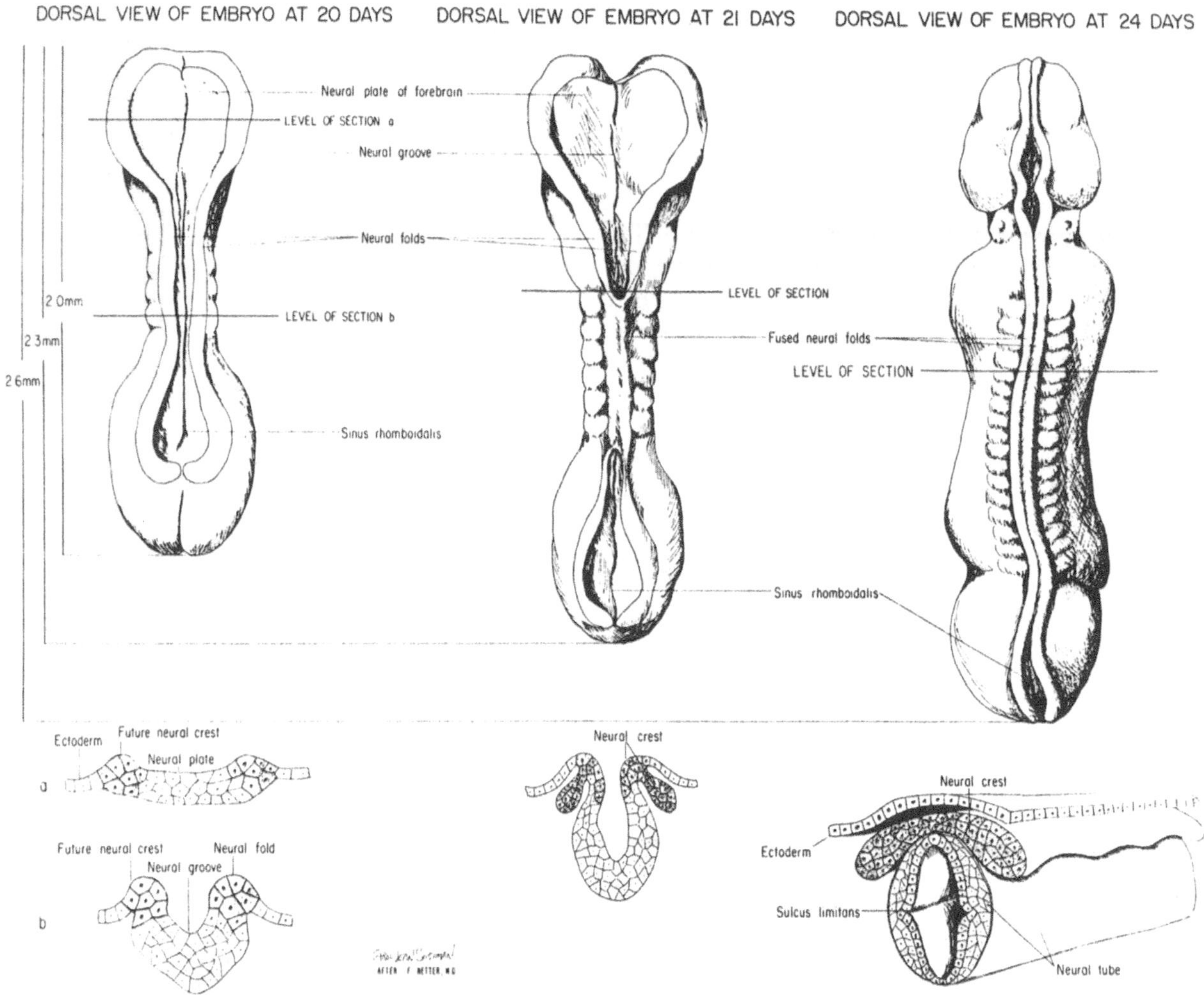

Figure 1. Neural tube (redrawn from *Clinical Symposia* (3) with permission).

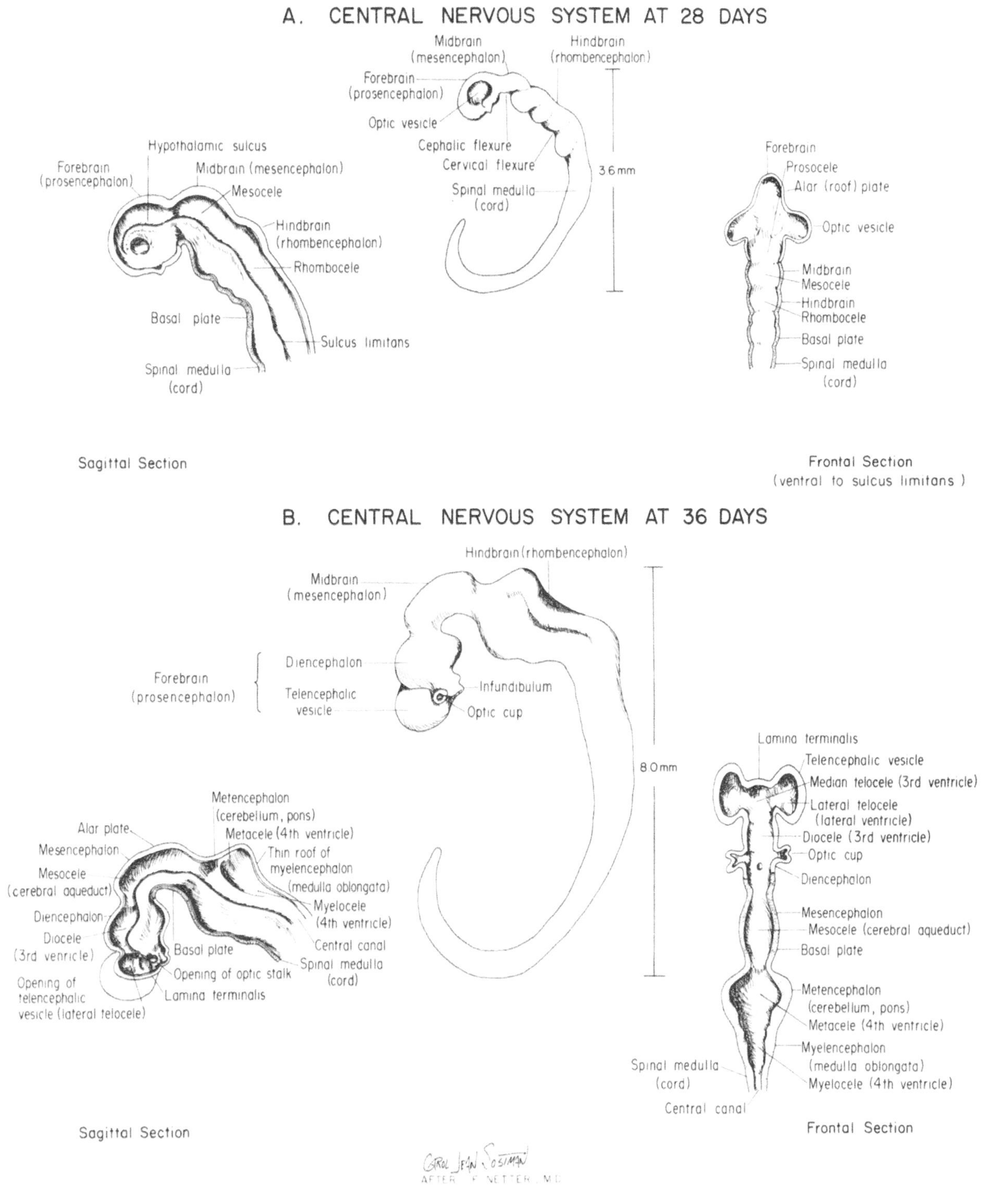

Figure 2. Developing central nervous system. (Redrawn from *Clinical Symposia* (3) with permission.)

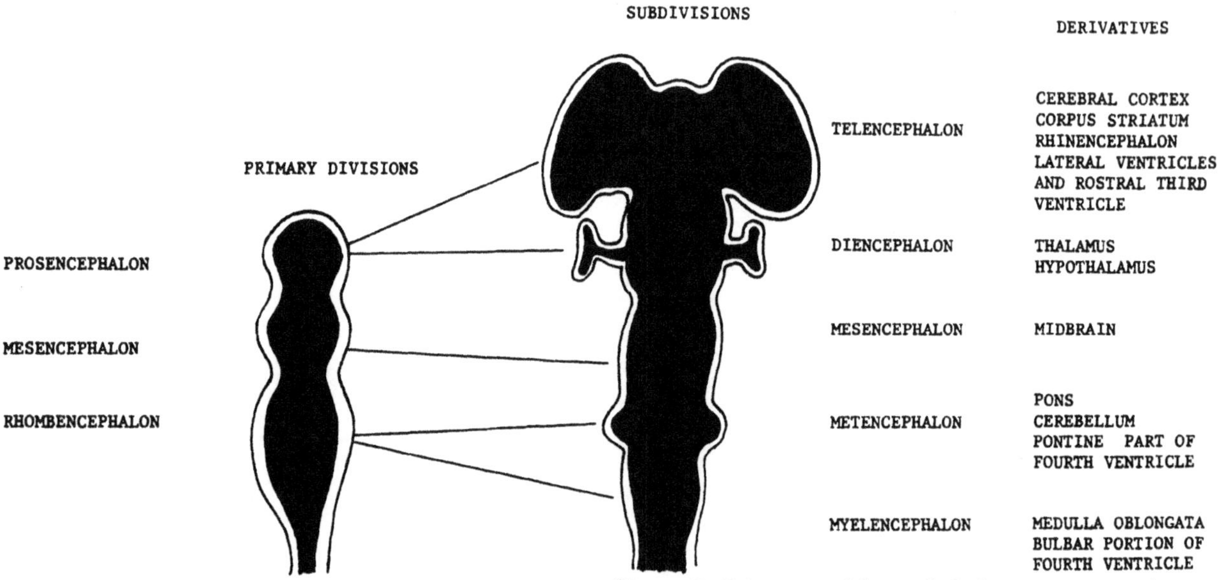

Figure 3. Primary vesicles and their secondary divisions and derivatives.

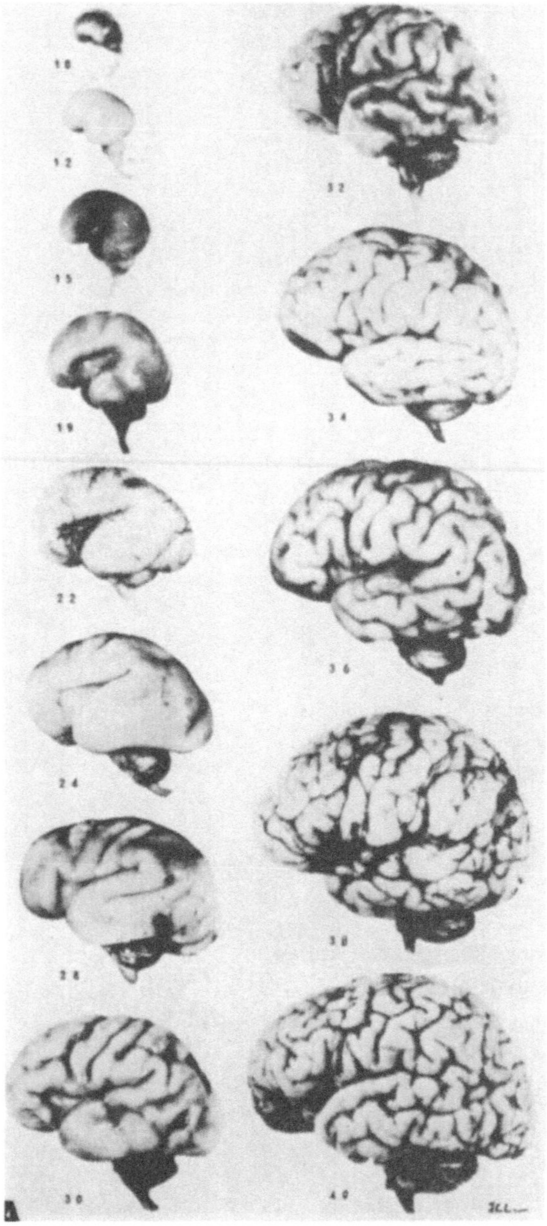

Figure 4. Developing brain. A) Lateral aspect of the developing brain from 10-40 weeks. (Taken from (5)

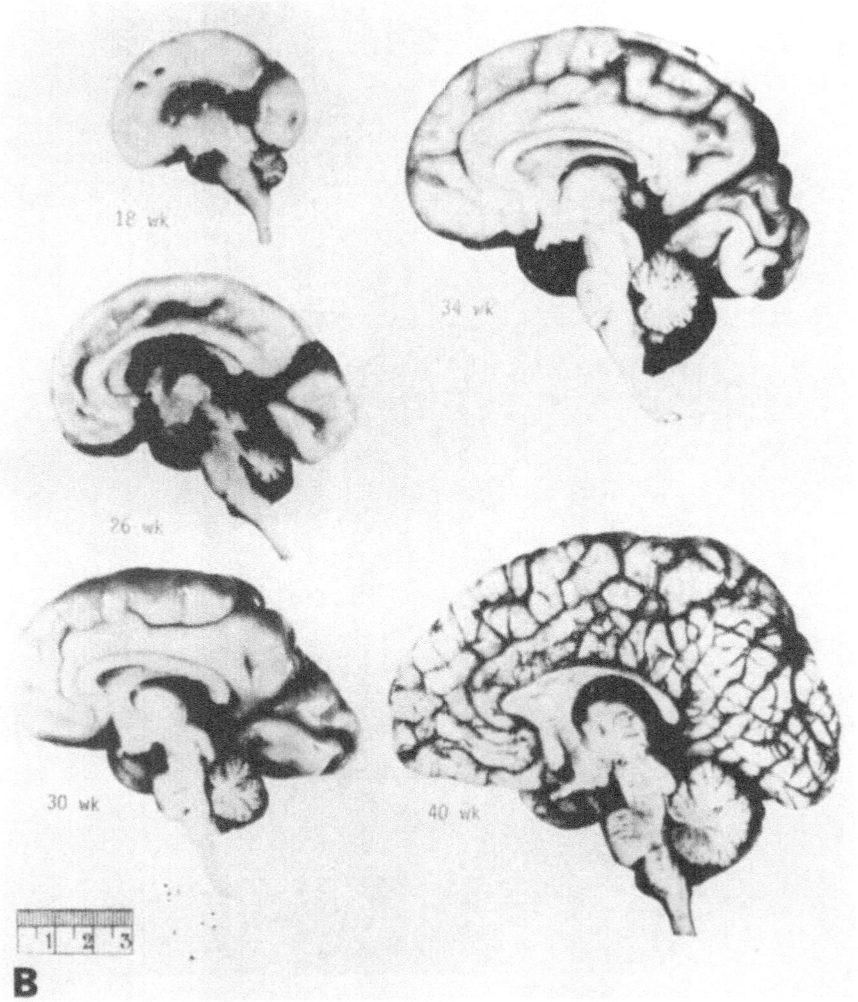

Figure 4. Developing brain. B) Medial aspect of the developing brain from 18–40 weeks. (Taken from (5) with permission.)

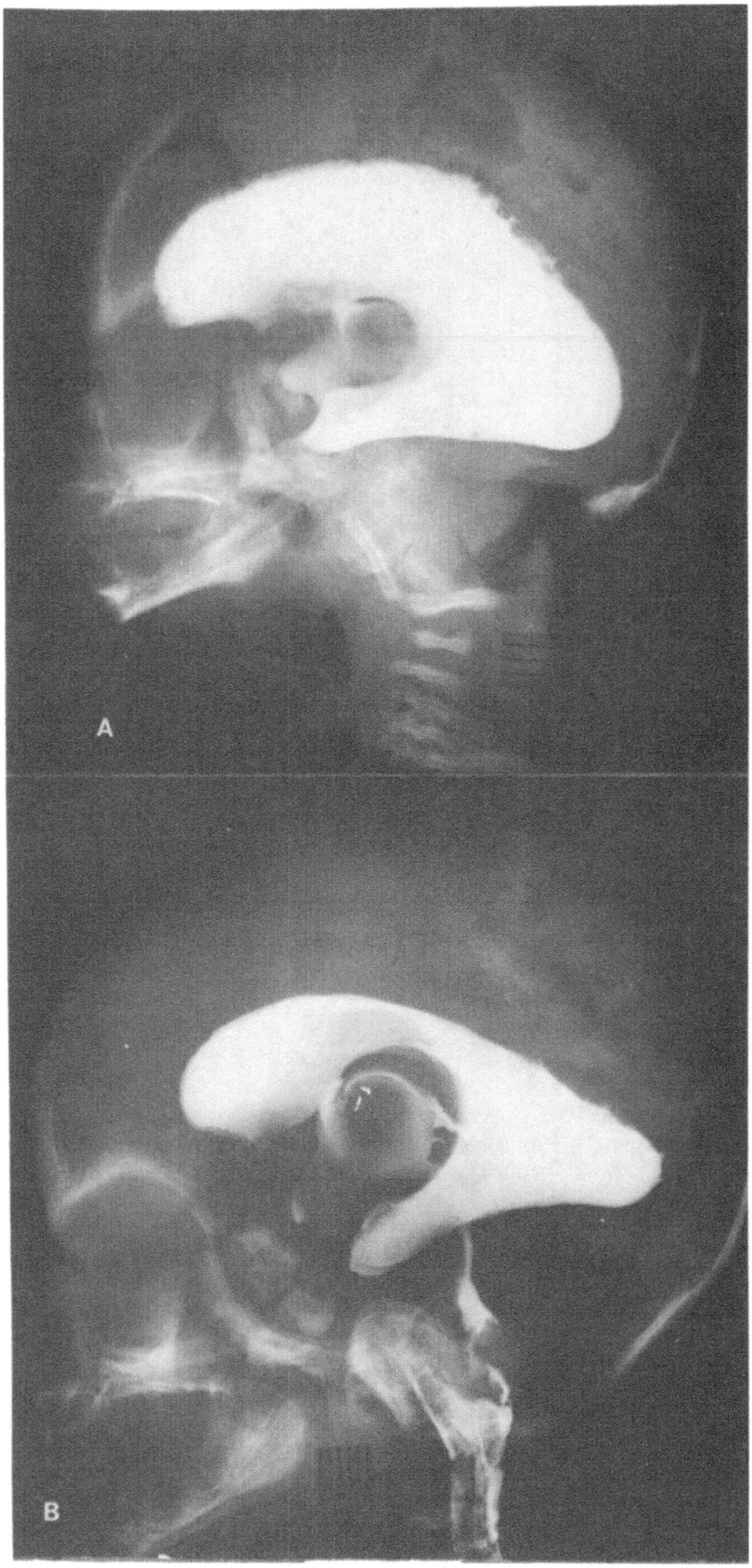

Figure 5. Barium-cast of the human ventricular system. A) 16-week fetus and B) 24-week fetus. Note that at 16 weeks gestation, lateral ventricles fill a far larger portion of the cranial cavity than at 24 weeks. The ventricular system gradually becomes smaller as the brain grows. (From Kier EL: The cerebral ventricles: A phylogenetic and ontogenetic study. In Newton TH, Potts DG, eds: *Radiology of the Skull and Brain, Vol. III. Anatomy and Pathology*, St. Louis, 1977, The C.V. Mosby Co., with permission.)

particularly well-developed along the frontal horns. These cells migrate to the periphery with each successive generation progressing further than the preceding one. The migration process occurs at a rate of 1/10mm per day and appears to be amoeboid. The complexity of neuronal organization can lead to developmental disorders of the cerebral cortex, which may be manifested in a variety of ways. Brain dysmorphogenesis may be caused by defects in gyration (micropolygyria), cortical organization (disruption of normal cortical lamination), cell migration (heterotopia of gray matter), and in cell proliferation (astrocytosis). Neuronal ectopias, although commonly seen in association with other CNS malformations, can be present in apparently normal brains.

The cerebral convolutions are nature's ingenious way of providing an area of about 2300 cm^2 to the cerebral cortex, which varies in thickness from 1.5 to 4mm (Fig. 6). The sylvian fissure is the first fissure to form; it develops by the tethering effect of the basal ganglia and is recognizable by the third gestational month. Secondary and tertiary sulci, peculiar to the human brain, develop in the final months of fetal life (Table I).

TABLE I
CHRONOLOGY OF FORMATION OF FISSURES

Fetal Months	Name of Fissure
3	Sylvian
4	Rhinal, hippocampal
5	Rolandic, calcarine, and parieto-occipital
6	Precentral, superior temporal, olfactory, orbital, and callosomarginal
7	Superior frontal, inferior temporal, and occipital
8-9	Secondary and tertiary sulci

While the primitive fissures – the Sylvian, hippocampal, parieto-occipital, calcarine and collateral sulcus – are formed by infolding of the entire hemispheric vesicle wall, the sulci that develop later are merely depressions in the surface of the cerebral hemisphere. Development of the sulci and gyri results in tortuosity of the originally straight cortical vessels. In addition to sulcal and gyral growth, overlapping of the fronto-parietal operculum produces the Sylvian triangle. Lack of undulations in the branches of the middle cerebral artery indicates defective gyral development - agyria (Lissencephaly = smooth brain). Failure of the cerebral hemispheric operculum to form results in unprotected insula. An open or gaping insula, therefore, indicates cerebral hypoplasia.

VENTRICULAR SYSTEM AND CHOROID PLEXUS

The interconnecting ventricular system is formed by modification of the primary lumen of the neural tube. Closure of the neuropores marks the earliest form of the ventricular system (Fig. 7). The thinned roof of the hindbrain at 26 days indicates the site of the fourth ventricle; within a week, the lateral recesses of the fourth ventricle become recognizable. The median aperture becomes differentiated and probably is functional by about 51 days. The third ventrical is defined gradually, beginning at about the 37th day. The interventricular foramina (IVF's) are recognizable by about the 41st day. The choroid plexus of the lateral ventricles begins to form at about 42-44 days of gestation. The IVF's become narrowed at about the seventh week. Whereas the V-shape of the lateral ventricles (as seen from the side) is obvious at about 12 weeks of gestation, the posterior horns develop late (18 weeks). The ventricles do not become slender until about 32 weeks. The definite shape and structure of the lateral ventricles is attained by the fifth to sixth month of prenatal life. The cavity of the midbrain (aqueduct) is relatively wide in the embryonic period, but becomes a narrow canal during the early fetal period.

"Physiologic hydrocephalus" (during vesicular stage) is gradually reduced due to increased thickness of the cerebral mantle (neocortex) – beginning mainly at about four months of gestation. In immature and very young infants, slightly dilated lateral ventricles, especially the temporal horns, do not imply atrophy, hypoplasia or hydrocephalus, but are a sign of immaturity of the brain. Occipital horns as distinct structures are present only in primates and in man. The size of the occipital horns is determined by the growth of the periventricular white matter which includes forceps major (tapetum) of corpus callosum and optic radiations. Their size also is influenced by the calcarine fissures, which are among the first to appear, together with the parieto-occipital fissures, at the 18th to 20th week of gestation. The choroid plexus is formed by invagination of the ependymal cells accompanied by the choroidal vessels and the adjacent pia mater.

BASAL GANGLIA AND THALAMUS

Generally, it is believed that the basal ganglia are entirely of telencephalic origin and that the thalamus is of diencephalic origin. Also, the globus pallidus is derived from the diencephalon.

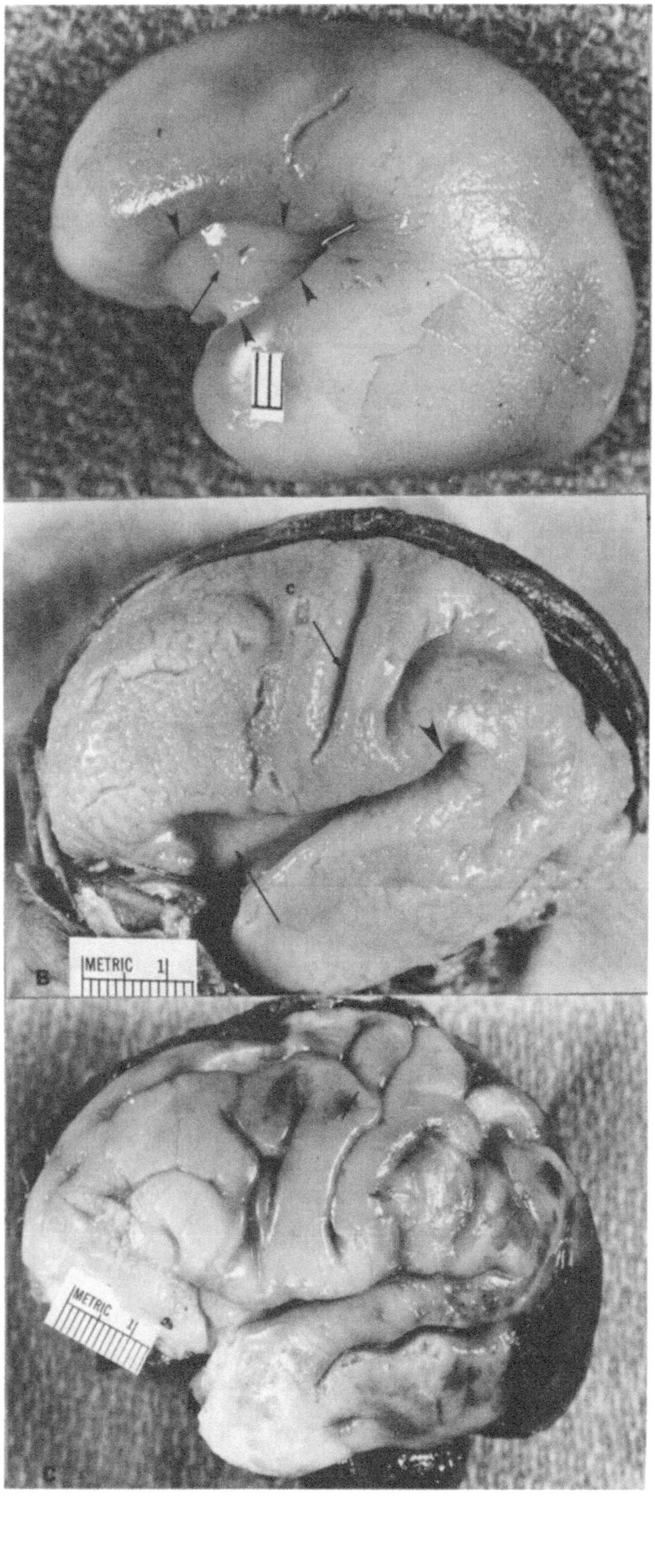

Figure 6. Lateral view of fetal cerebral hemispheres demonstrating formation of the fissures and sulci and opercularization of the sylvian fossa. A) 17-week fetus. The external surface of the cerebral hemisphere is smooth. The insula (**arrow**) can be seen through the wide open sylvian fossa (**arrowheads**). B) 24-week fetus. The insula (**arrow**) is now partially overlapped, mainly by the parietal operculum. The posterior portion of the sylvian fossa is now transformed into the sylvian fissure (**arrowhead**). C = Central Sulcus C) 32-week fetus. The insula is now almost totally covered by the parietotemporal opercula. The frontal operculum develops completely postnatally. (From Kier EL: Development of cerebral vessels. Section 1. Fetal cerebral arteries: a phylogenetic and ontogenetic study. In Newton TH, Potts DG, eds: *Radiology of the Skull and Brain. Vol. II. Angiography.* St. Louis, 1974, The C.V. Mosby Co., with permission.)

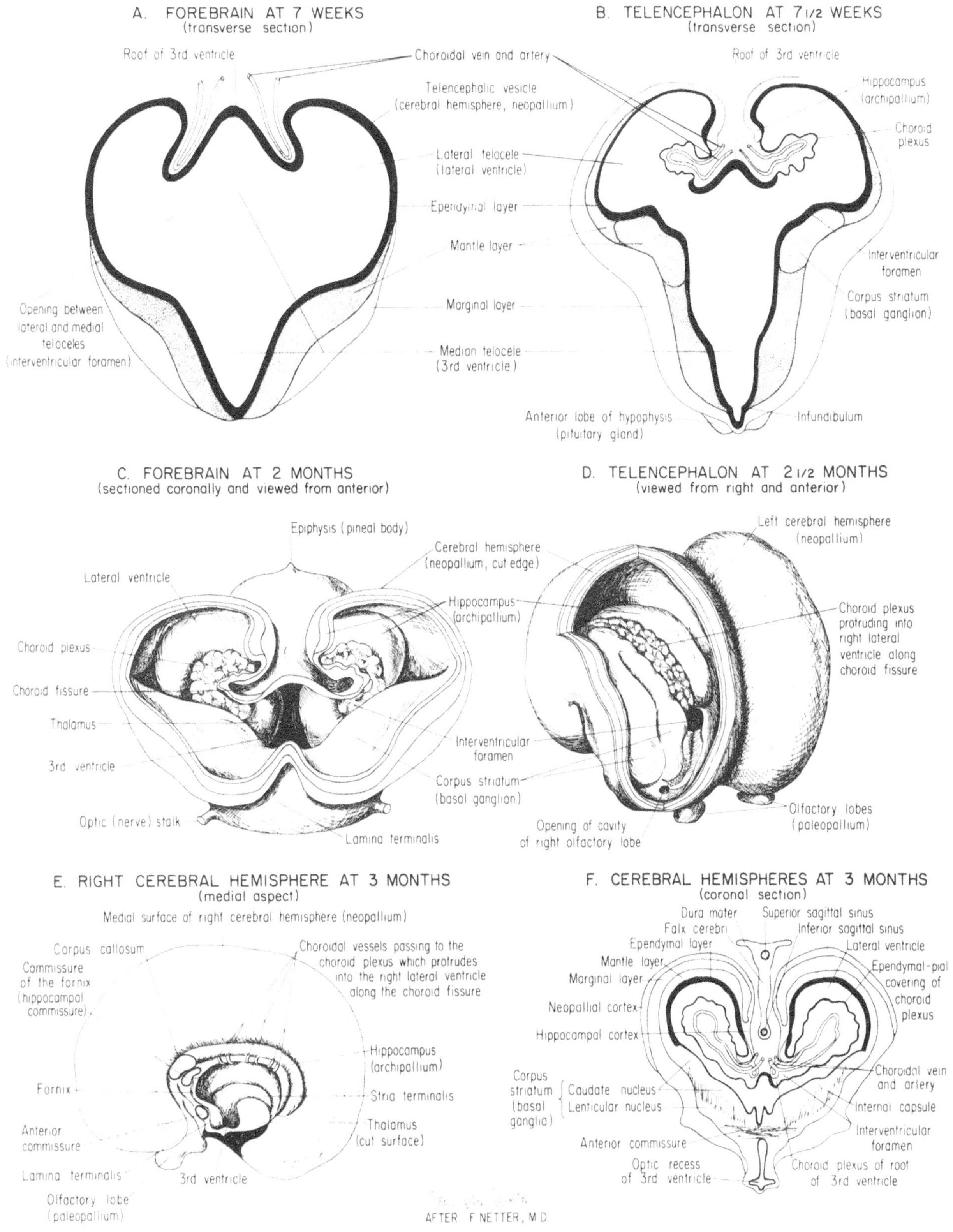

Figure 7. Developing telencephalon. (Redrawn from *Clinical Symposia* (3) with permission.)

BRAINSTEM AND CEREBELLUM

The brainstem and the spinal cord grow much more rapidly in the first half of prenatal life; the converse is true of the cerebellum. Growth of the cerebellum is completed by about 1.5-2 years of life after birth (cf: maturation of the cerebral cortex is relatively delayed, extending well into the postnatal period). Cerebellar primordia are paired structures; they soon coalesce at the midline: The medial portions form the vermis, and the cerebellar hemispheres expand rapidly on either side of the vermis. During the fourth to fifth month of gestation, the superficial parts of the cerebellum grow profusely, accounting for the numerous lobules and fissures (Fig. 8). The horizontal fissure (at fourth month of gestation) divides the cerebellar hemispheres transversely. The pons is intimately related structurally and functionally to these structures; it develops secondarily in the ventrolateral margins of the original rhombencephalon. Early in the embryo stage, its location is indicated by the pontine flexors.

Table II summarizes the main events of brain development.

TABLE II
OUTLINE OF NEUROEMBRYLOGIC DEVELOPMENT

Weeks	Length	Body Weight (in grams)	
3.5	2.5mm		Optic vesicles and auditory placodes present.
4	5mm		1) Neural tube closed. 2) Three primary brain vesicles present. 3) Olfactory placodes present.
5	8mm		Five brain vesicles.
6	12mm		Three primary flexors present
7	27mm		1) Cerebral hemispheres enlarging. 2) Prominent basal ganglia and thalami. 3) Choroid plexi forming.
8	23mm		Meninges distinct.
12	56mm		1) Confluence of sinuses attains normal location. 2) Cerebellum developed.
16	112mm		Myelination begins.
24	32cm	800	Typical layers in cerebral cortex.
28	38.5cm	1100	Cerebral fissures and convolutions.

RATE OF BRAIN GROWTH

At birth, the brain weighs 400-450 gm. It doubles its weight in one year and triples it at three to five years of age. After age five, the brain growth slows considerably; the adult weight is attained by about 7-12 years of age (Fig. 9 and 10).

DEVELOPMENTAL HISTOLOGY AND CELLULAR PROLIFERATION AND MIGRATION

The nerve cells, which themselves do not divide, originate from the periventricular (neuroepithelial) **germinal cells** (these cells form the loosely arranged periventricular germinal matrix). Germinal cells may be considered the precursors of all types of cells. Located at the ventricular surface, germinal cells give rise to neurons, while the more externally placed spongioblasts give rise to neuroglia. It is believed that germinal cells and spongioblasts are the same type of cells but that they have moved different distances from the ventricular wall during the various phases of the mitotic cycle.

An intricate system of mutually inductive processes between the three germ layers leads to formation of the brain. The major inductive processes are complete by about 30 days of gestation when cellular differentiation begins. The young neurons, which arise from the germinal cells, migrate peripherally from the ventricular surface in a radial pattern using the glial fibers as guides. Each successive neuron moves to the outside of its predecessor ("inside-out" rule). Cell migration produces white and gray matter. It follows, therefore, that CNS malformations may originate at the time of migration or during any process that impairs the migratory pattern or development of the synaptic mechanisms.

By about 25 weeks of gestation, the adult number of neurons is achieved; from thereon there is minimal, if any, further cellular proliferation. At the same time, neuronal electrical activity becomes identifiable. The process of formation of neuronal (synaptic) processes – dendrites and axons – rapidly ensues. The synaptic development continues into the second year after birth. At the time of birth, the oligodendroglia show great activity presaging postnatal myelination. By about the 12th week, the cerebral cortex is highly cellular, and programmed cell death occurs in those structures that are destined to disappear.

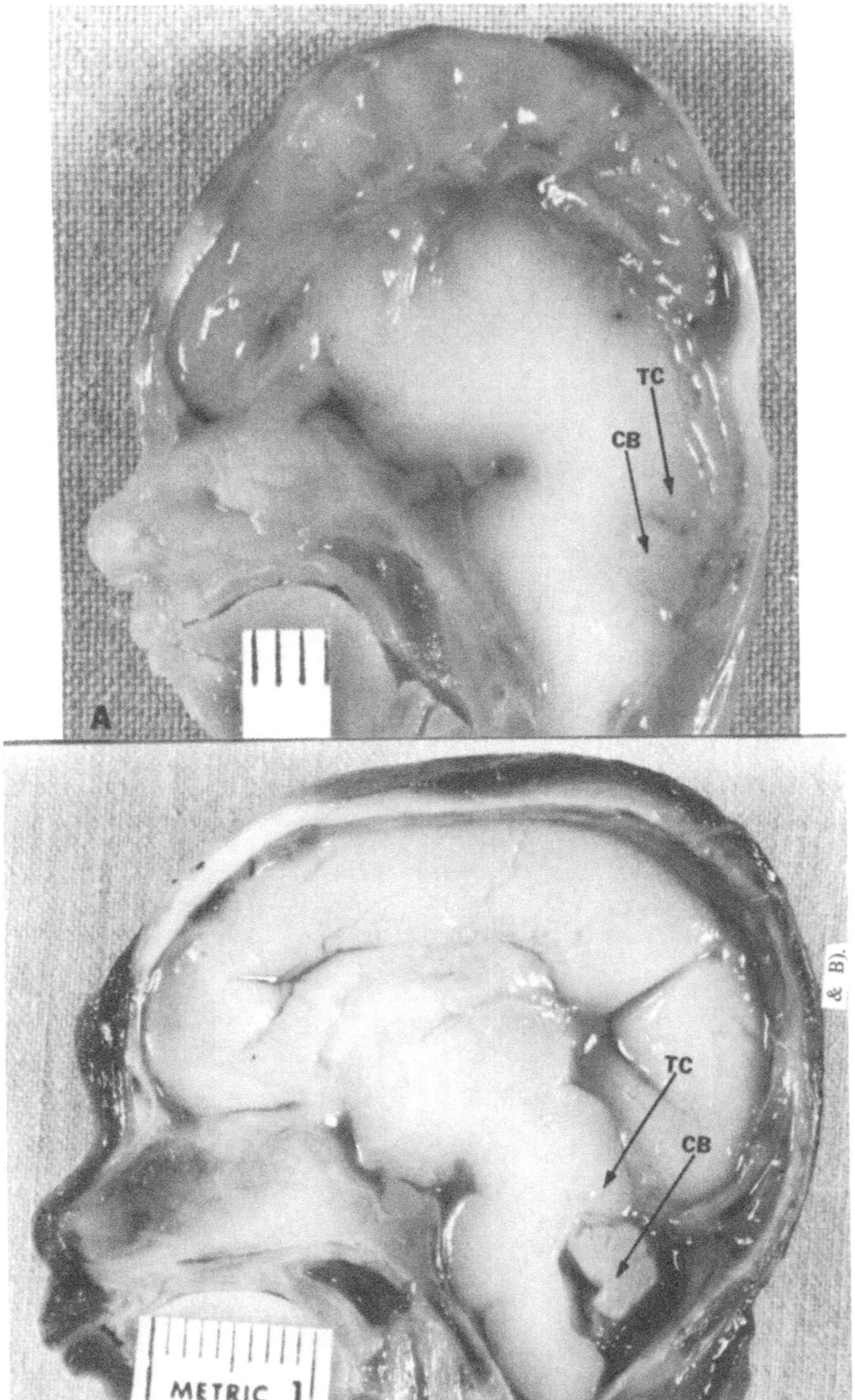

Figure 8. Sagittal sections of human fetal heads showing progressive development of the cerebellum. A) 11-week fetus; B) 15-week fetus; C) 24-week fetus; D) 30-week fetus. From its rudimentary status in A, the cerebellum (CB) attains considerable size and folial formation by 30 weeks as seen in D. The brainstem is relatively larger than the cerebrum and cerebellum in the early fetal period. Note how the tectum (TC) overlaps the cerebellum at 11 weeks and 15 weeks of gestation (A & B). The corpus callosum (CC) is recognizable at 24 and 30 weeks of gestation (C & D). Note also the progressive growth of the cerebrum (From Kier EL: The cerebral ventricles: a phylogenetic and ontogenetic study. In Newton TH, Potts DG, eds: *Radiology of the Skull and Brain. Vol. III. Anatomy and Pathology,* St. Louis, 1977, The C.V. Mosby Co., with permission.)

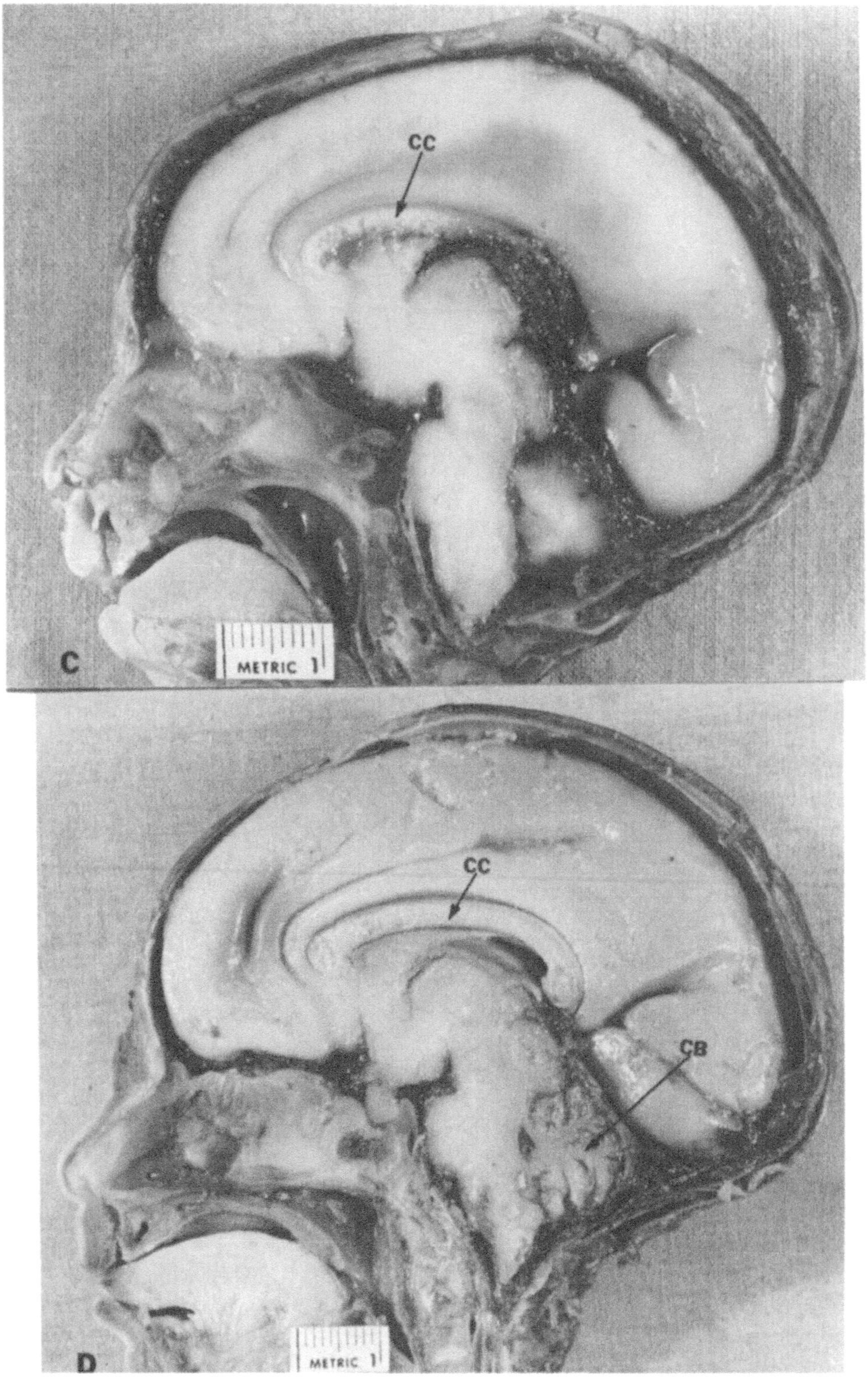

Figure 8. Sagittal sections of human fetal heads showing progressive development of the cerebellum. C) 24-week fetus, and D) 30-week fetus.

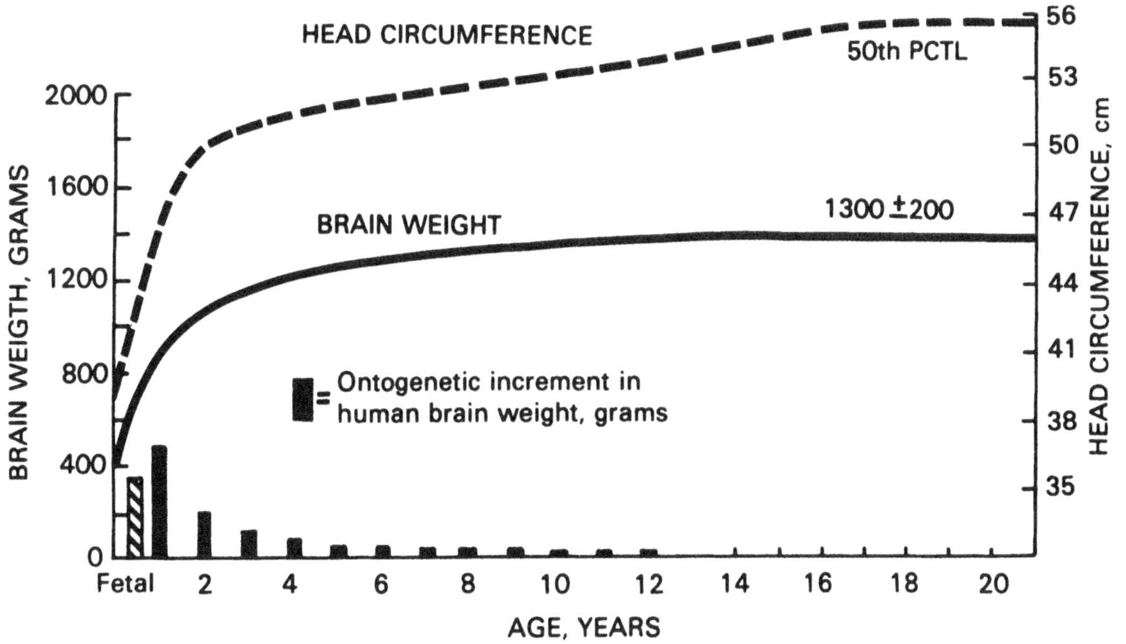

Figure 9. Early rapid growth of the brain. (From Momose JK: *Rad Cl N·Amer* 9:101, 1971, with permission.)

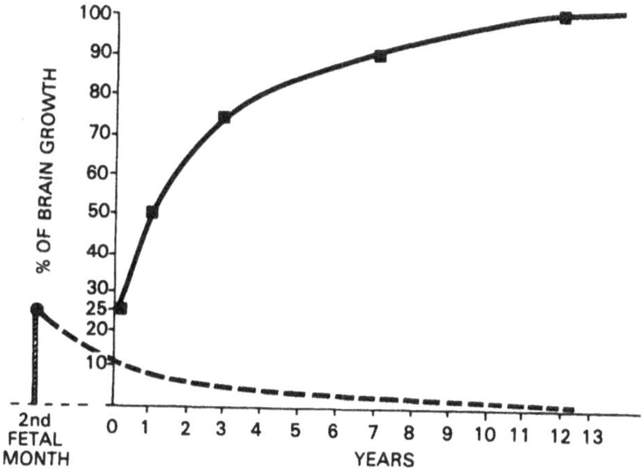

Figure 10. Brain growth. The solid line shows percent of brain growth in relation to age in years. Note its early rapid growth. The interrupted line shows that percent of brain weight compared to body weight decreases with advancing age. In other words, the brain attains maturation earlier than rest of the body.

MYELINATION

At birth and in the perinatal period, most of the white matter of the cerebral hemispheres of the full term newborn is deficient in myelin. The exceptions are a small number of fibers of the primary afferent projection system – e.g., somatic sensory fibers from the ventral posterolateral nucleus of the thalamus to the postcentral and precentral cortex and the visual and auditory fibers from the geniculate bodies to their respective cortical areas. At the end of the first month in the full term infant, nascent deposition of myelin in the corticospinal tract is recognizable. Simultaneously, a considerable number of commissural fibers of the corpus callosum become myelinated. The frontotemporal pontine fibers and the long association tracts, such as the superior occipital frontal fasciculum and cingulum, contain only a small trace of myelin sheaths at birth and in early infancy. The process of myelination, although more pronounced in the first two years after birth, continues into the early adult life. The chronology and pace of myelination of different fiber tracts is closely related to their function – i.e., the ability of the infant to acquire progressive control of its muscular movement in the first and second year of life bears close relationship to the relatively rapid pace of myelination in the latter part of the first and early part of the second postnatal year.

REFERENCES

1. Arey JB: *Developmental Neuroanatomy.* Philadelphia, Saunders, 1954.
2. Cowan WM: The development of the brain. *Scientific American* 241:113-133, 1979.
3. Crelin ED: Development of the nervous system. A logical approach to neuroanatomy. *CIBA Clinical Symposium 26:*No. 2, 1974.
4. Kier EL: The cerebral ventricles: A phylogenetic and ontogenetic study. In: Newton TH, Potts DG, eds: *Radiology of the Skull and Brain. Anatomy and Pathology.* p.2787. St. Louis, CV Mosby Co, 1977.
5. Larroche J-C: *Developmental Pathology of the Neonate.* Amsterdam, Excerpta Medica, 1977.
6. Lemire RJ, Loeser JD, Leech RW, Alvord EC, Jr: *Normal and Abnormal Development of the Human Nervous System.* Hagerstown, Harper and Row, 1975.
7. Patten BM: *Human Embryology.* 3d ed. New York, Blakiston Division, McGraw - Hill, 1968.

3

Dysgenesis of the Corpus Callosum

INTRODUCTION (1-3)

The corpus callosum is the largest commissure connecting the neopallial cortex of the cerebral hemispheres. It occupies about 11% of the supratentorial neural tissue and constitutes an important mode of cross-talk between the cerebral hemispheres. Its defective development results in a variable degree of neurologic dysfunction that often is difficult to detect clinically without sophisticated neuropsychiatric testing. Reil has been credited with first describing dysgenesis of the corpus callosum (DCC) in 1912. However, the earliest comprehensive review of the subject was provided by Bruce in 1899. Since then considerable literature has accumulated on the clinical, pathologic and radiologic aspects of this congenital malformation. Because some fiber tracts of the corpus callosum are present in all cases, the term "dysgenesis" is preferable to "agenesis." Imperfect development may involve different portions of the corpus callosum; partial dysgenesis commonly (about 70%) occurs posteriorly.

A review of the embryology and pathogenesis of the corpus callosum is essential to an understanding of the morphologic alteration and the neurologic dysfunction present in this disorder.

EMBRYOLOGY AND PATHOGENESIS (3-10)

The corpus callosum evolves as a new commissure in placental mammals and is related to an enlarged mammalian cortical mantle (neopallium). It develops from the lamina reuniens of His (the dorsal part of the anterior telencephalic wall located above the lamina terminalis). This lamina thickens (beginning at 6-8 weeks of gestation) and folds into a median groove. Juxtaposition and fusion of the lips of the groove lead to the definitive development of massa commissuralis by 9-10 weeks of gestation. The pioneer fibers of the corpus callosum then appear in the massa commissuralis (located ventral to the lamina reuniens) at 11-12 weeks of gestation; the corpus callosum is almost completely formed by 13-20 weeks. Its development proceeds rostro-caudal (from front to back) thus explaining the rarity of dysgenesis of only the anterior corpus callosum. When such dysgenesis does occur, often it is secondary (e.g., associated with lipoma of the corpus callosum, embryonal tumors and infarction). The corpus callosum malformation occurs around the 12th to 14th week of gestation.

The septum pellucidum seems to result from thinning of the lamina terminalis as the corpus callosum grows in an upward arch. Because the corpus callosum is composed of fibers emanating from the isocortex (neopallium), its formation is related closely to cortical development. The complexity of this entity explains its association with other anomalies, particularly those related to the defective development of telencephalon (i.e., holoprosencephaly complex, microgyria, gray matter heterotopia, Arnold-Chiari malformation, Dandy-Walker syndrome, encephalocele, micrencephaly, interhemispheric arachnoid cyst and septo-optic dysplasia). As indicated, seldom is the corpus callosum completely absent; some portion usually is formed. It is the commissural fibers that are missing; the decussating fibers are present invariably to some degree (e.g., the Probst's bundle, which consists of an anteroposterior oriented fiber tract). Defective development of fiber tracts (white matter) in other cerebral lobes that normally connect with corpus callosum fiber tracts is concomitant with dysgenesis of the corpus callosum.

Of the associated lesions, lipoma of the corpus callosum and interhemispheric arachnoid cyst are of particular interest. This lipoma originally was described by Rokitansky in 1856 and is associated with DCC in 30-50% of cases (11,12). Quite possibly, lipoma of the corpus callosum is a congenital lesion that either inhibits development of this commissure or destroys it after its formation. Lipoma causes almost total disruption and destruction of the callosal fibers; most cases show a variable degree of calcification. Choroid plexus lipoma in association with lipoma of the corpus callosum has been described (12). Hypertelorism may be associated with both the lipoma and DCC.

Frontal dysrhaphism in association with lipoma of the corpus callosum, an uncommon occurrence, has been described (13). This dysraphism is characterized by a frontal bony defect through which an encephalocele/ encephalomeningocele, and embryonic tumor (e.g., lipoma) or some other soft tissue mass containing an abnormal neural tissue protrudes. These frontal bone defects have been reported in 7.5 percent of lipomas of the corpus callosum (11).

Interhemispheric arachnoid cysts are rare lesions, and the majority of reported cases have been associated with DCC. If one recognizes that DCC is a manifestation of defective development of the telencephalic midline structures, then its association with interhemispheric arachnoid cyst can be understood. Dilatation of the diencephalic roof plate by hydrocephalus or intrinsic tissue failure may produce a midline cystic structure that can extend dorsally in the roof of the third ventricle. This explains the filling of the interhemispheric arachnoid cyst through the third ventricle observed during pneumoencephalography. The cyst may be partially responsible for further defective development of the corpus callosum.

ETIOLOGY

The cause of DCC remains unknown in the majority of the human cases. Experimentally, DCC has been produced in mice and rats in early gestation by maternal exposure to irradiation and by maternal diet deficient in riboflavin. In humans, it has been reported in association with X-linked recessive genes, trisomy 13-15, occasionally trisomy 18, and the Aicardi Syndrome. Vascular, traumatic, toxic, or infectious lesions have been considered as causative in some cases. Encephaloclasia in perinatal hypoxic-ischemic encephalopathy may result in some acquired callosal defect.

CLINICAL SYMPTOMATOLOGY

The clinical symptoms of DCC vary. The usual clinical examination may not demonstrate any neurologic dysfunction in the presence of isolated DCC. However, sophisticated neuropsychiatric testing can reveal interhemispheric dissociation. Its absence in some cases of DCC probably is due to the highly developed functional capability of the anterior commissure (which indeed may be larger in such cases) and ipsilateral motor pathways (14). Common clinical symptomatology consists of seizures and mental retardation. The somewhat generalized defective development of the white matter implied by DCC certainly adds to the neurologic dysfunction associated with this lesion. The presence of other associated anomalies (e.g., Arnold-Chiari malformation and Dandy-Walker syndrome) further contribute to the clinical symptomatology. Diencephalic epilepsy (15), periodic hypothermia (16) and infantile spasms (17) have been reported in association with DCC.

In our experience, DCC is more common than generally recognized in children who present with a variable degree of mental retardation and seizure disorder. This higher incidence, of course, is due to the fact that CT scanning is now employed far more frequently in the evaluation of such children.

CT SCANNING OF DCC

Technical Considerations

In a severe case of DCC, the CT scan findings are typical and readily recognizable. However, the mild to moderate forms may escape detection if closely approximated CT scan slices are not obtained at the third and lateral ventricles level. It is, therefore, recommended that in a child under 3 years of age presenting with psychomotor retardation and/or seizure disorder, or in whom DCC is clinically suspected, the CT scan slices at ventricular level should be obtained at 3-5mm intervals. In older children and adults, 8-10mm thick slices are usually adequate to make the diagnosis. However, if the findings are doubtful, 5-10mm slices must be obtained. Whereas axial CT scans usually permit a correct diagnosis of DCC, coronal CT scan slices can add significant corroborative evidence, especially with regard to the location of the third ventricle, which may not be enlarged. Sagittal reformatted images can add another dimension to the morphology of this disorder, but probably are not needed routinely. Contrast CT scans usually are not necessary for diagnosing DCC, but can provide additional structural evidence of this malformation.

CT SCAN FINDINGS

CT scan findings (Figs. 1-7) in a typical case of DCC include a) abnormal proximity of the commonly prominent interhemispheric fissure to the anterior part of the third ventricle, b) separation of the usually dilated lateral ventricles, c) interpostion of the dilated and upwardly herniated third ventricle between them, and d) variable enlargement and abnormal separation of the interventricular foramina (Fig. 8). The first sign is the most common and the most reliable direct CT finding of DCC. The others are indirect signs of DCC. For this sign to be present, the abnormal proximity of the IHF to the third ventricle must be present in all contiguous CT slices and certain caveats observed (Figs. 9,10).

Not only are the dilated lateral ventricles in DCC separate (normally, the medial borders of the dilated lateral ventricles unassociated with DCC appose each other), they are abnormally shaped. In the majority of cases, the frontal horns are pointed and the occipital horns disproportionately enlarged (Figs. 5,11). The medial borders of these ventricles are relatively parallel to each other.

EXPLANATION OF AND COMMENT ON THE CT SCAN FINDINGS

VENTRICULOMEGALY seen in DCC is mostly on a developmental (cerebral hypoplasia) basis, mainly due to hypoplasia of white matter. (In the pneumoencephalography era, demonstration of an obstructive lesion was rare.) Embryologically, the size of the occipital horns is determined by normal development of the calcarine cortex and the forceps major of corpus callosum. Hypoplasia or aplasia of the latter in DCC explains **disproportionate enlargement of the occipital horns.** (One must recognize that we all pass through a stage of physiologic hydrocephalus. It is the growth of the neural tissue, particularly of the cerebrum, which results in shrinkage of the ventricular size. This state of physiologic hydrocephalus will persist as generalized or focal ventriculomegaly according to whether the impaired brain growth is generalized or focal.)

SEPARATION OF THE LATERAL VENTRICLES is not easily explained on an embryologic basis. Infolding of the neural tissue on the medial aspects of the cerebral hemispheres where the gyri are radially arranged (a well-known gross pathologic feature of DCC) may prevent ventricular apposition (Fig. 12). Also, excessive tissue formation (polymicrogyria also is a well-recognized gross pathologic feature of DCC) or reduced tissue elimination during brain organization at the medial aspects of the lateral ventricles, especially near frontal horns, may account for their separation and usually observed narrowness anteriorly. The frontal horns may assume a bulbous configuration due to considerable hypoplasia of the adjoining white matter.

In contrast to the normal horizontal arrangement of the collosal fibers, they are predominantly longitudinal in DCC, an arrangement that probably explains the SMOOTHNESS AND ROUGHLY PARALLEL APPEARANCE OF THE MEDIAL BORDERS OF THE LATERAL VENTRICLES seen in this disorder.

ENLARGEMENT AND ELEVATED POSITION OF THE THIRD VENTRICLE (Fig. 12) is very likely explained by poor development of the diencephalon, especially its roof (an aspect of DCC that makes it part of the spectrum of holoprosencephaly complex). The roof of the third ventricle is lined by a thin membrane.

THE ENLARGED INTERHEMISPHERIC fissure (Fig. 12) is probably a result of hypoplasia of the adjoining neural tissue, mainly of white matter.

ASSOCIATED LESIONS

THE INTERHEMISPHERIC ARACHNOID CYST appears as a large CSF-containing lesion arising at the superior aspect of the third ventricle, with which it usually communicates, and interposed between the lateral ventricles. Absence or hypoplasia of the falx can allow this cyst to straddle the midline (Figs. 13,14). The pathogenesis of this cyst is not fully explained, although it is unlikely to be porencephalic. It may result from defective development of the roof of the third ventricle creating an accumulation and loculation of CSF in the midline (Fig. 15). Alternatively, the cyst is a manifestation of an associated meningeal abnormality.

CALCIFIED LIPOMA OF THE CORPUS CALLOSUM appears as a lesion of fat density commonly located in the anterior to midpart of the corpus callosum and surrounded by linear areas of calcification (Fig. 16). Other described lesions associated with corpus callosum lipoma also can be recognized readily (Fig. 17,18).

CONTRAST CT SCAN IN DCC

Although the contrast CT scan usually is not required in reaching the diagnosis of DCC, it may provide some additional information regarding the status of the internal cerebral veins. These veins normally lie above the roof of the third ventricle and are close together except in their posterior parts where they separate somewhat in cistern velum interposition before joining the vein of Galen. IN DCC, THESE VEINS ARE

ABNORMALLY SEPARATED AND LIE AT THE WALLS OF THE DILATED THIRD VENTRICLE (Fig. 3). On sagittal images, their higher location and flattening of the curve of the vein of Galen can be appreciated as this curve is formed normally by the splenium of the corpus callosum.

The loss of normal curvature of the PERICALLOSAL ARTERIES and their assumption of an undulating course can be appreciated on high resolution reformatted sagittal images. Also, an azygos (unpaired) anterior cerebral artery, which is overrepresented in DCC, may be recognized on coronal and/or sagittal images.

The choroid plexi normally converge at the interventricular foramina, usually forming an angle of from 45-70 degrees (Fig. 19). However, in DCC THE CHOROID PLEXI BECOME LESS CONVERGENT and tend to adopt a more parallel orientation, the resulting angle thus usually measuring less than 35-40 degrees (Figs. 3,20).

PARTIAL DYSGENESIS OF CORPUS CALLOSUM

This is usually seen at the posterior part of the corpus callosum, since normally the corpus callosum develops rostro-caudal (that is, if the anterior part does not develop, the posterior cannot be expected to develop). However, the anterior part can be secondarily destroyed by a vascular, inflammatory or some other type of cerebral insult.

CT scan diagnosis of partial dysgenesis of the corpus callosum is difficult to make with confidence.

DIFFERENTIAL DIAGNOSIS

Usually, the CT scan features of DCC are quite typical and no difficulty should be encountered in reaching the correct diagnosis. However, occasionally, an associated large interhemispheric arachnoid cyst may be mistaken for DORSAL SAC OF HOLOPROSENCEPHALY. In such a case, the presence of interhemispheric fissure and recognition of separated lateral ventricles as such should prevent such a misinterpretation (Fig. 21). Also, invariably, there will be associated facial anomalies in holoprosencephaly.

Extensive ISCHEMIC-HYPOXIC ENCEPHALOPATHY AND RESULTANT WIDESPREAD LEUKOMALACIA involving the corpus callosum as well might cause confusion, particularly when the interhemispheric fissure also is enlarged. In such a situation, careful evaluation of CT scan and clinical history of a known devastating illness (Fig. 22) may provide a clue to the appropriate diagnosis.

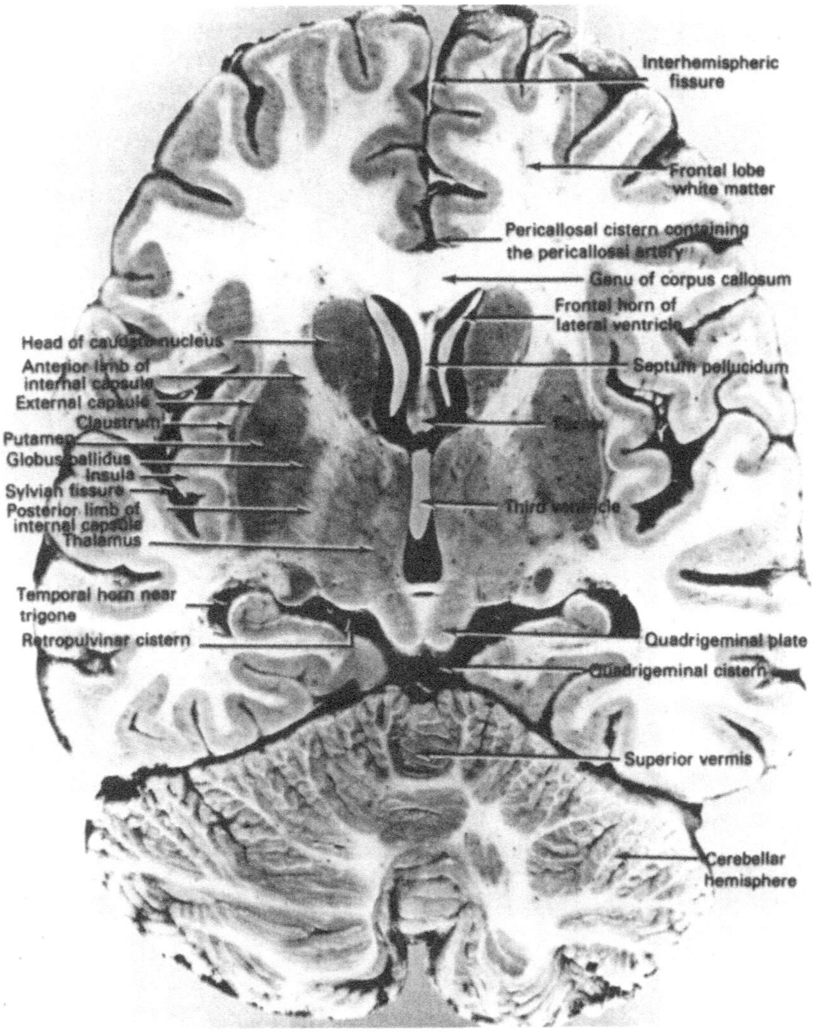

Figure 1. Axial brain section at third ventricle level to show separation of the interhemispheric fissure from the third ventricle by the corpus callosum and the adjoining midline structures. In dysgenesis of the corpus callosum, the interhemispheric fissure comes to lie abnormally close to third ventricle.

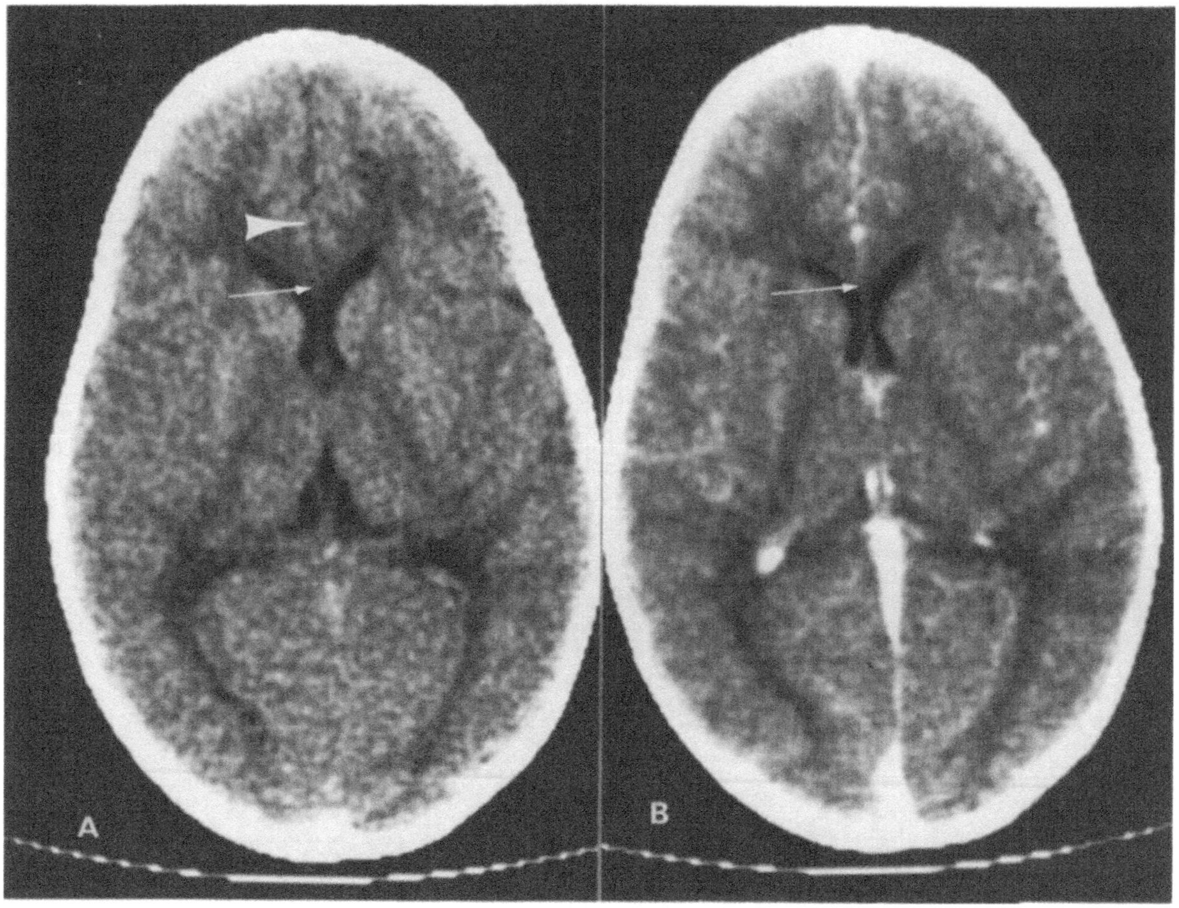

Figure 2. Normal non-contrast (A) and contrast (B) CT scan at third ventricle level. The interhemispheric fissure (**arrowhead**) is separated from the third ventricle by the corpus callosum and the neighboring midline structures. On the contrast CT, the pericallosal arteries outline the surface of the corpus callosum.

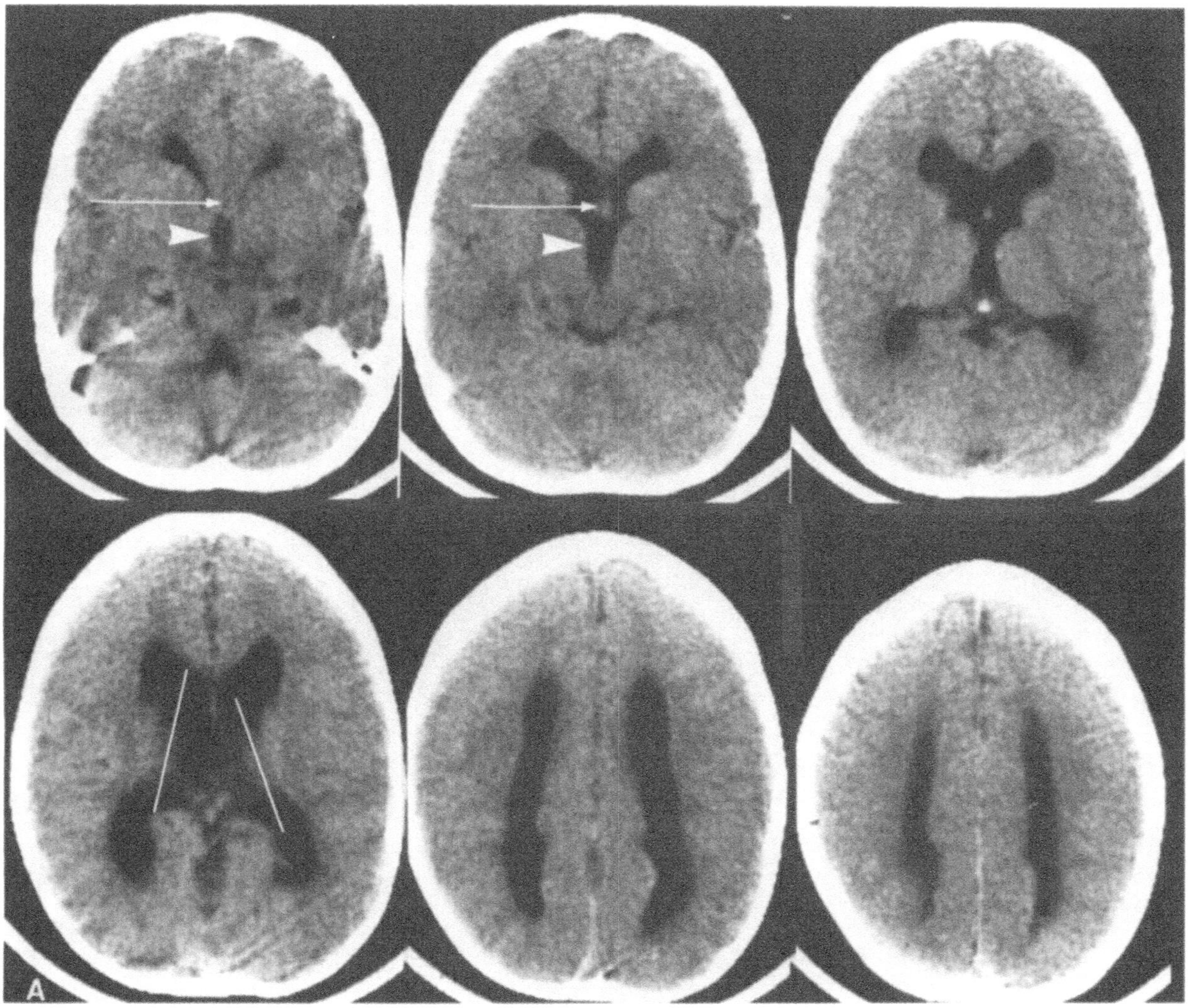

Figure 3. Dysgenesis of corpus callosum.
A. Non-contrast CT scan. Note continuation of the interhemispheric fissure (**arrow**) to the anterior wall of the third ventricle (**arrowhead**). The third ventricle is moderately dilated and the interventricular foramina are more separated than normal. The lateral ventricles are separated from each other on higher CT slices. The lines drawn along choroid plexi do not meet at interventricular foramina and form an angle of about 35 degrees.

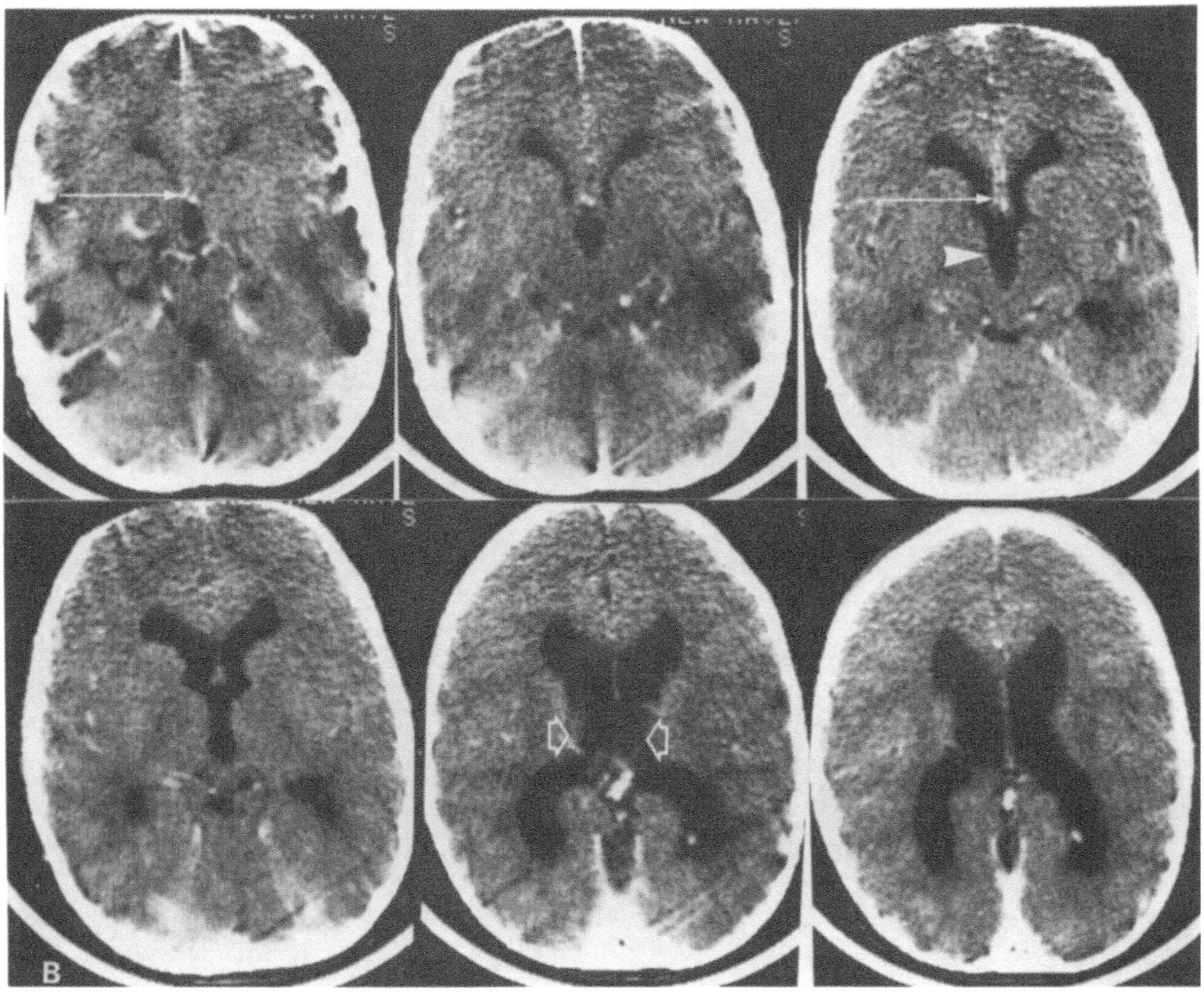

Figure 3. Dysgenesis of corpus callosum.
B. Contrast CT scan. Note close approximation of the pericallosal arteries (**closed arrows**) to anterior wall of the third ventricle (**arrowhead**) (normally they should be a little distance away as they lie on the corpus callosum which separates them from the third ventricle). The internal cerebral veins (**open arrows**) are abnormally separated and lie on the side of the third ventricle rather than above it.

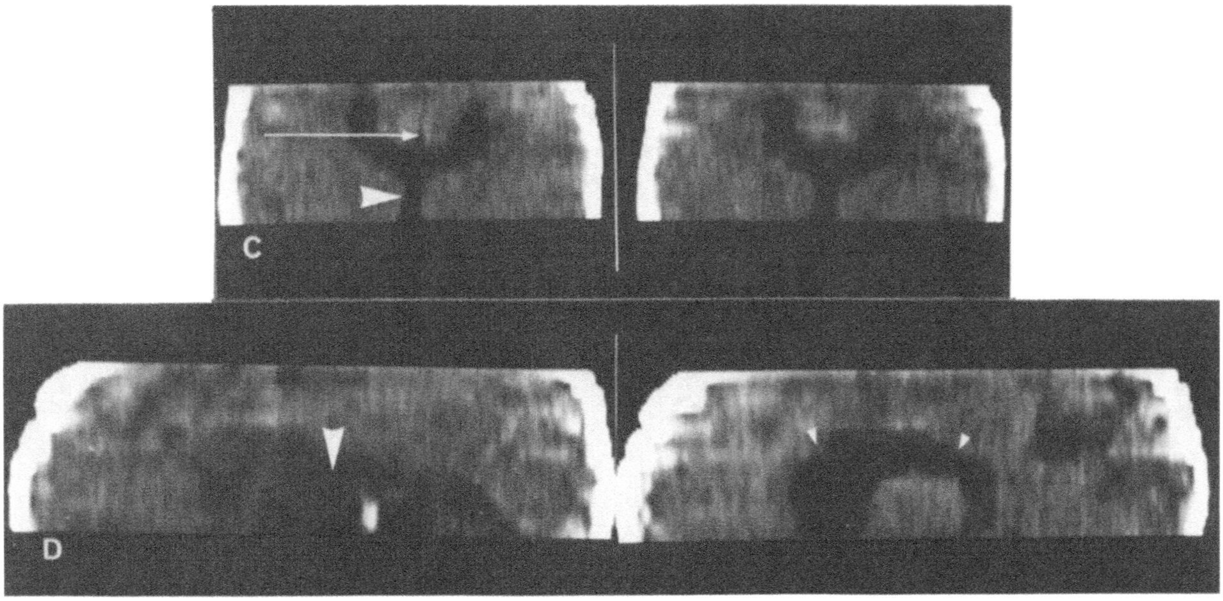

Figure 3. Dysgenesis of corpus callosum.
C. Reformatted coronal CT scan. Again, the interhemispheric fissure (**arrow**) can be traced to roof of third ventricle (**arrowhead**). Note bulbar configuration of the frontal horns.
D. Reformatted sagittal CT scan. Note abnormal elevation of the dilated third ventricle (**large arrowhead**). Irregularity of roof of the lateral ventricle very likely is caused by heterotopic gray matter (**small arrowheads**). Same heterotopias probably explain irregularity of lateral ventricle walls seen on axial images.
This 6-year-old girl had presented with learning disability and did not have seizure disorder.

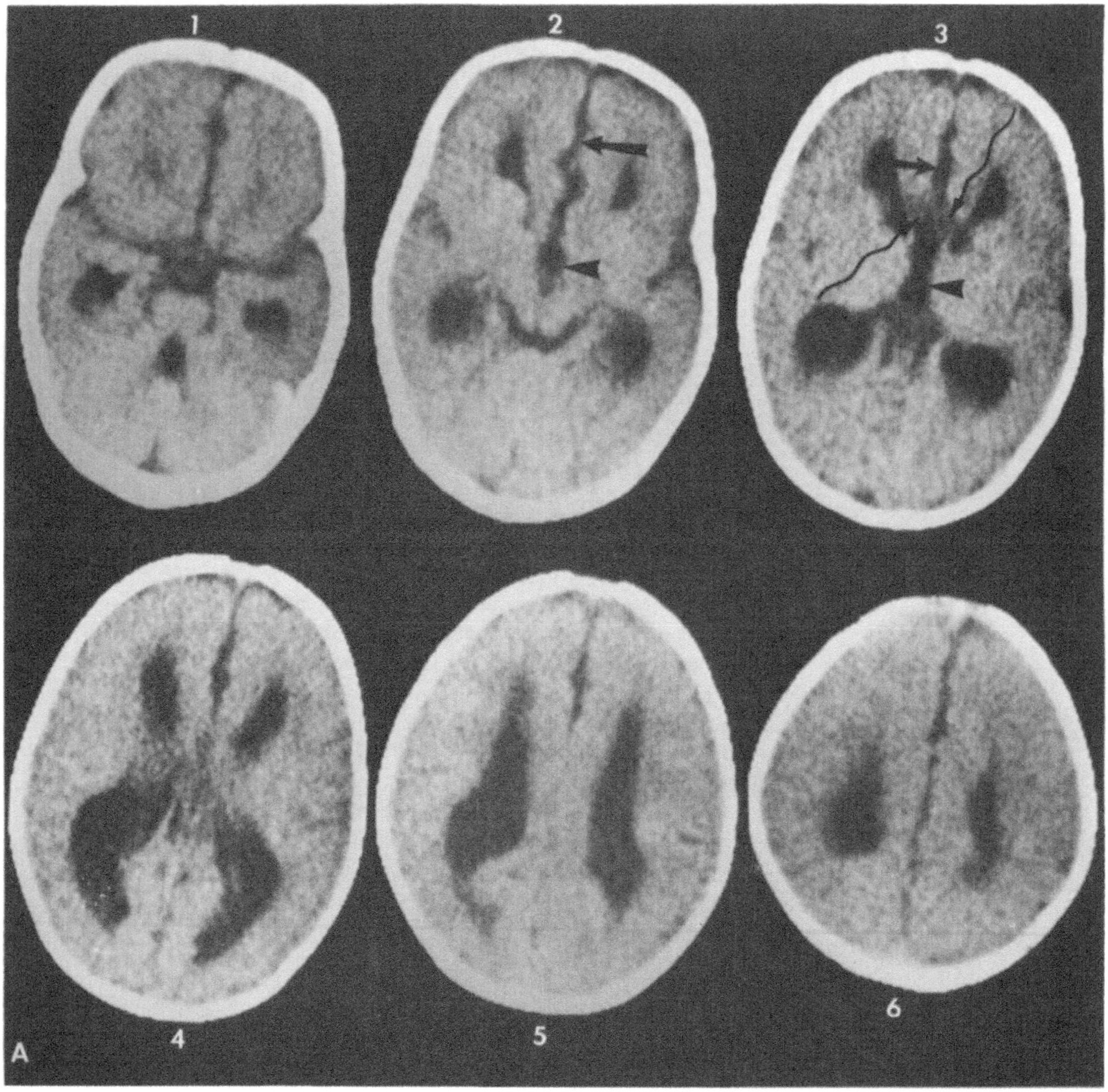

Figure 4. Dysgenesis of corpus callosum.
A. Axial CT scan images. 1-6 are sequential slices. Note continuation of the prominent interhemispheric fissure **(straight arrow)** to the anterior aspect of the dilated third ventricle **(arrowheads).** Normally, it would be interrupted by the anterior part of the corpus callosum. Inability to see the interhemispheric fissure on slice 5 indicates that some of the corpus callosal tissue was present at that level (if it were absent, the entire interhemispheric fissure would have been continuous from top to bottom). **Zig-zap arrows** = Anteriorly placed and abnormally separated interventricular foramina.

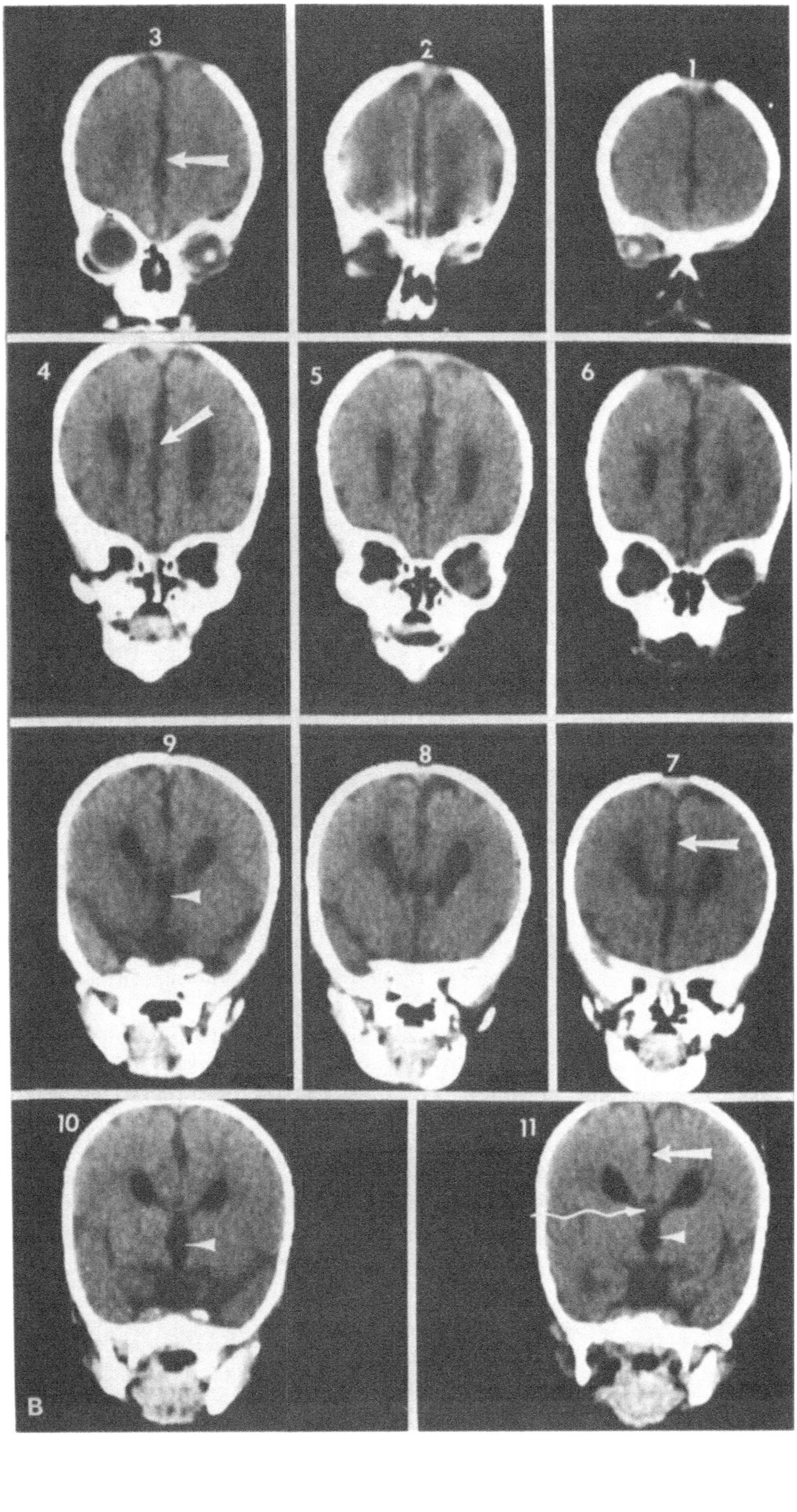

B. Coronal reformatted images. 1-11 are sequential images from front to back of the head. Note that the interhemispheric fissure **(arrows)** is a continuous structure except in slices 10 and 11 (corresponding to slice level 5 on axial images). The dilated and elevated third ventricle **(arrowhead)** resides between lateral ventricles. Please consult normal sectional anatomy atlas of brain to appreciate the changes described here.

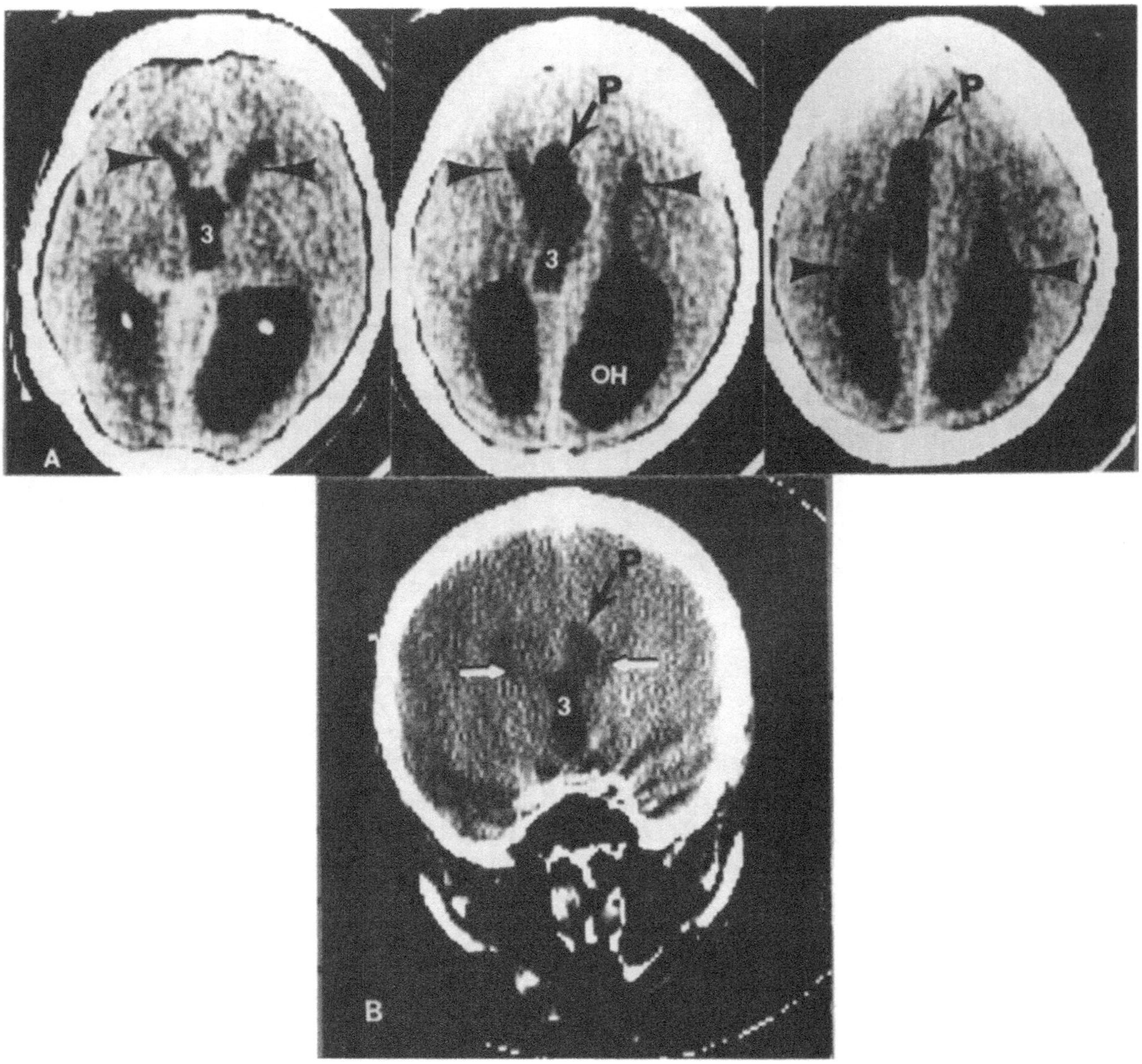

Figure 5. Dysgenesis of corpus callosum and associated porencephaly of undetermined cause.

A. Axial CT scans. There is separation of lateral ventricles (**arrowheads**). Dilated and elevated third ventricle (3) resides between the lateral ventricles and medial to the porencephalic cyst (P). Observe pointing of the frontal horns and disproportionate distension of the occipital horns (OH).

B. Coronal CT scan. Side reversed. Third ventricle (3) is located between separated lateral ventricles (**unlabelled arrows**). Note that the hemisphere ipsilateral to porencephalic cyst (P) is smaller than its companion.

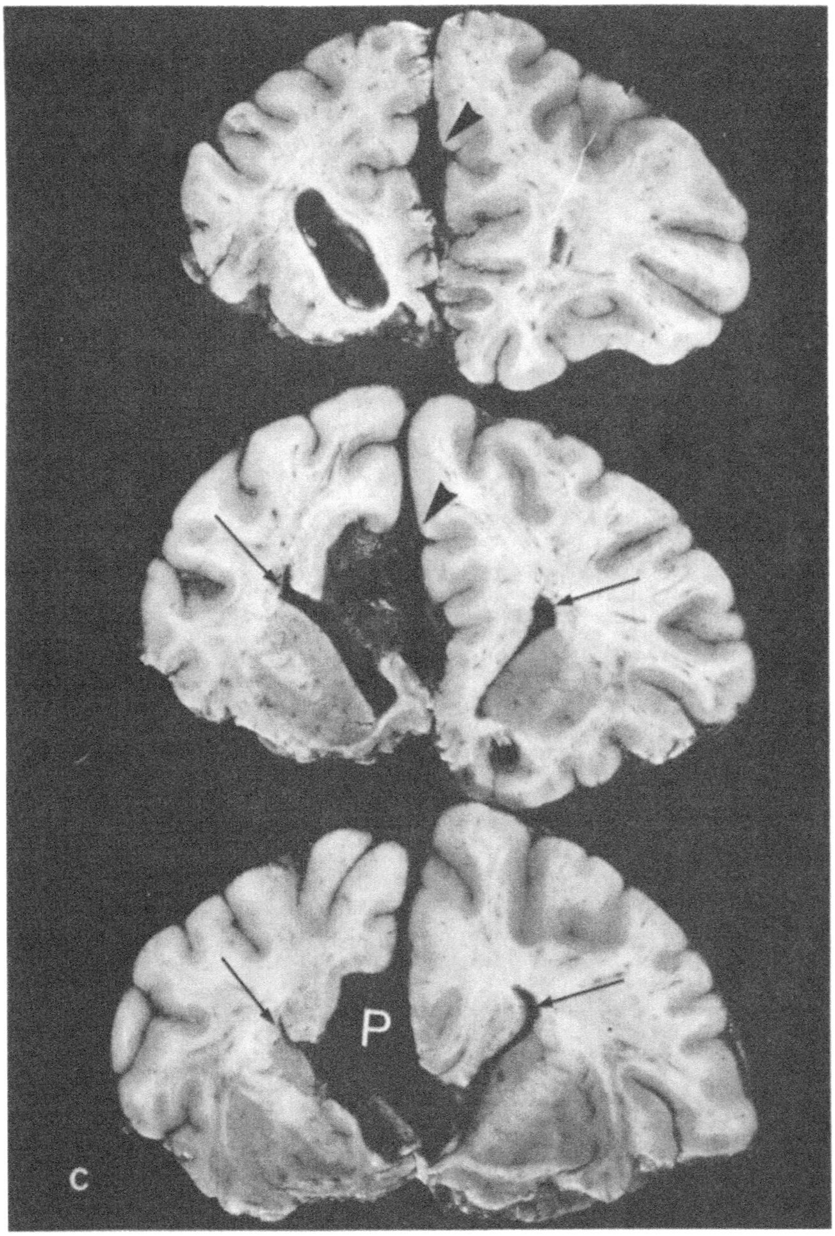

C. Pathologic specimen. Coronal sections. Front to back sections are arranged bottom to top in this illustration. Note separation of the lateral ventricles **(arrows)**. The anterior aspects of the lateral ventricles are narrow compared to the posterior parts as shown on CT scan. The interhemispheric fissure **(arrowheads)** is large. Note rolling in of the cerebral tissue adjacent to the interhemispheric fissure. The porencephalic cyst (P) communicates with the neighboring lateral ventricle.

This 55-year-old female had presented with subarachnoid hemorrhage. Angiogram revealed two aneurysms: one at internal carotid-posterior communicating artery and the other at an anterior temporal branch of middle cerebral artery.

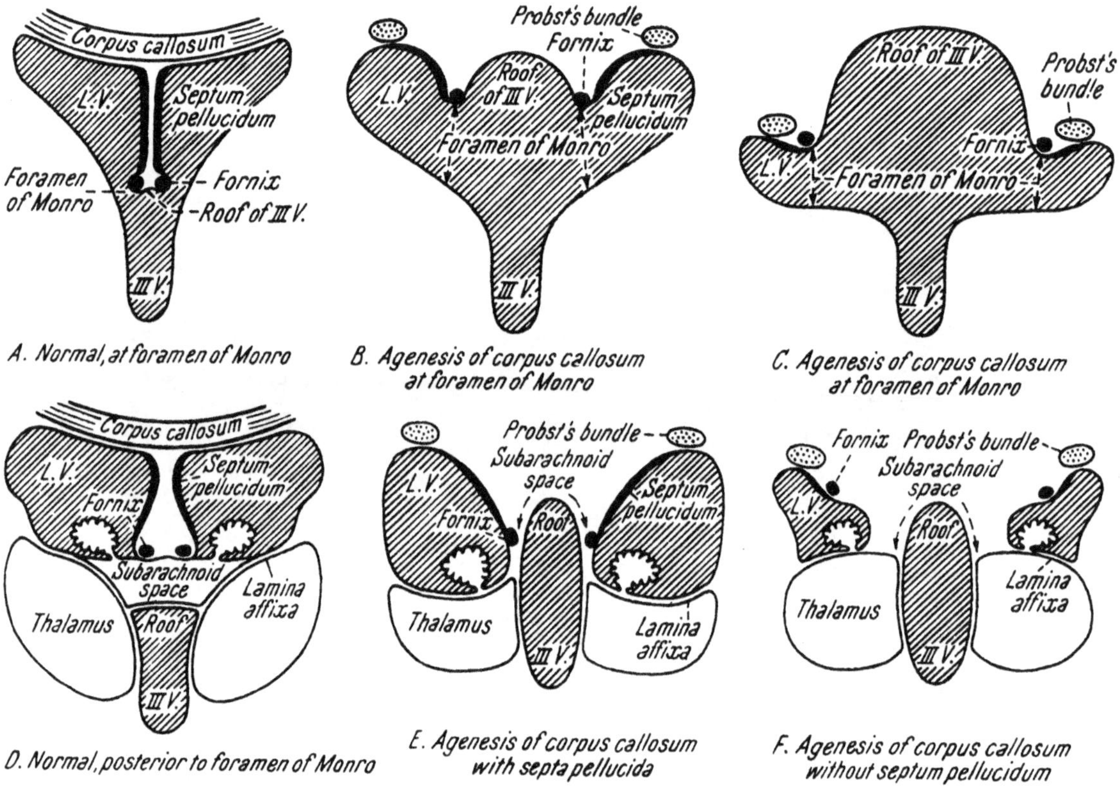

Figure 6. Diagrammatic representation of normal and abnormal relationships of structures at and about level of roof of third ventricle (from (4) with permission).

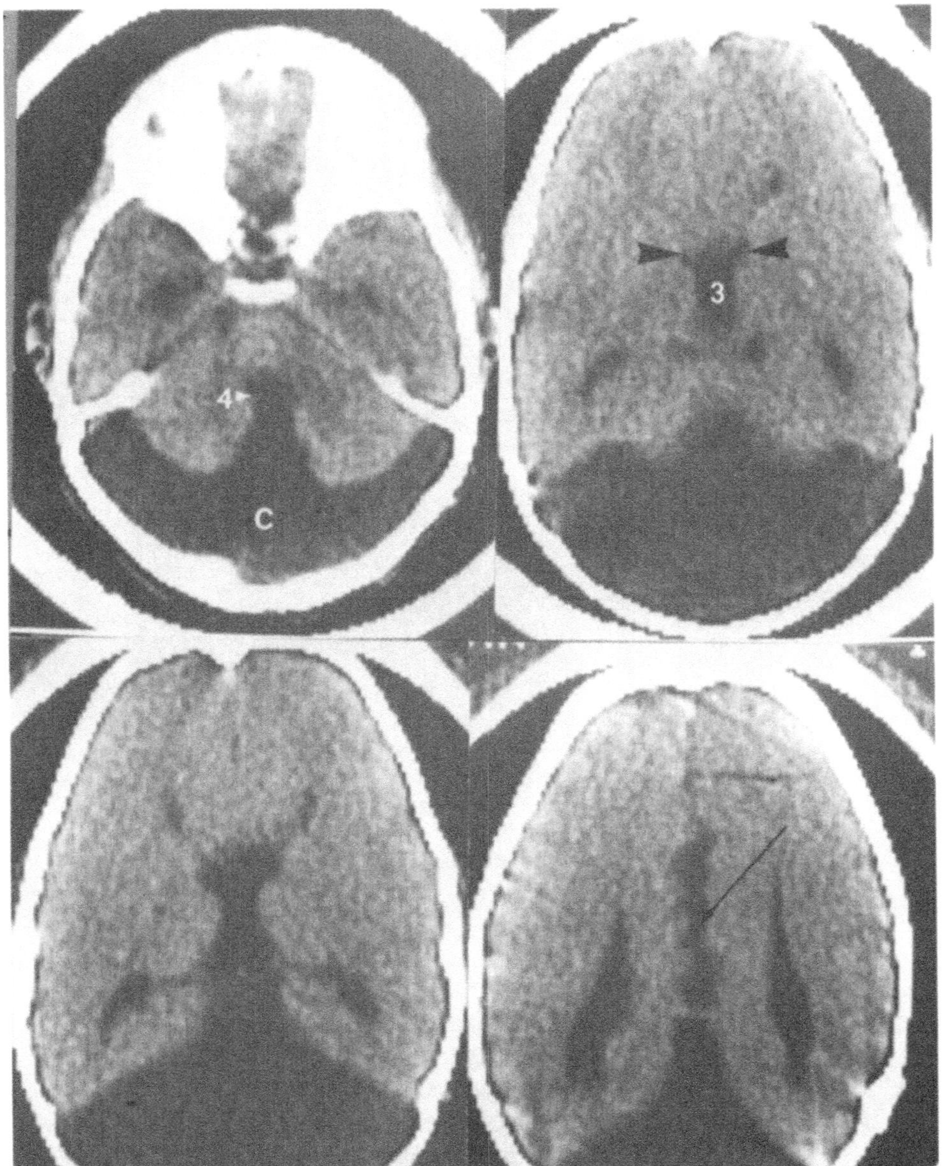

Figure 7. 12-year-old child with Dandy-Walker Syndrome and concurrent dysgenesis of corpus callosum. Note that the cyst (C) communicates with the dorsal aspect of the enlarged fourth ventricle (4). The vermis is absent. The cerebellar hemispheres are present. Lateral ventricles are separated; note their pointed anterior ends. Third ventricle (3) is dilated and the interventricular foramina (**arrowheads**) are abnormally separated. The interhemispheric fissure (**arrow**) also is very prominent.

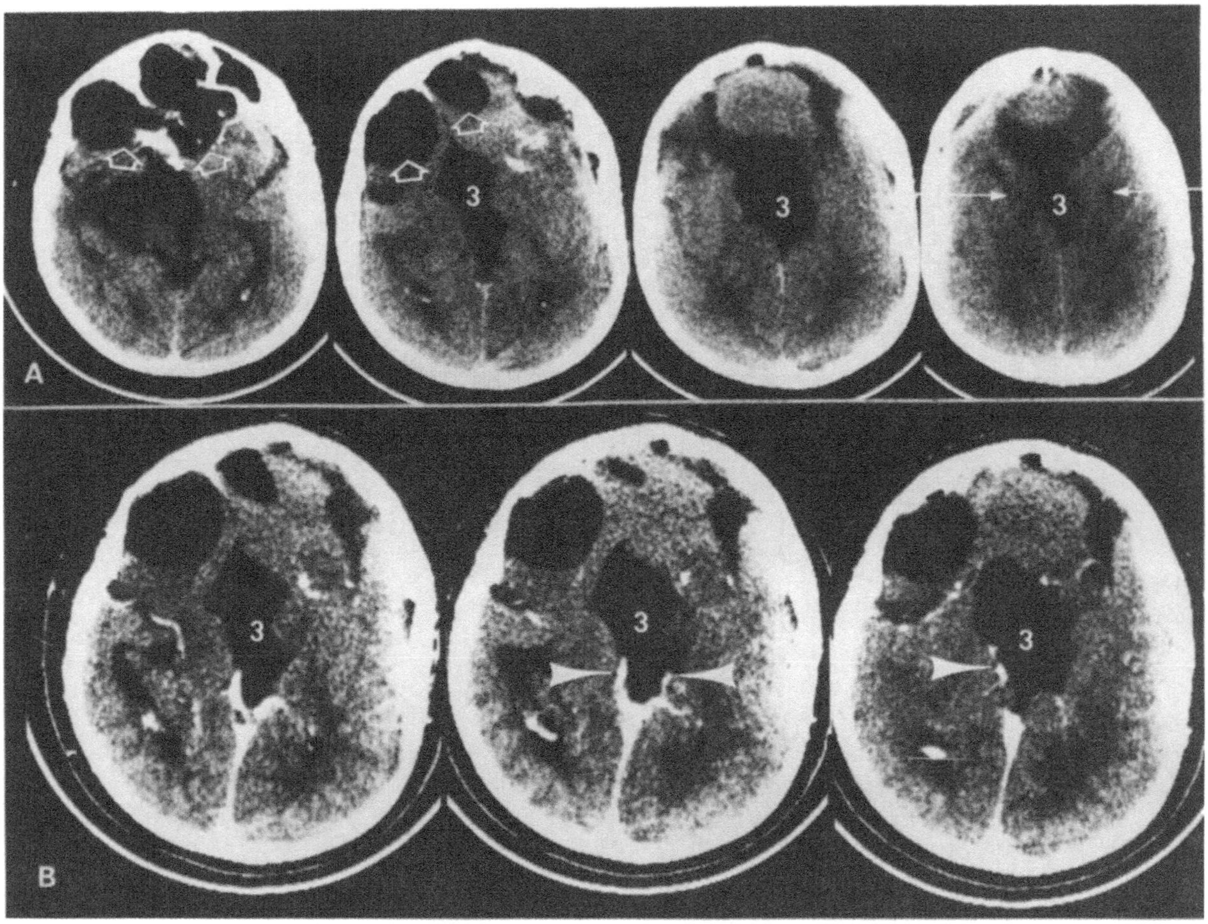

Figure 8. a 25-year-old female who presented with seizure disorder. She had skull base teratoma removed at age 9 months. A) non-contrast and B) contrast CT. There is still residual/recurrent partly calcified tumor **(open arrows)**. The patient also has dysgenesis of the corpus callosum. The lateral ventricles are slit-like and markedly separated **(closed arrows)**. The dilated third ventricle (3) has a bizarre shape and extends considerably higher to interpose between the lateral ventricles. The interventricular foramina are markedly separated. The internal cerebral veins **(arrowheads)** are abnormally separated. Part of the frontal lobe lucencies are related to prior surgery.

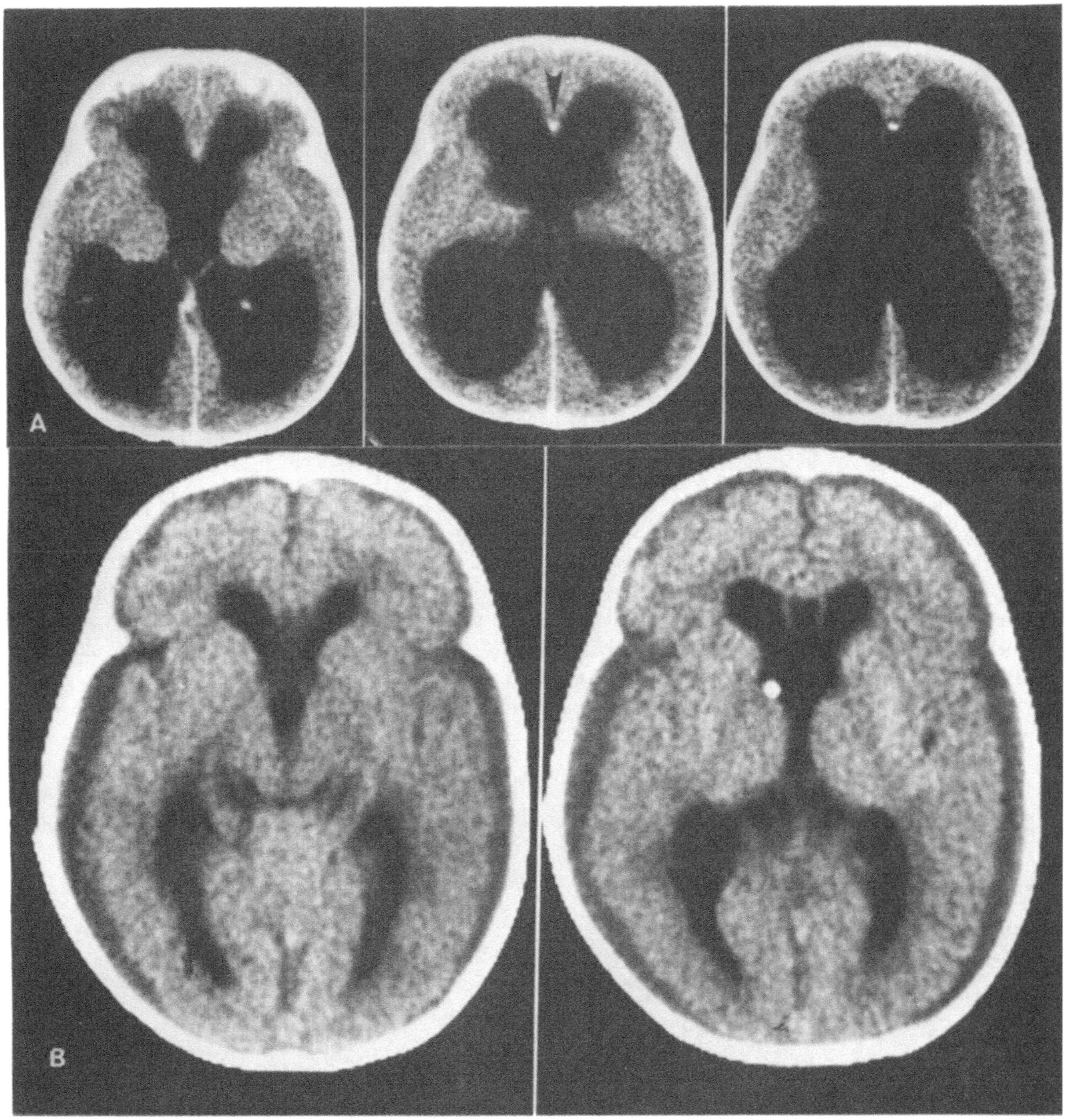

Figure 9. In massive ventriculomegaly the interhemispheric fissure may become so much compressed that it may not be recognizable. On the contrast CT, however, the pericallosal arteries become closely applied to the arteriomedial walls of the lateral ventricles as shown on the contrast CT scan (A) where arrowhead points to the pericallosal arteries. This situation may falsely suggest dysgenesis of the corpus callosum. The CT obtained after ventricular shunting clarifies the situation, however, when the interhemispheric fissure becomes recognizable, as shown on the non-contrast CT done after the ventricular shunt placement. In other words, the interhemispheric fissure sign of dysgenesis of corpus callosum is best studied on the post-shunted CT.

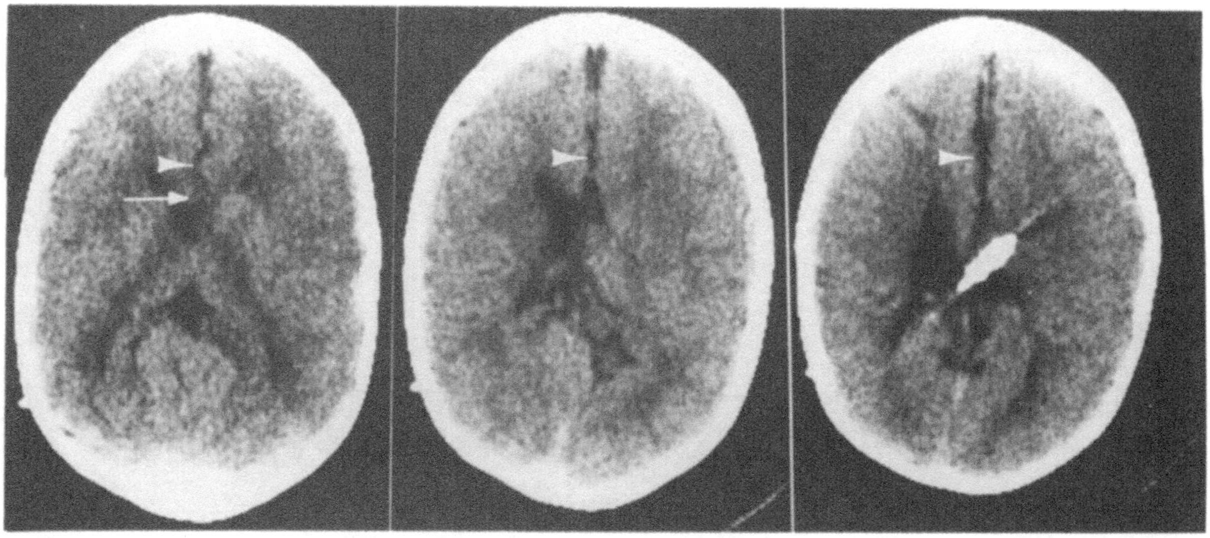

Figure 10. In Chiari II malformation, the interhemispheric fissure is commonly enlarged on the post-shunted CT. On the higher CT slices, such an enlarged interhemispheric fissure (**arrowheads**) can spuriously suggest dysgenesis of corpus callosum as shown here in the middle and right hand CT scan slices. However, on the CT slice at third ventricle, the interhemispheric fissure is shown to be separated by the corpus callosum (**arrows**) from the third ventricle. In other words, concomitant presence of dysgenesis of the corpus callosum with Chiari malformation type II should not be suggested on CT unless the interhemispheric fissure is shown unequivocally to be abnormally close to the third ventricle on CT scan slices at level of the third ventricle.

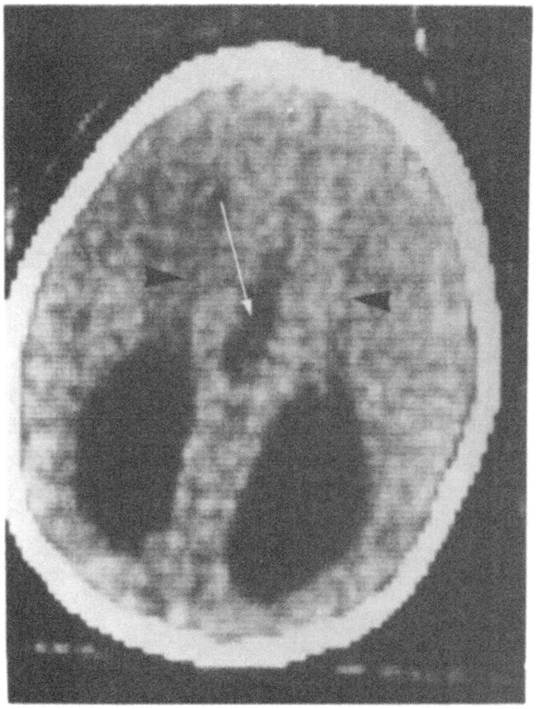

Figure 11. Dysgenesis of corpus callosum associated with cyst. Note pointed frontal horns (**arrowheads**). The occipital horns are bulbous. This 30-year-old man presented with headaches only. **Arrow** = Upwardly herniated and dilated third ventricle.

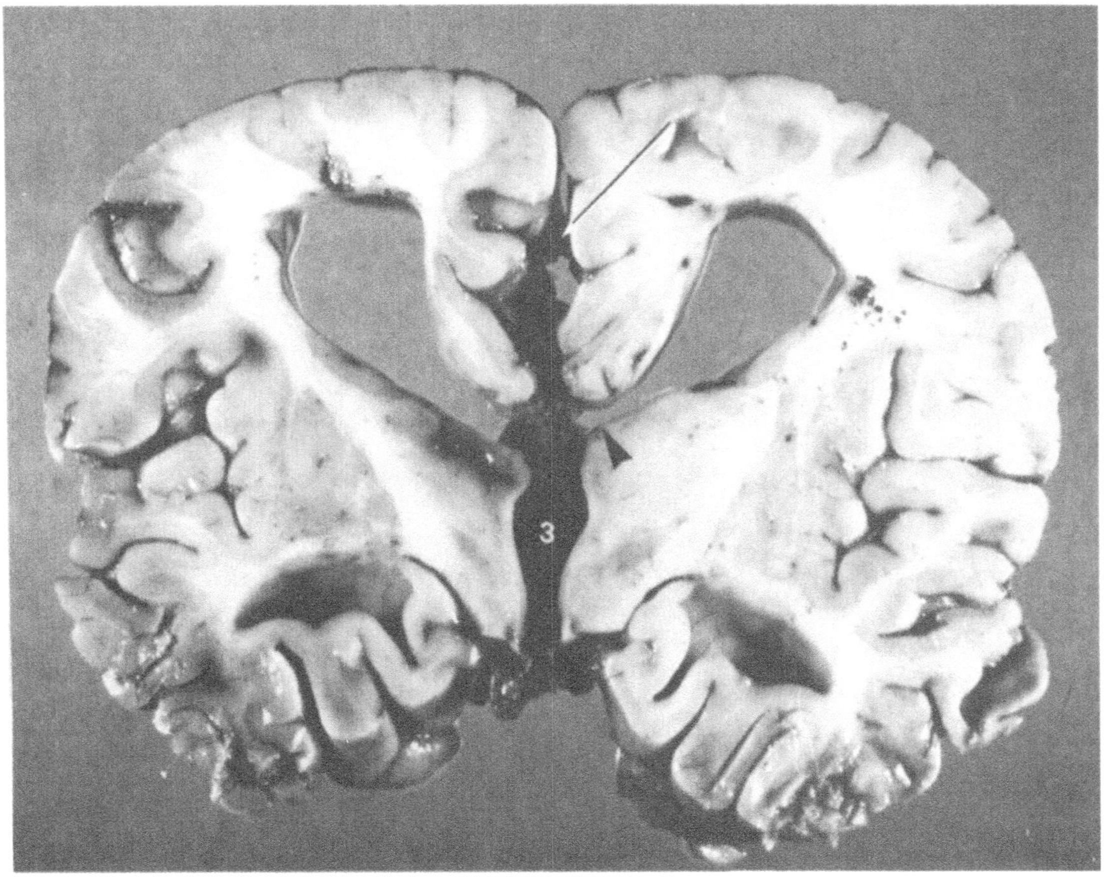

Figure 12. Coronal section of brain showing dysgenesis of the corpus callosum. Third ventricle (3) is dilated and separated from the markedly enlarged interhemispheric fissure (IHF) **(arrow)** by a membranous structure. The interventricular foramina **(arrowhead)** are larger. Corpus callosum is not recognizable. Note rolling in of the brain tissue adjoining the IHF. The frontal horns are bulbous due to white matter hypoplasia, which is generalized. Compare this brain section with one at same level in an anatomy atlas to better appreciate these abnormalities.

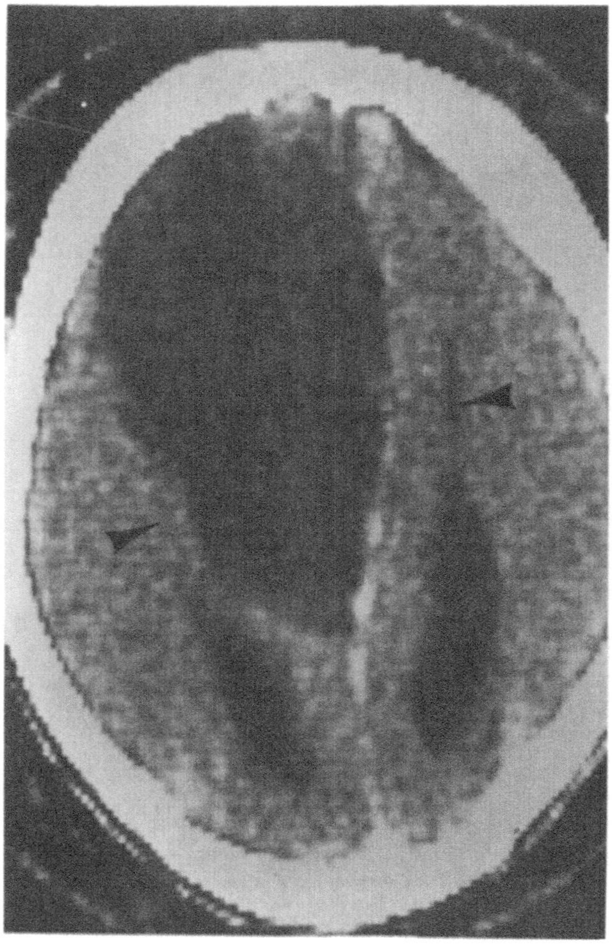

Figure 13. Dysgenesis of corpus callosum associated with cyst. Note narrowness (**arrowheads**) of the frontal horns.

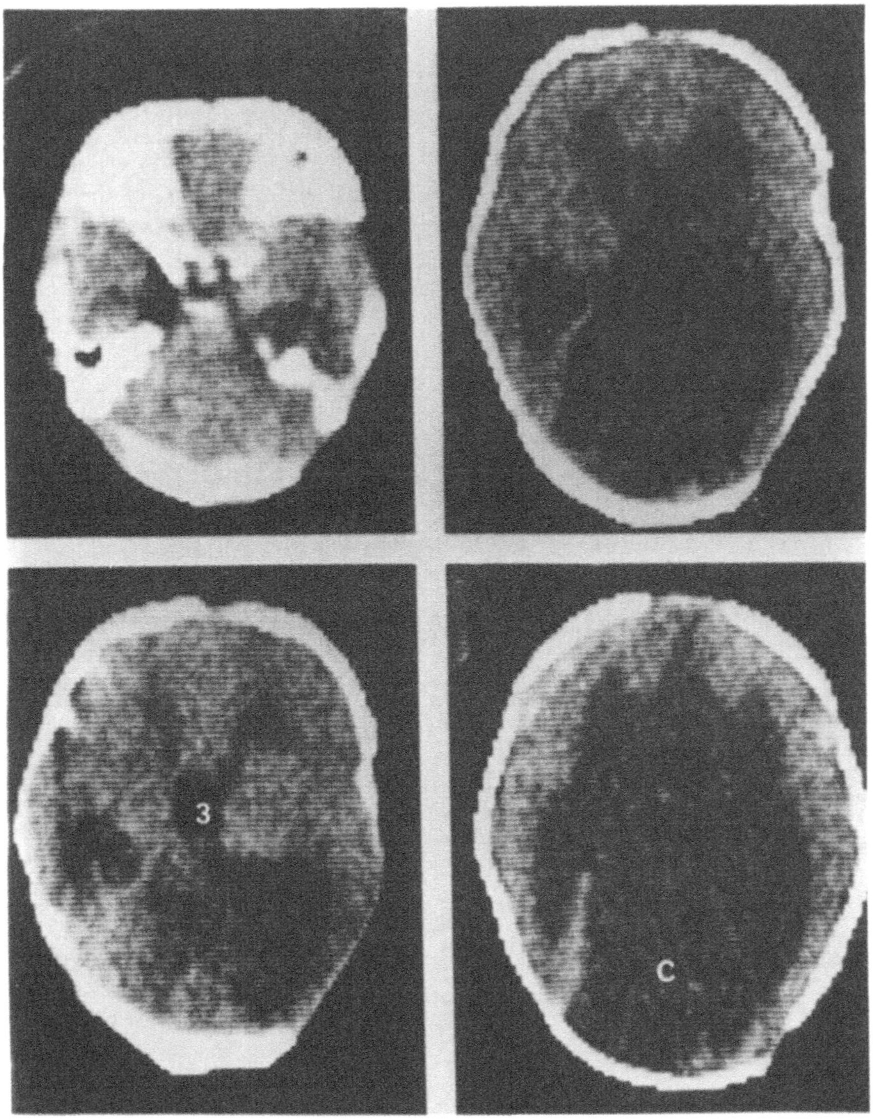

Figure 14. Dysgenesis of corpus callosum associated with midline cyst (C). Third ventricle (3) is markedly enlarged and lateral ventricles are separated.

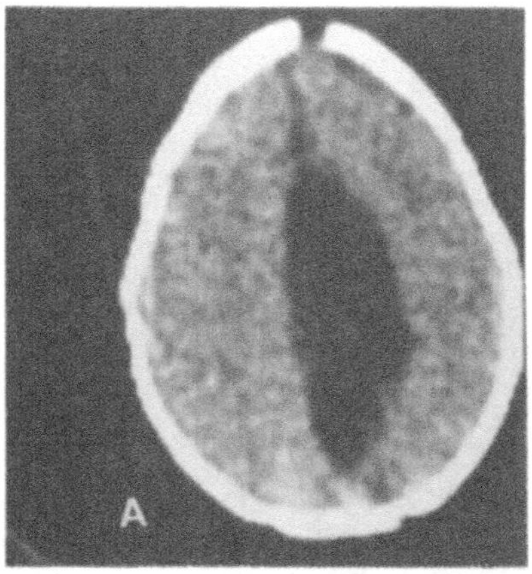

Figure 15. A young child with dysgenesis of the corpus callosum and associated interhemispheric cyst.
A. Higher CT scan slice showing the cyst.

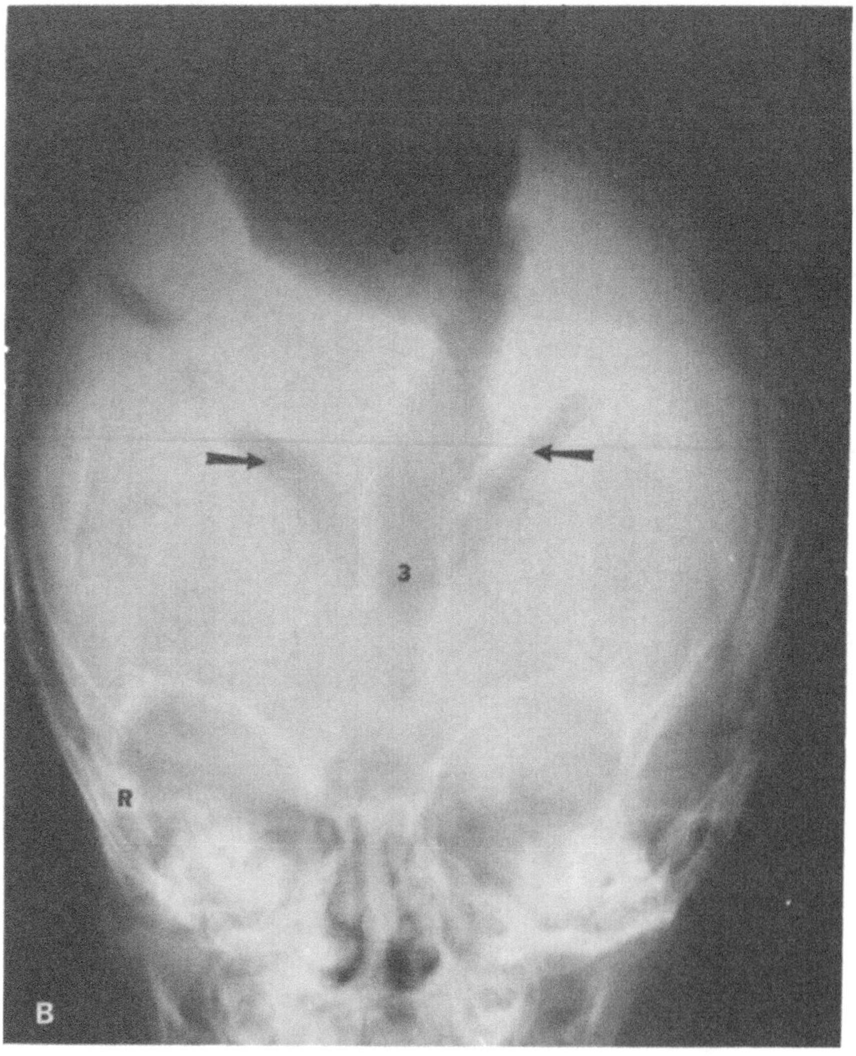

B. Pneumoencephalogram. Note communication of the dilated and upwardly placed third ventricle (3) with the cyst (C). Arrows are at separated lateral ventricles.

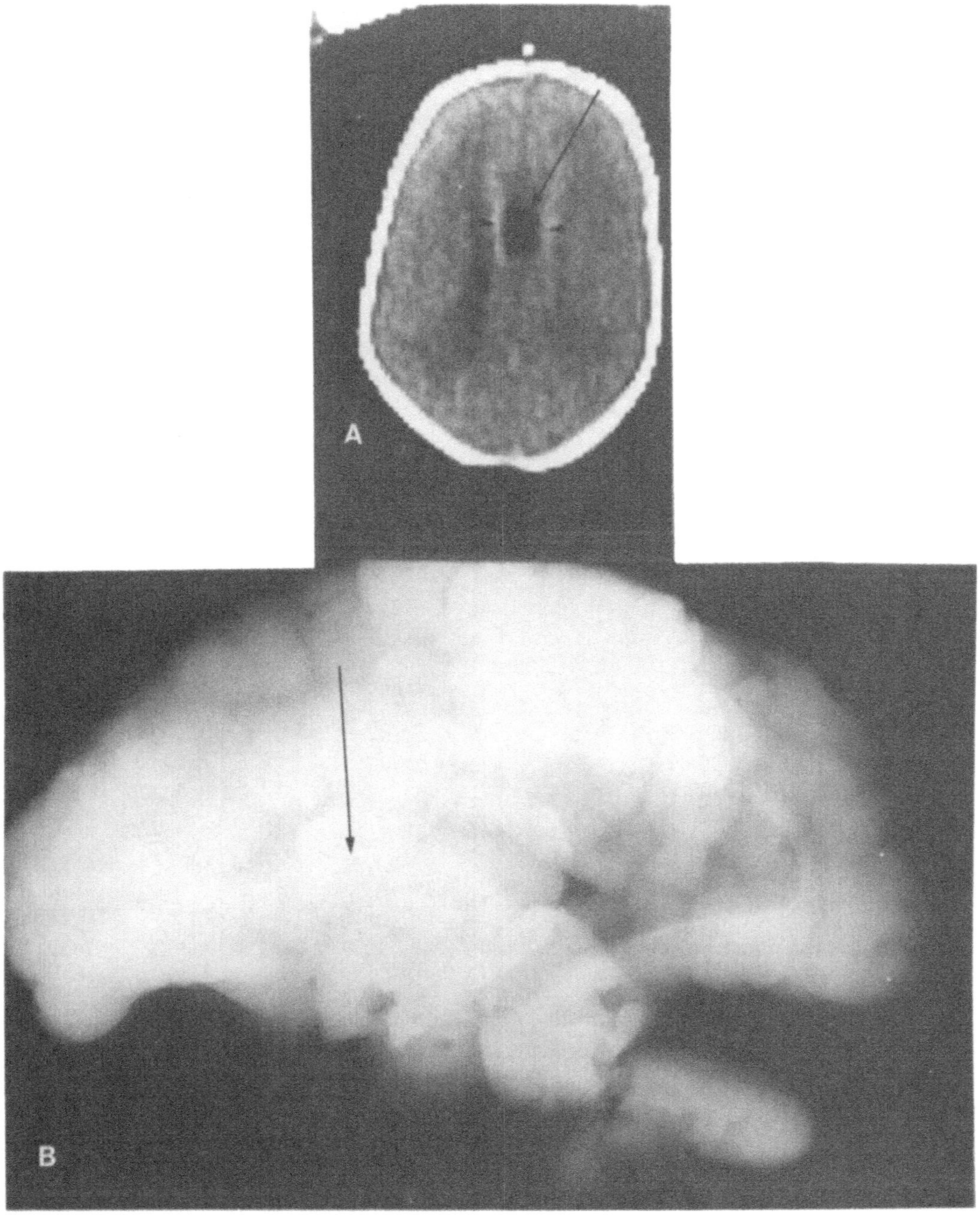

Figure 16. Calcified corpus callosum lipoma.
A. CT scan. Note fat density of the lipoma (**arrow**) rimmed by calcification (**arrowhead**).
B. Radiograph of the pathologic specimen. Arrow is at calcification related to the lipoma.

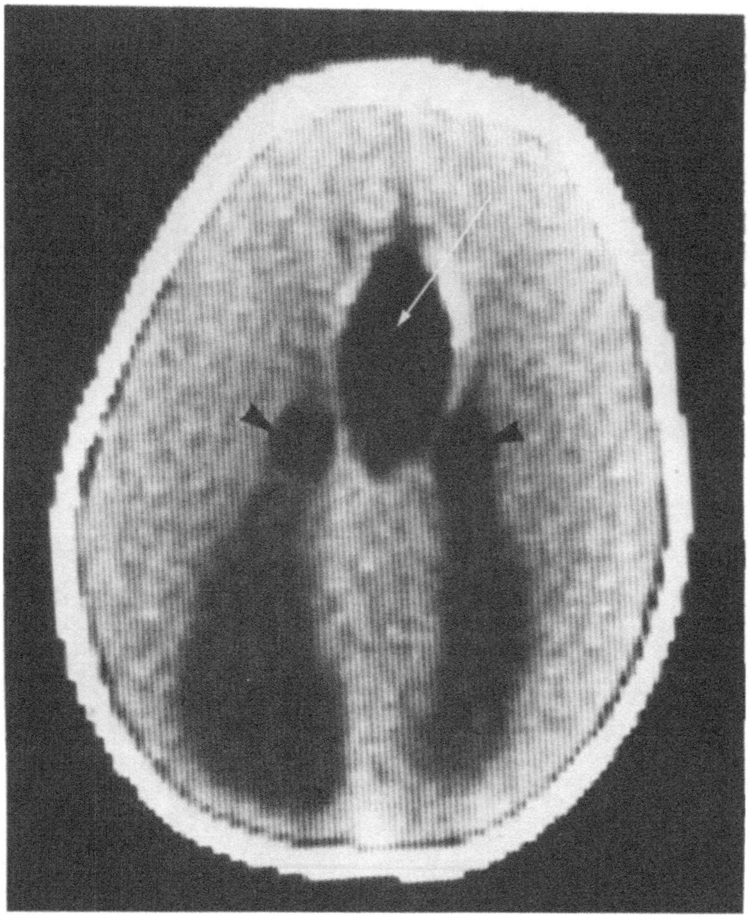

Figure 17. Calcified corpus callosum lipoma (**arrow**) associated with bilateral choroid plexus lipoma (**arrowhead**). (From [12] with permission.)

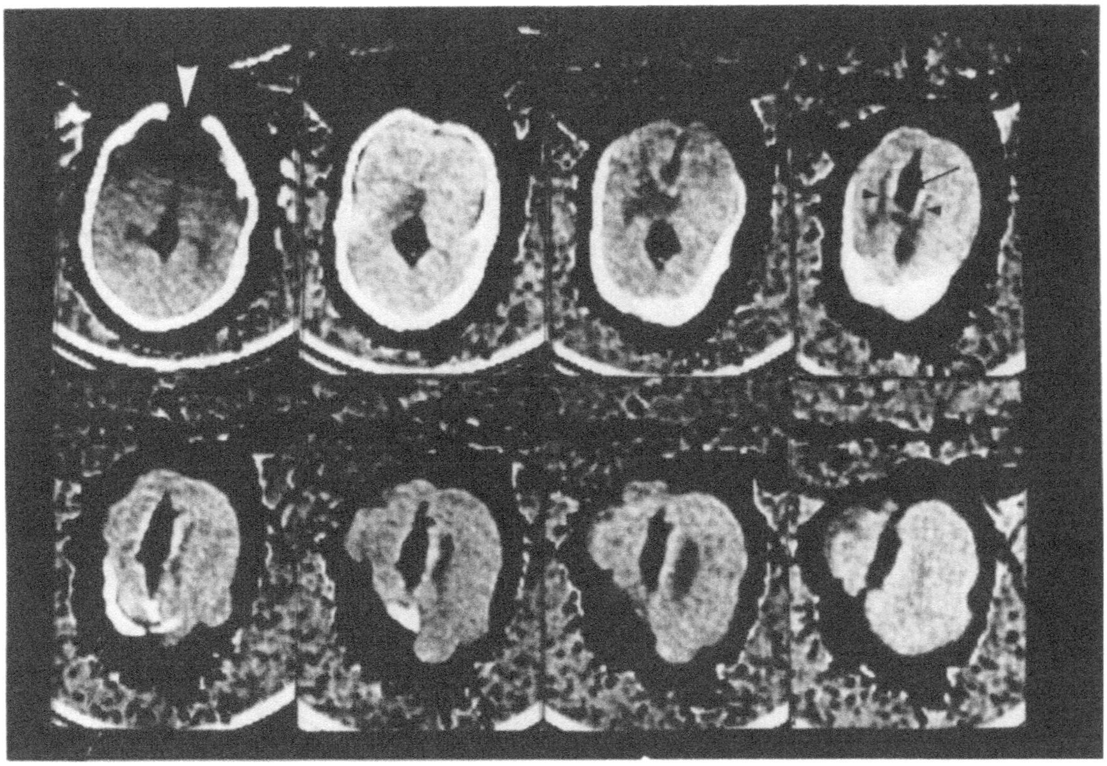

Figure 18. Calcified lipoma of the corpus callosum (**arrow**) associated with frontal dyraphism (**white arrowhead**). An encephalocele had protruded through it. Note separation of lateral ventricles (**small black arrowheads**). (From [13] with permission.)

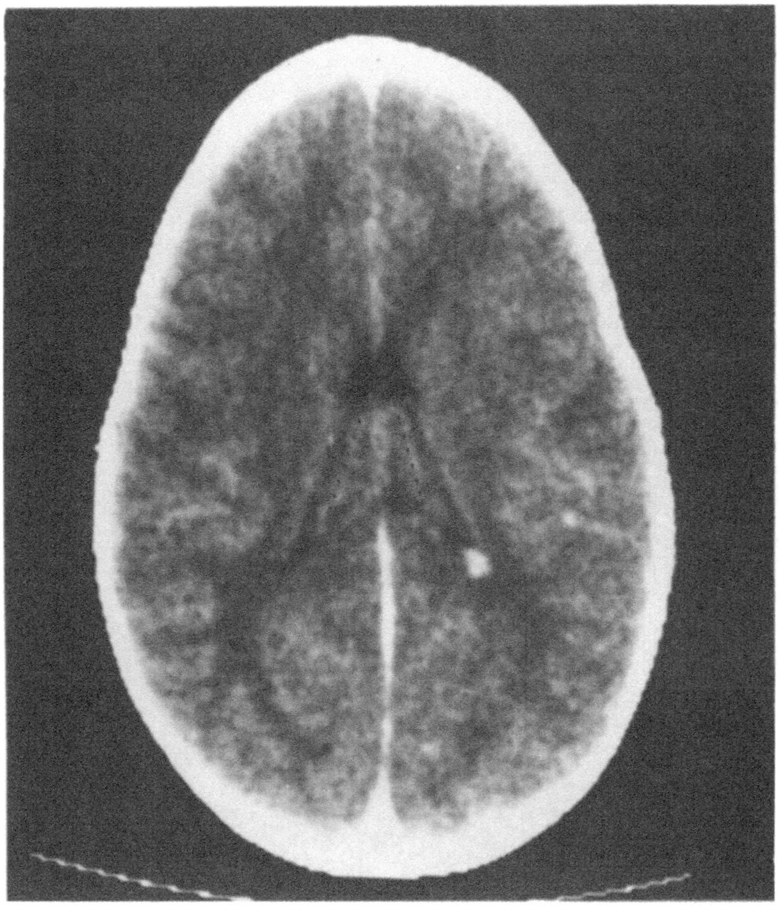

Figure 19. Contrast CT scan at choroid plexus level to show that angle formed by lines drawn along the choroid plexi usually measures more than 45 degrees.

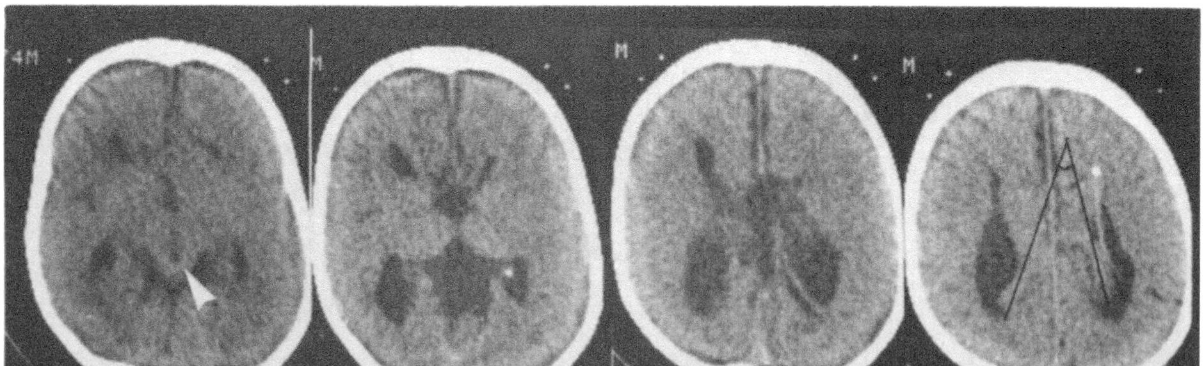

Figure 20. Dysgenesis of corpus callosum and associated Arnold-Chiari malformation type II. Note that the angle formed by lines down along choroid plexi is 35 degrees which is less than in normal cases. Also, note continuation of interhemispheric fissure to anterior wall of third ventricle. There is mesencephalic beaking (**arrowhead**) seen in Arnold-Chiari malformation type II.

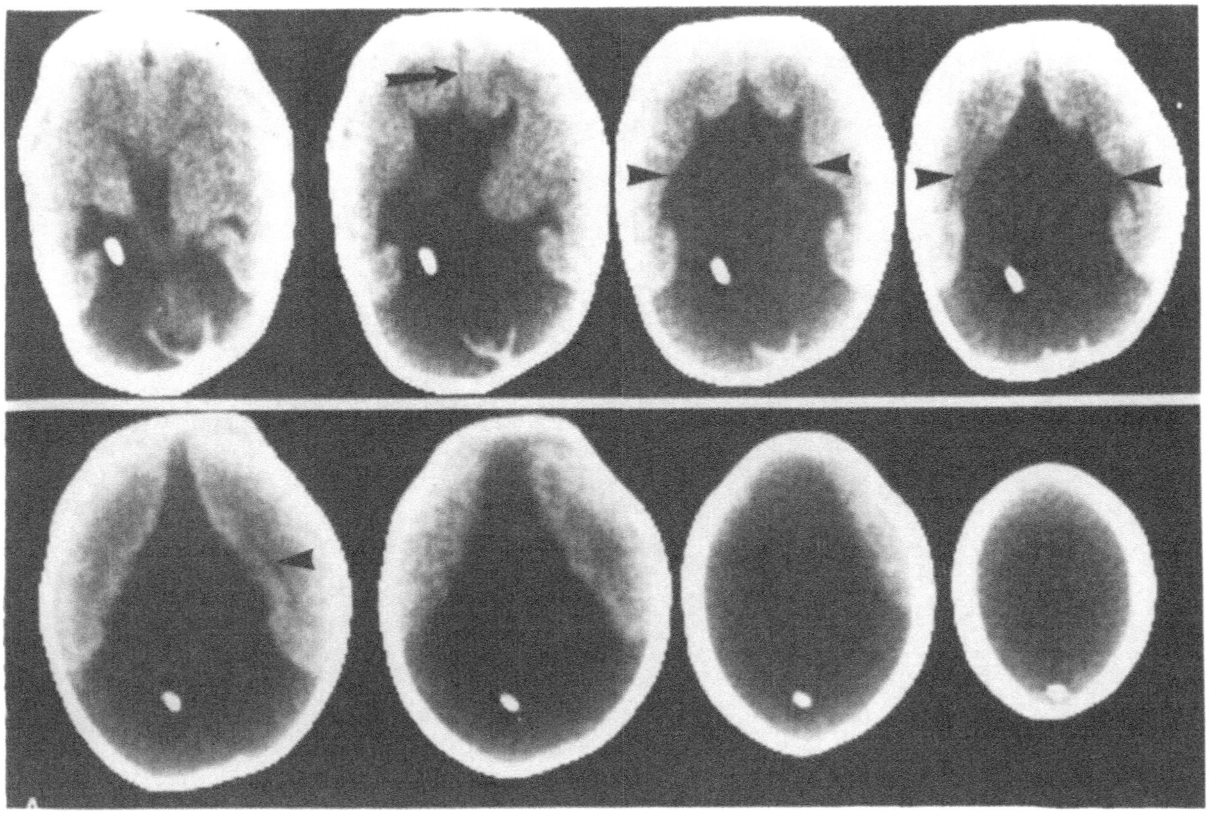

Figure 21. A. Dysgenesis of corpus callosum and associated cyst extending to either side of the midline indicating concurrent dysplasia of the falx. Presence of the interhemispheric fissure (**arrows**) and ability to recognize separated lateral ventricles (**arrowheads**) should avoid misdiagnosis with alobar holoprosencephaly and associated dorsal sac.

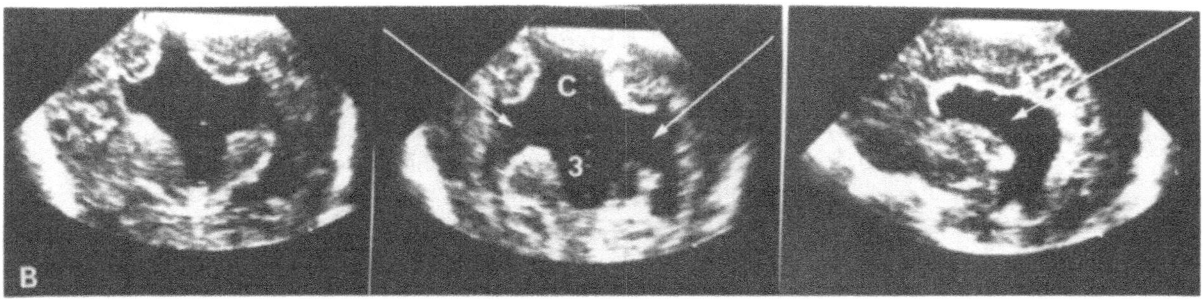

B. Ultrasonogram. Dilated third ventricle (3) and its continuation into the cyst (C) is shown. The lateral ventricles are separated and easily recognized (**arrows**).

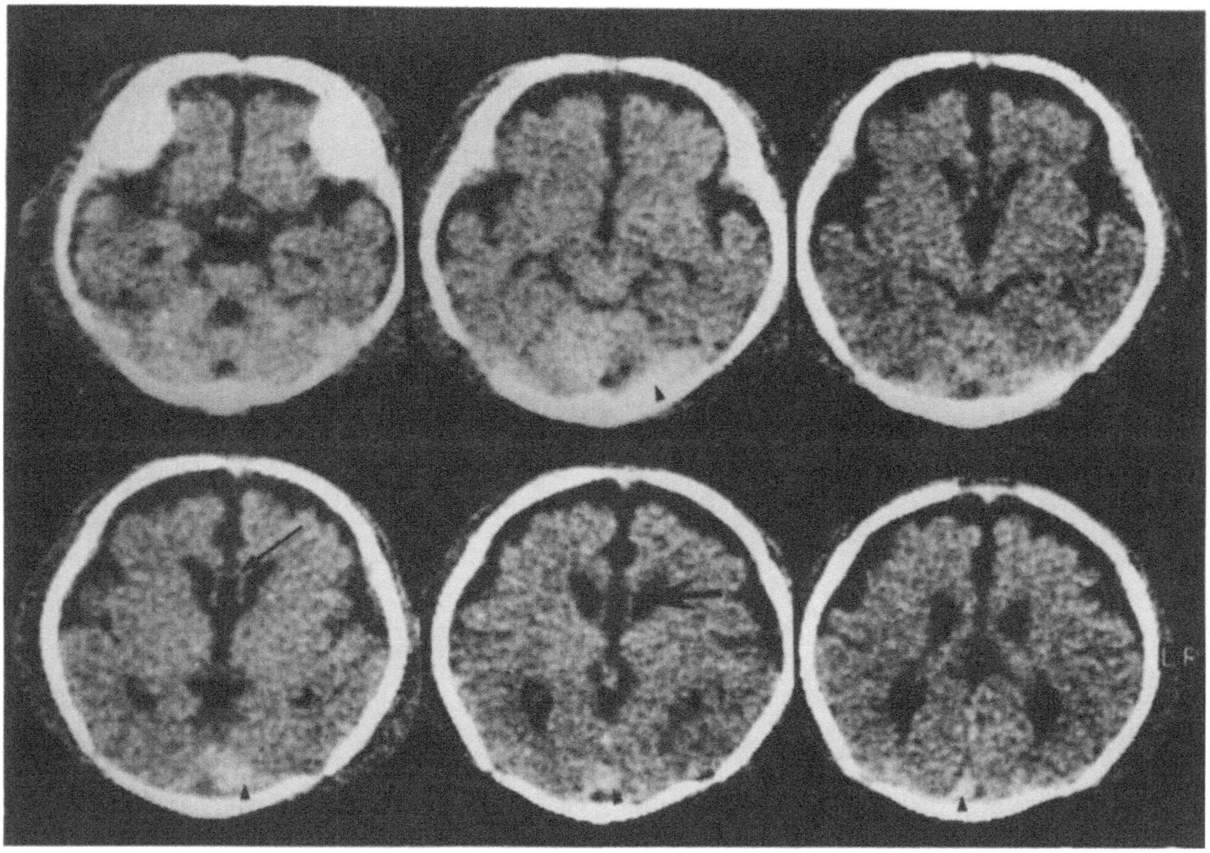

Figure 22. A newborn premature with birth weight 1.7 lb. He had superior vena cava obstruction, cerebral venous sinus thrombosis **(arrowheads)** and hypoxic ischemic encephalopathy. Prominent subarachnoid spaces are manifestation of external hydrocephalus.
Note apparent approximation of the interhemispheric fissure to the third ventricle suggesting dysgenesis of corpus callosum. However, the following negate such a consideration: 1) Presence of cavum septum pellucidum **(thick arrow)** which should not be seen as such in dysgenesis of corpus callosum, 2) normal distance between the interventricular foramina, 3) visualization of a small part of genu of corpus callosum **(thin arrow)**, and 4) normal convergence of choroid plexi.

REFERENCES

1. Bruce A: On the absence of the corpus callosum in the human brain, with the description of a new case. *Brain* 12:171, 1889.
2. Bull J: The corpus callosum. *Clin Radiol* 18:2-18, 1967.
3. Ettinger G: Agenesis of the corpus callosum. In: *Handbook of Clinical Neurology, Congenital Malformations of the Brain and Skull,* Part I. Eds: Vinken PJ, Bruyn GW. North-Holland Publishing Co., Amsterdam, New York, Oxford. P 285-297, 1977.
4. Loeser JD, Alvord Jr, EC: Agenesis of the corpus callosum. *Brain* 91:533-570.1968.
5. Loeser JD, Alvord Jr, EC: Clinicopathological correlations in agenesis of the corpus callosum. *Neurology* 18:745-756, 1968.
6. Lemire RJ, Loeser JD, Leech RW, Alvord Jr, EC: *Normal and Abnormal Development of the Human Nervous System.* Harper and Rowe, Hagerstown, Maryland PP265-272, 1975.
7. Probst FP: Congenital defects of the corpus callosum. *Acta Radiologica,* Supplement 331, 1973.
8. Rakic P, Yakovlev Pl: Development of the corpus callosum and cavum septi in man. *J Comp Neurol* 132:45-72, 1968.
9. Solt LC, Deck JHN, Baim RC, TerBrugge K: Interhemispheric cyst of neuroepithelial origin in association with partial agenesis of the corpus callosum. Case report and review of the literature. *J Neurosurgery* 52: 399-403, 1980.
10. Brun A, Probst F: The influence of associated cerebral lesions on the morphology of the acallosal brain. A pathological and encephalographic study. *Neuroradiology* 6:121-131, 1973.
11. Kushnet MW, Goldman RL: Lipoma of the corpus callosum associated with the frontal bone defect. *AM J Roentgenol* 131:517, 1978.
12. Yock Jr, DH: Choroid plexus lipoma associated with lipoma of the corpus callosum. *J Comput Assist Tomog* 4:678-683, 1980.
13. Zee C-S, McComb JG, Segall HD, Tsai FY, Stanley P: Lipomas of the corpus callosum associated with frontal dysraphism. *J Comput Asst Tomog* 5:201-205, 1981.
14. Gott PS, Sand RE: Agenesis of the corpus callosum: Limits of functional compensation. *Neurology* 28:1272-1279, 1978.
15. Carr-locke D, Millac P: Diencephalic epilepsy in a patient with agenesis of the corpus callosum confirmed by computerized axial tomography. *J Neurol Neurosurg Psychiat* 40: 808-814, 1977.
16. Summers GD, Young AC, Little RA, Stoner HR, Forbes WS, Jones RA: Spontaneous periodic hypothermia with lipoma of the corpus callosum. *J Neurol Neurosurg Psychiat* 44:1094-1099, 1981.
17. Singer WD, Haller JS, Sullivan LR et al: The value of neuroradiology in infantile spasms. *J Pediatrics* 100:47-50, 1982.
18. Byrd SE, Harwood-Nash DC, Fitz CR: Absence of the corpus callosum: computed tomographic evaluation in infants and children. *J Can Assoc Radiol* 29:108-112, 1978.
19. Guibert-Tranier F, Piton J, Billerey J, Caille JM: Agenesis of the corpus callosum. *J Neuroradiology* 9:135-160, 1982.
20. Fitz CR: Midline anomalies of the brain and spine. *Rad Clin N Amer* 20:95-104, 1982.

4

Holoprosencephaly (Prosencephaly)

HISTORY, DEFINITION AND GROSS MORPHOLOGY (1-5)

Initially described by Rudius in 1588 (4), holoprosencephaly comprises malformation of the brain and the face. **Arhinencephaly**, the original name coined by Kundrat in 1882 (5), is not appropriate since it implies maldevelopment of only the olfactory bulbs and tracts, whereas this disorder involves almost all supratentorial compartment structures.

The term "holoprosencephalon" means the "entire prosencephalon" (holo = entire); that is, the prosencephalon remains as a whole. Normally, the prosencephalon is created by ballooning of the rostral end of the neural tube (figs. 1 and 2); it then forms diverticulae, which include those destined to form the cerebral hemispheres (telencephalon), neurohypophysis and the optic bulbs (diencephalon).

If the telencephalic (cerebral hemispheric) diverticlae do not develop, one on each side (Figs. 1 and 2), a **holosphere** forms. The holosphere either fails to cleave or cleaves imperfectly in the sagittal plane and has a single ventricle (monoventricle), which represents the third and lateral ventricles and communicates with the aqueduct.

Failure of the diencephalon to cleave results in nondivision of its derivatives so that the thalami remain fused as, quite frequently, do mamillary bodies; the midbrain also may fail to divide into halves. The optic nerves usually are formed, although hypoplastic, but are absent in the cyclops.

The final external shape of the holosphere depends on the degree to which its margins enfold to enclose the monoventricle (Fig. 3) (1), a variable process. a) If the holosphere margins do not cover the monoventricle, the thin membranous ventricular roof expands superiorly and dorsally to form the DORSAL SAC (Fig. 4). This sac sometimes pulls back the cerebral mantle to leave a large extracerebral space anteriorly. In this situation, the head can be abnormally large – although this is unusual in holoprosencephaly complex, since **micrencephaly** is most common. The cerebral tissue then becomes applied in the anterior cranial fossa assuming the appearance of a *pancake* or a horseshoe. b) If the holosphere margins roll over somewhat further, the external appearance resembles a *cup*. c) If this enfolding process continues, ultimately the monoventricle will be completely covered and resemble a *ball*. In such a situation, the holosphere is located in the middle fossa and is covered by fluid.

Three varieties of holoprosencephaly occur depending on the degree of separation between the cerebral hemispheres (1).

1) **Alobar Holoprosencephaly**
This is the most severe form. There are no separate cerebral hemispheres, no interhemispheric fissure (IHF) and no falx (Fig. 5). Olfactory bulbs and tracts are absent in virtually all cases, and only a single ventricle is present.

2) **Semilobar Holoprosencephaly.**
Fusion of the frontoparietal lobes accounts for the absence of IHF anteriorly; this fissure is present posteriorly. Olfactory bulbs and tracts usually are absent or may be hypoplastic.

3) **Lobar Holoprosencephaly.**
Cerebral hemispheres either are normally formed (Fig. 6) or show some continuity of the cingulate gyri deep within IHF. Olfactory bulbs and tracts are aplastic or hypoplastic.

The association between malformations of the brain and face can be traced to their closely related embryologic origin. According to Johnston *et al.* (6), the facial skeleton in the median plane (derived from the frontonasal prominence) arises from the **prechordal mesoderm augmented by the neural crest cells** (Fig. 7). This mesenchymal analogue of the median facial skeleton also is responsible for inducing the rostral end of the neural tube to develop the cerebrum.

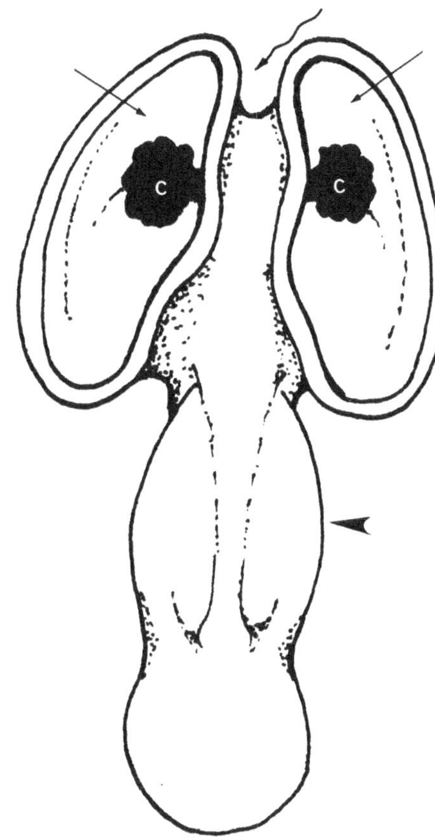

Figure 1. Human brain with part of the wall removed at six weeks gestation. Note the telencephalic vesicles **(straight arrows)**. **Arrowhead** = Diencephalon. **Wavy arrow** = Interhemispheric fissure. **C** = Choroid plexus.

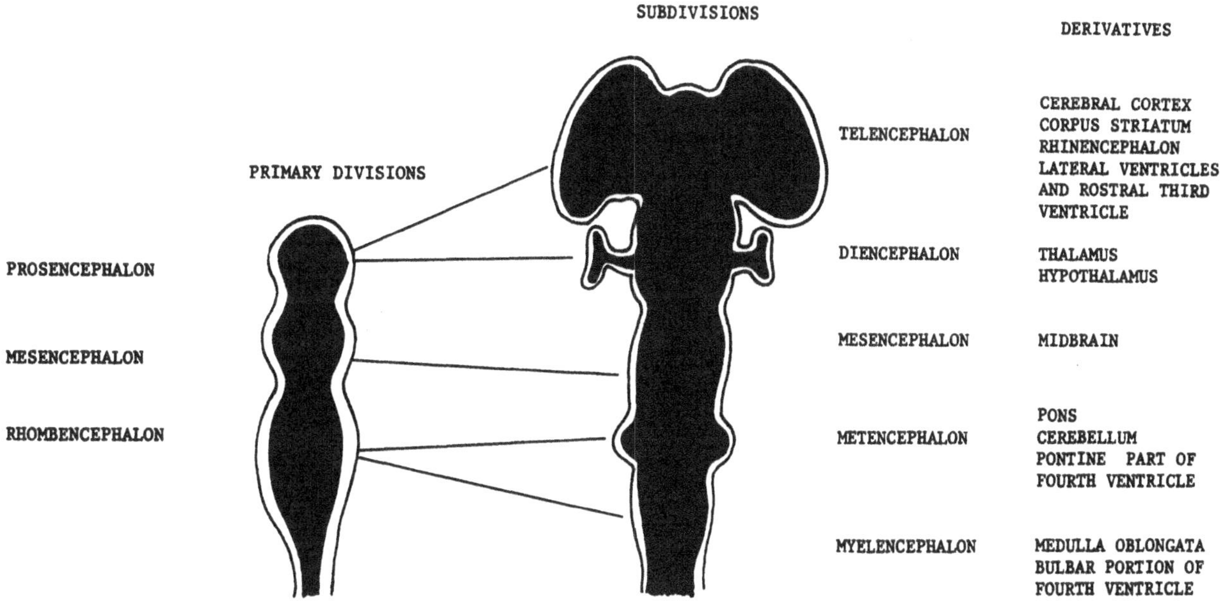

Figure 2. Subdivisions of the brain at three and five vesicle stages and their derivatives.

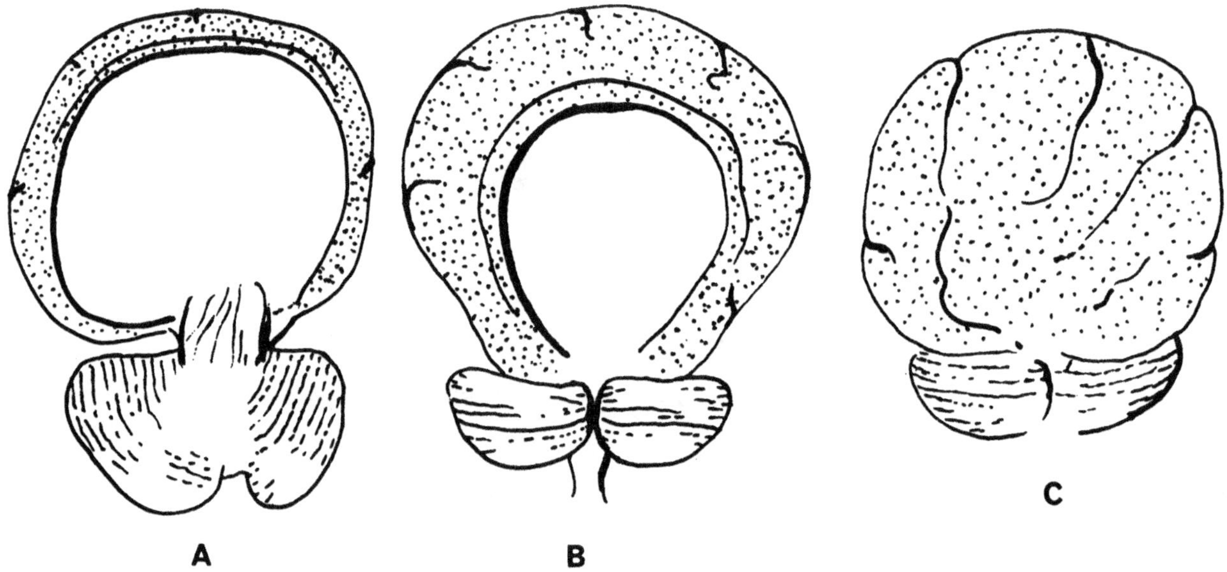

Figure 3. Depending on the degree to which the holotelencephalon rolls over to cover the membranous ventricular roof, alobar holoprosencephaly may have one of three external configurations: A) Pancake-like, B) cup-like, and C) ball-like. [Redrawn from (1).]

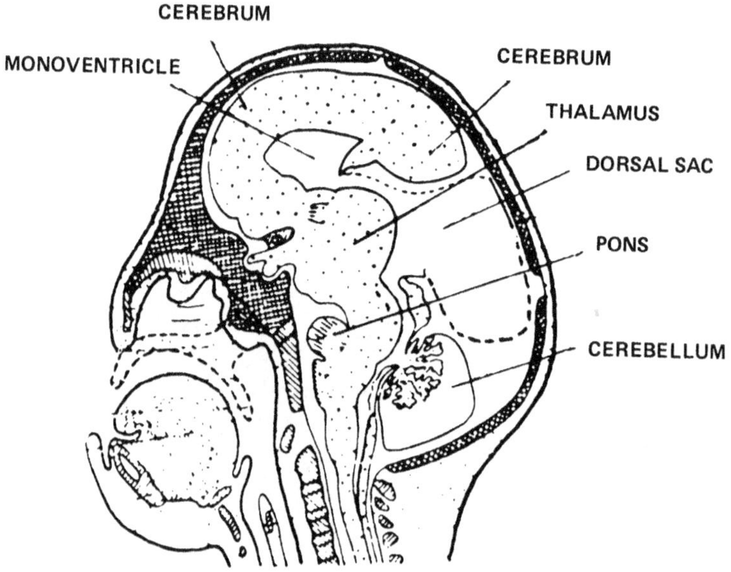

Figure 4. Alobar holoprosencephaly. Schematic presentation of the brain and dorsal sac. [From (3) with permission.]

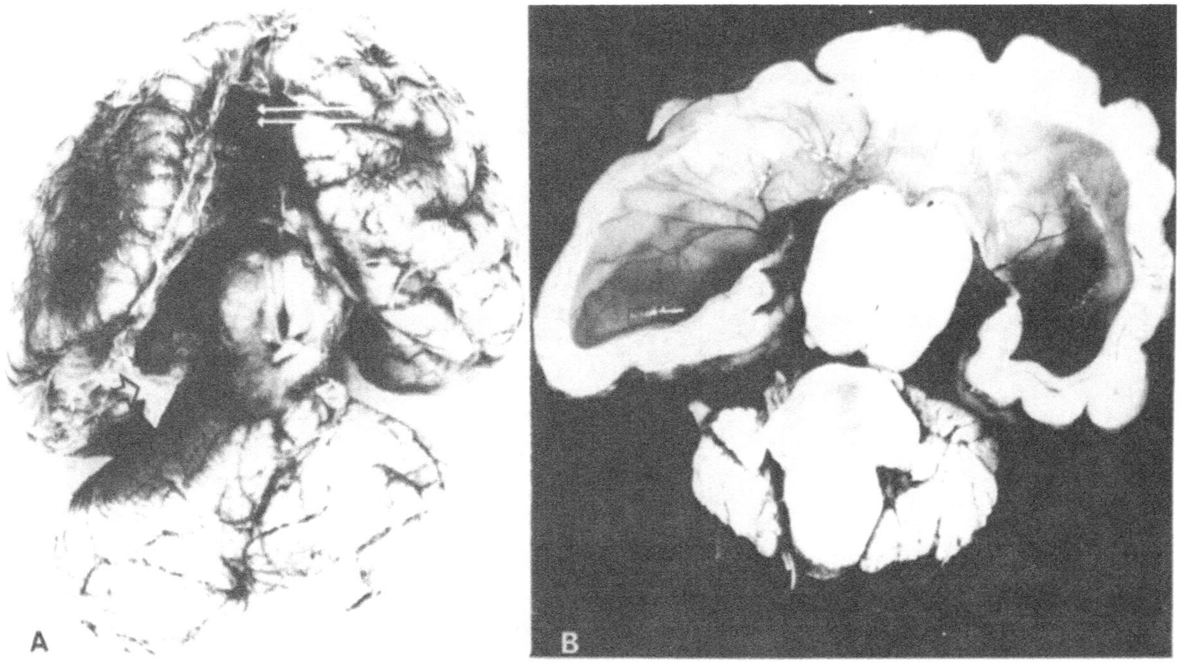

Figure 5. Pathologic specimen of alobar holoprosencephaly in a one-day-old girl.

A. Dorsal view of the brain showing the dorsal sac extending anteriorly over the cerebrum (**closed arrows**). The torn wall of the dorsal sac is indicated by an open arrow at lower left.

B. Coronal section of the brain. There is no interhemispheric fissure. Lateral ventricles are undivided (nonventricle). [From (3) with permission.]

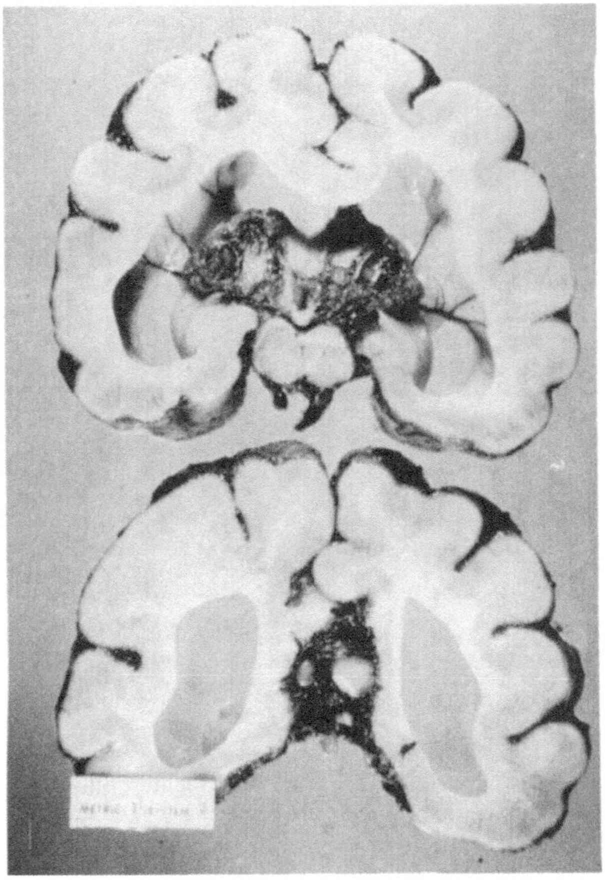

Figure 6. Pathologic specimen of a semilobar to lobar holoprosencephaly. Note monoventricle in the upper coronal brain section. The interhemispheric fissure is present. There is macrogyria. The choroid plexi are unusually prominent. [Courtesy W.F. McCormick M.D., with permission.]

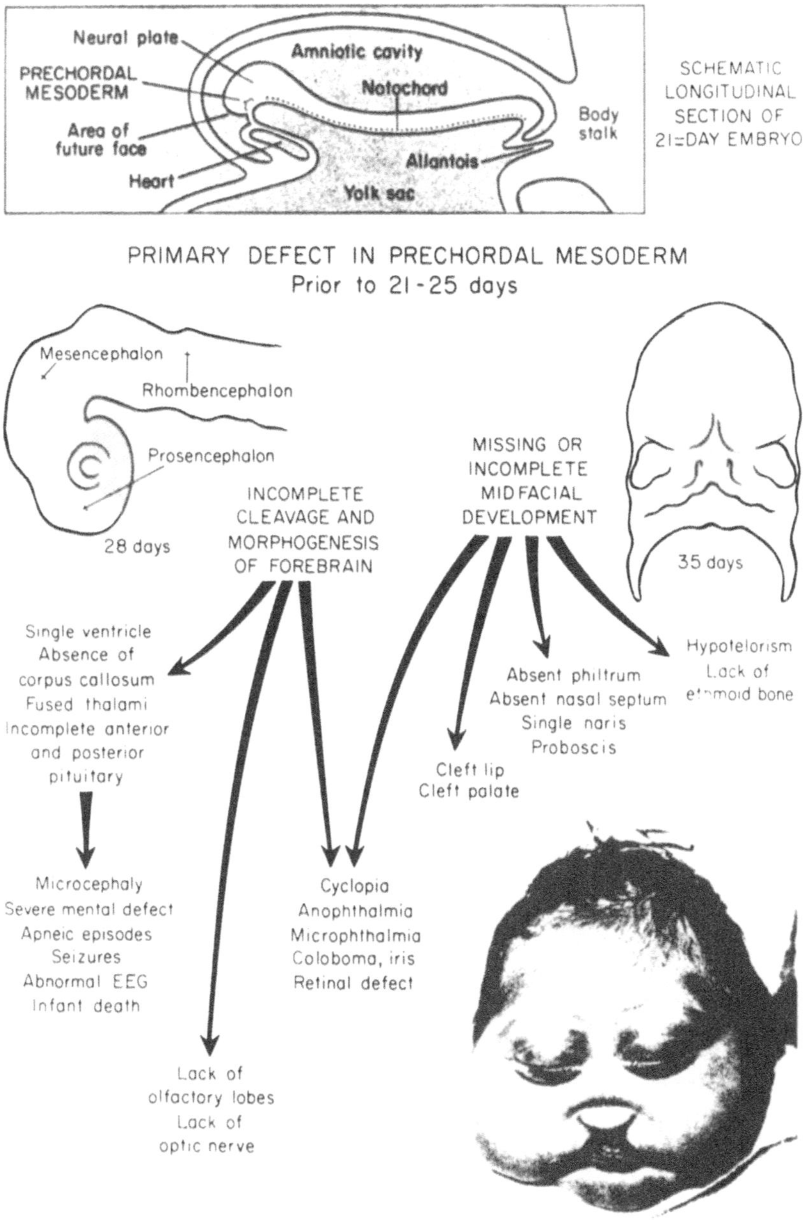

Figure 7. Developmental pathogenesis of the holoprosencephaly malformation [From Smith DW: *Recognizable Patterns of Human Malformation.* W.B. Saunders Co., Philadelphia, 1976, p 367, with permission.]

The **facial anomalies (1,7-9) are classified** as follows (Fig. 8):

1) ***Cyclopia**
The orbits are fused in the midline and contain one or two closely approximated or partially fused eyeballs. A small proboscis (elephant trunk) projects from the forehead above the orbits. There is no nose.

2) **Ethmocethely**
There are two eyes each with its own orbit. A median proboscis resides between them. Median facial bones of frontonasal process origin are absent or hypoplastic.

3) **Cebocephaly**
There are two eyes and two orbits and a proboscis-like nose with a single aperture which ends blindly. There is no cleft lip.

4) **Median cleft lip with hypotelorism**
The nasal bridge is flat. There are nasal alae but no nasal septum.

5) **Intermaxillary rudiment with hypotelorism**
(Philtrum – premaxilla anlage)

Common to all these facies is **aplasia or hypoplasia of the medial facial skeleton** (ethmoid, nasal and premaxillary bones, vomer and nasal septum) of frontonasal prominence origin. This results in excessive approximation of the orbits – **hypotelorism** – which is virtually a constant feature of holoprosencephaly complex.

DeMyer (1) states that Facies I - 4 (Fig. 8) predict holoprosencephaly, usually of alobar type. However, if alobar holoprosencephaly is considered the independent variable, some patients may have a normal or nondiagnostic face (1). In very mild forms, the face may be normal or so subtly abnormal that the disorder escapes clinical recognition. There is less correlation between face and brain malformations at the mild to normal end of the spectrum. An occasional patient may have hypertelorism rather than hypotelorism.* A good rule is to search for holoprosencephaly complex in a patient with **hypotelorism and midline facial anomaly**. This type of malformation is extremely uncommon in a patient with **hypertelorism and midline facial defect**; if a brain anomaly does exist in the latter situation, it usually consists of dysgenesis of the corpus callosum. **Trigonocephaly** (due to premature closure of the metopic suture) also is a fairly common accompaniment of holoprosencephaly complex.

Holoprosencephaly may rarely be associated with other brain malformations including dysgenesis of the corpus callosum (10), encephalocele (11), and Dandy-Walker malformation (12). On occasion, trigonocephaly may be seen concomitant with this disorder. Its familial occurrence (13) and concurrence with chromosomal aberrations (Trisomy 13-15) have been reported (14), and it has been observed both in monozygotic and dizygotic twins (15).

According to Osaka (3), holoprosencephaly is the most common malformation of the central nervous system. Rarely is it seen clinically since many cases are aborted and an adequate pathologic examination is not permitted or performed.

Most patients with alobar holoprosencephaly die in infancy. Longer survival, but with varying degree of neurologic deficit, is possible in milder forms of the disorder.

CT SCAN FINDINGS (16-19)

The combination of facial and brain anomalies greatly facilitates the diagnosis of holoprosencephaly. These facial abnormalities are especially useful when CT scan findings are atypical, confusing or equivocal.

1) Alobar Holoprosencephaly

In this most severe form of holoprosencephaly, the hallmark of CT scan findings is total absence of the interhemispheric fissure and falx. Lateral ventricles are not identifiable as two separate structures; instead, monoventricle represents both the lateral and third ventricles (Figs. 9-11). The cerebral tissue is recognizable anteriorly and superiorly. The dorsal sac, when present, can be seen as a cerebrospinal fluid (CSF) containing structure posterosuperiorly. The fused thalami are seen in the midline as a solid mass of dystrophic tissue. The posterior fossa structures are normal.

The most severe forms of facial anomalies are present in alobar holoprosencephaly. Hypotelorism, absence of the ethmoids and of the crista galli, as well as midline facial anomalies can be recognized on the coronal CT scans viewed with the reverse mode and with window level and window width set for viewing the bone. Associated anomalies such as microphthalmia, anophthalmia, micrognathia and trigonocephaly (Fig. 12) also can be recognized.

**Note: Cyclopia: In Greek mythology this term was used for a race of giants with a single eye in the middle of the forehead. It is the most common malformation in the pig.*

These midline facial anomalies should not be confused with* **Median Cleft Face Syndrome *which is an entirely different disorder. See page*

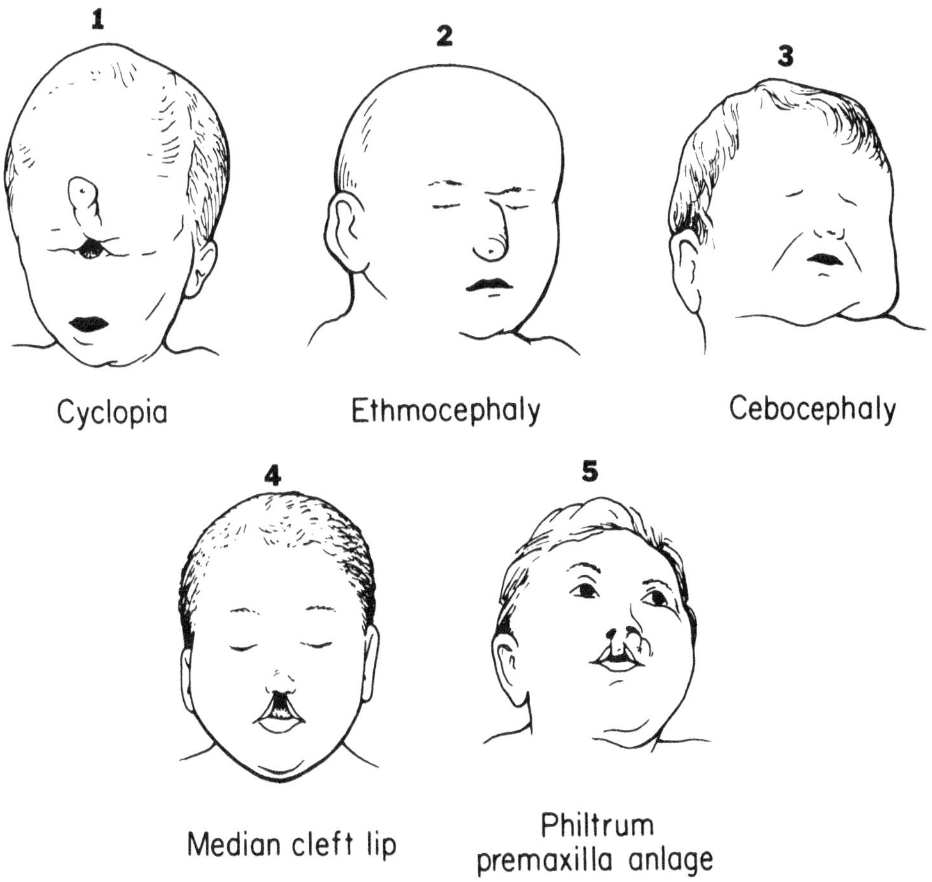

Figure 8. Facies in holoprosencephaly. [Redrawn from (9).]

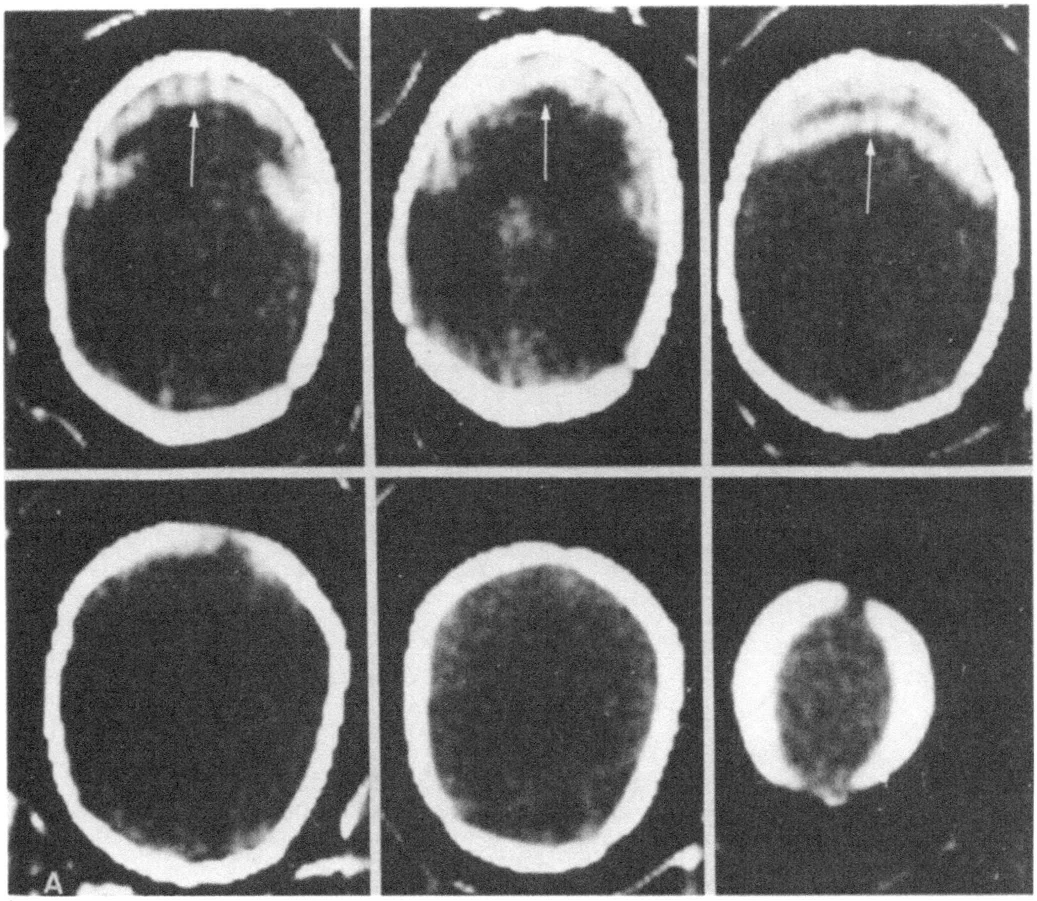

Figure 9. Alobar holoprosencephaly in an infant.

A. CT scan. Note that the cerebral tissue is predominately recognizable only anteriorly (**arrows**). There is monoventricle and the falx is absent.

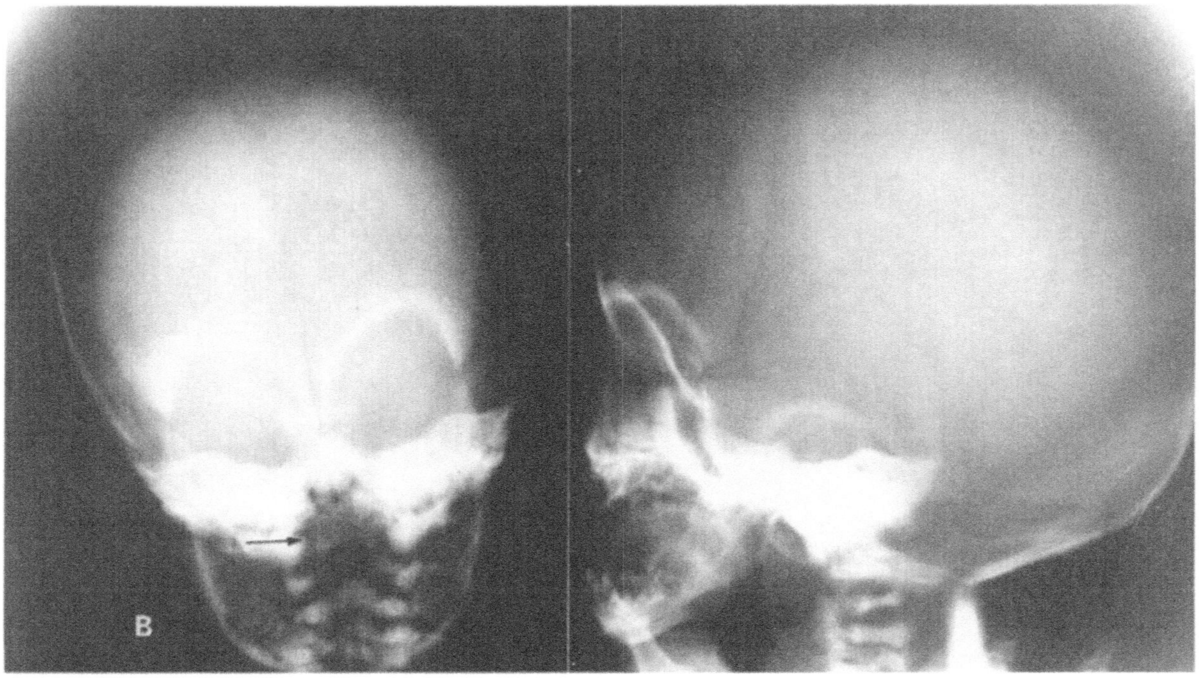

Figure 9. Alobar holoprosencephaly in an infant.

B. Skull films. Midline bony structures are absent (**arrow**), and there is hypotelorism with absence of crista galli. The skull is microcephalic. Absence of sella turcia indicates concomitant pituitary aplasia.

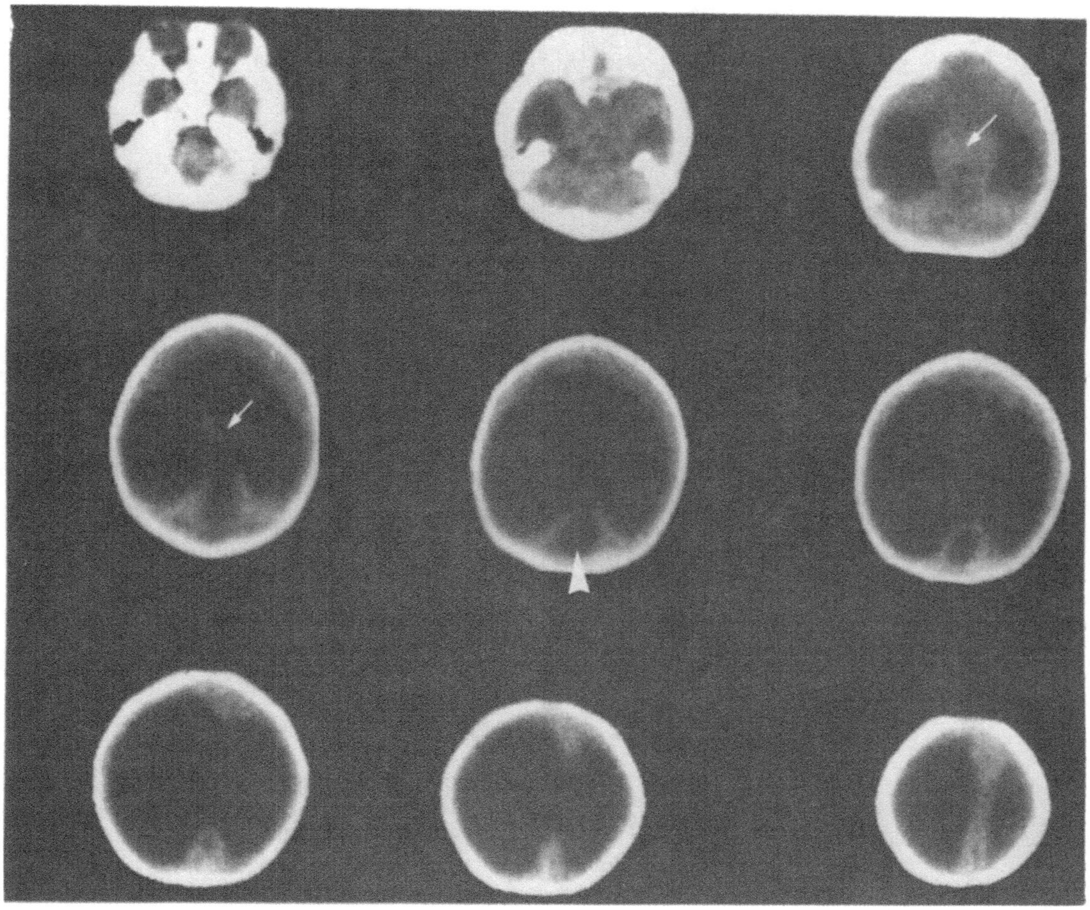

Figure 10. A microcephalic infant with alobar holoprosencephaly. There is monoventricle; the dorsal sac **(arrowhead)** is merely its posterior extension. The thalami **(arrow)** are fused and there is no third ventricle. The interhemispheric fissure and falx are absent. There is hypotelorism.

TABLE I
DIFFERENTIAL DIAGNOSIS OF HOLOPROSENCEPHALY

A. CLINICAL FEATURES

	Holoprosencephaly	*Hydrocephalus*	*Hydrencephaly*	*Massive Bilateral Chronic Subdural Hematoma or Hygroma*	*Interhemispheric Arachnoid Cyst Associated with Dysgenesis of Corpus Callosum*
1. Various facial anomalies	+	–	–	–	Midline facial anomalies, mainly cleft lip and palate, may be present. Nò severe form like cyclopia.
2. Hypotelorism	+	–	–	–	Instead, there may be hypertelorism.
3. Head	Small	Large	NL or Small	Large	Normal or large due to the presence of the arachnoid cyst.

+ = Present — = Absent

B. CT SCAN FEATURES

	Falx	*Interhemispheric Fissure*	*Cerebral Lobes*	*Ventricular System*
Alobar Holoprosencephaly	–	–	Neural tissue present at periphery, though most noticeable anteriorly on axial images. Fused thalami.	–
Hydrencephaly	+	–	Absent, except for central cerebral tissue (basal ganglia).	–
Hydrocephalus	+	+	+	+
Massive Bilateral Chronic Subdural Hematomas or Hygromas	+	+	+	+

+ = Identifiable — = Unidentifiable

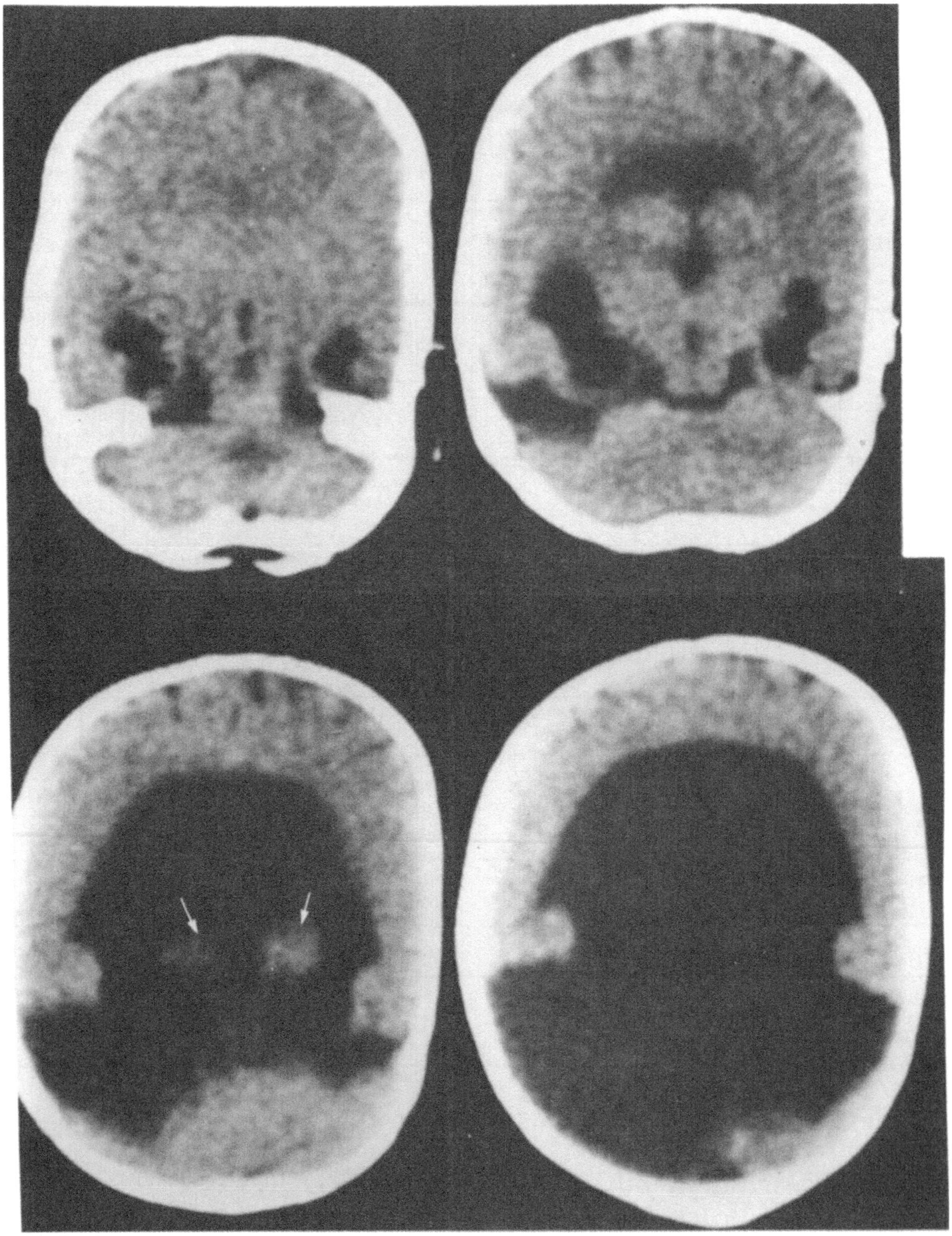

Figure 11. Alobar holoprosencephaly in an 18-month-old boy with hypotonicity. There is no interhemispheric fissure. Cerebral tissue is present all around the monoventricle, more so anteriorly. The posterior fossa structure are small, although normally formed. **Arrows** = Thalami. [Courtesy Dr. Guinto.]

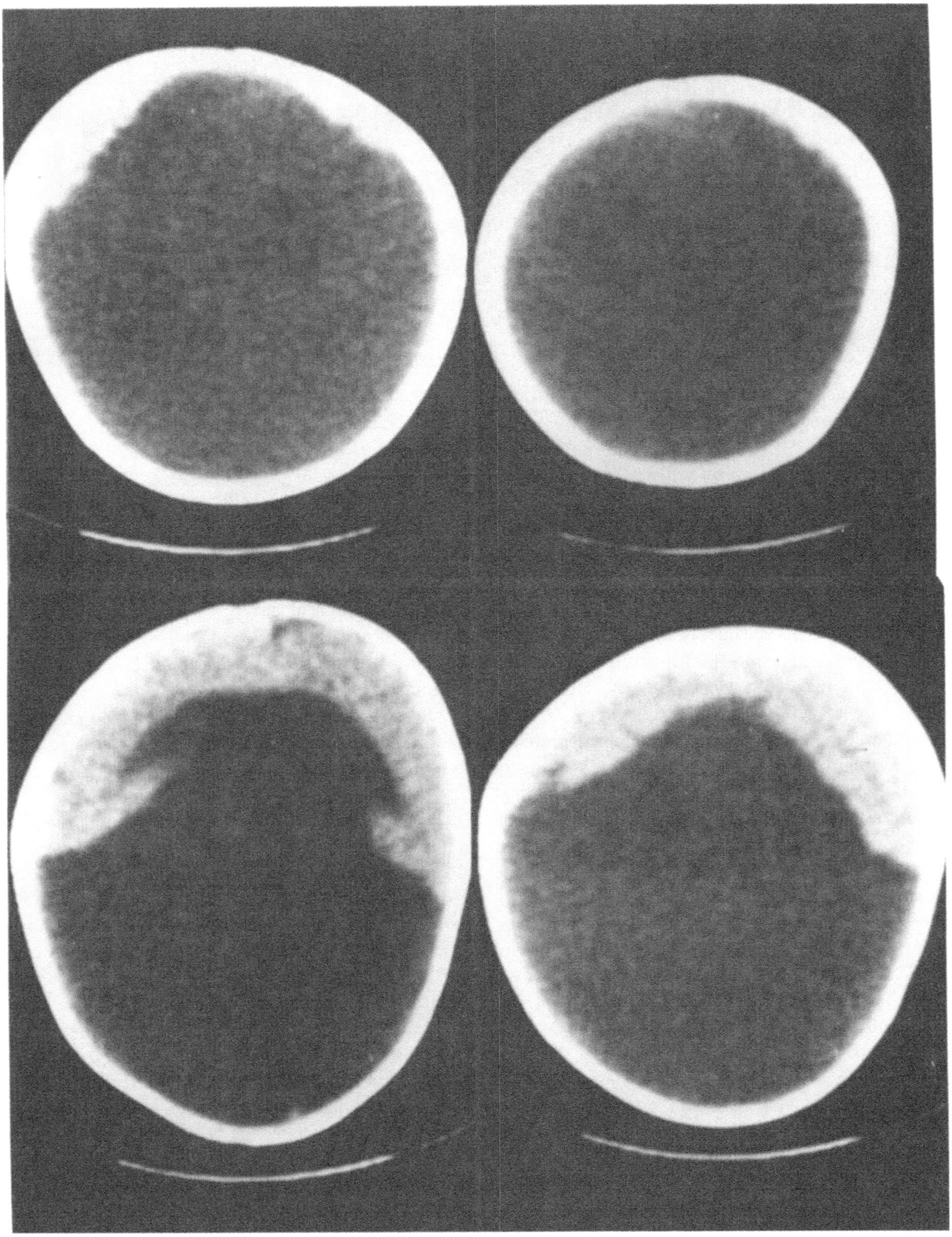

Figure 11. Continued

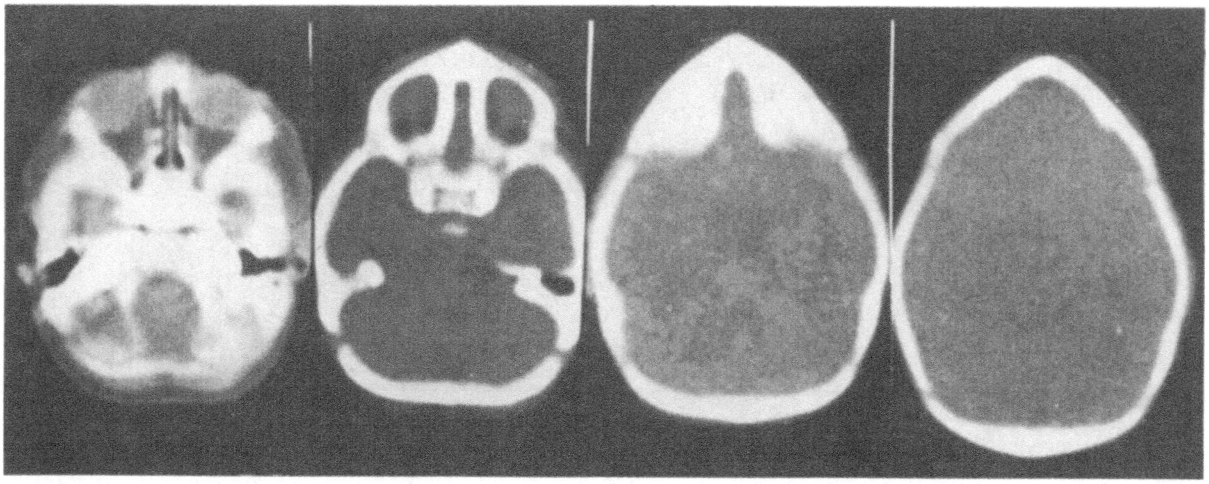

Figure 12. Trigonocephaly in a 6-week-old infant with metopic synostosis. Note the pointed forehead. There was no associated holoprosencephaly.

2) Semilobar and Lobar Holoprosencephaly

Less severe forms of holoprosencephaly include semilobar holoprosencephaly (intermediate) and lobar holoprosencephaly (mild).

In **semilobar holoprosencephaly** (Fig. 13-15), the monoventricle is not as large as in alobar, and more cerebral tissue is present. Partial formation of the occipital horn may be evident. The associated facial anomalies are less severe.

Children afflicted with **lobar holoprosencephaly** can survive into adulthood, although they are usually mentally retarded. In this mild form, the cerebral lobes are fairly well-developed and recognizable (Fig. 16). The frontal horns are squared off with a flat roof; the septum pellucidum is absent; and the third ventricle is in a normal position. The lateral ventricles are slightly dilated due to cerebral hypoplasia. The interhemispheric fissure is fairly well defined, although with high resolution CT scanning some contiguity of the cerebral tissue may be evident anteriorly as interdigitations of the cerebral lobes. The facial anomalies are either very mild or not clinically evident.

As a matter of fact, any peculiarly formed, slightly dilated ventricular system should prompt a detailed study of the anterior interhemispheric fissure to assess continuity of the cerebral tissue. Thin section CT scanning is particularly useful for such an evaluation. Such a detailed and careful study is especially warranted in the presence of a very minimal or suspicious midline facial anomaly and hypotelorism.

Frequently, it may be quite difficult to differentiate semilobar from lobar holoprosencephaly on CT criteria alone.

DIFFERENTIAL DIAGNOSIS OF HOLOPROSENCEPHALY

1. Absence of the septum pellucidum.
2. Massive hydrocephalus.
3. Hydrencephaly.
4. Massive chronic bilateral subdural hematomas or hygromas.
5. Multicystic encephalomalacia and polyporencephaly.
6. Interhemispheric arachnoid cyst associated with dysgenesis of the corpus callosum.
7. Septo-optic dysplasia.

An **absent septum pellucidum** as a sole finding is not considered part of the holoprosencephaly complex. Absent septum pellucidum may be a simple variant of normal or an acquired condition due to rupture in hydrocephalus. In contrast to findings in mild forms of holoprosencephaly complex, the lateral ventricles maintain their normal shape in simple absence of septum pellucidum.

Even in **marked hydrocephalus**, some rim of cortical tissue as well as IHF and falx can be recognized (Fig. 17), and, of course, there is macrocephaly, which is only an occasional feature of holoprosencephaly.

In **hydrencephaly**, the falx usually can be recognized. Even if the CSF-containing cavity is erroneously considered to be monoventricle (implying holoprosencephaly), absence of facial anomalies should suggest a diagnosis of hydrencephaly.

In **massive chronic bilateral subdural hematomas or hygromas**, macrocephaly is present, and the compressed ventricular system and the cerebral hemispheres are seen afloat in the center. (Fig. 18).

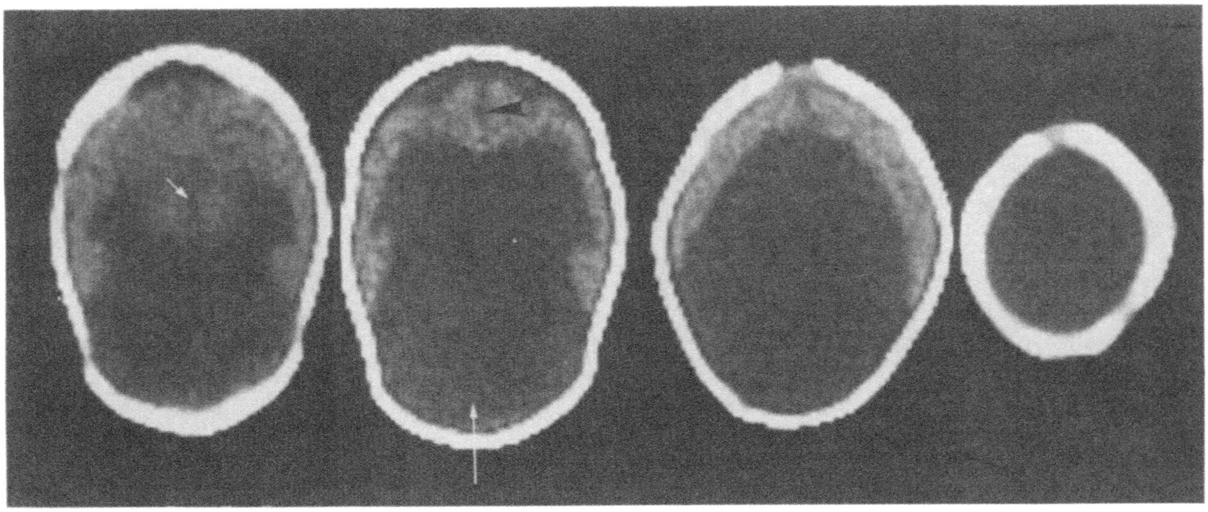

Figure 13. Semilobar holoprosencephaly. Note that the lower part of the frontal interhemispheric fissure (**arrowhead**) is present. The thalami are partly fused and the third ventricle is partly recognizable (**short arrow**). The dorsal sac (**long arrow**) pulls back the frontal cerebral tissue resulting in the creation of a capacious subarachnoid space between the neural tissue and the bone.

This micrencephalic seven-week-old infant had unilateral cleft lip and palate and hypotelorism. He had hypothalamic dysfunction manifested by dysregulation of temperature; his temperature would rise to between 105 and 107°F and was difficult to control.

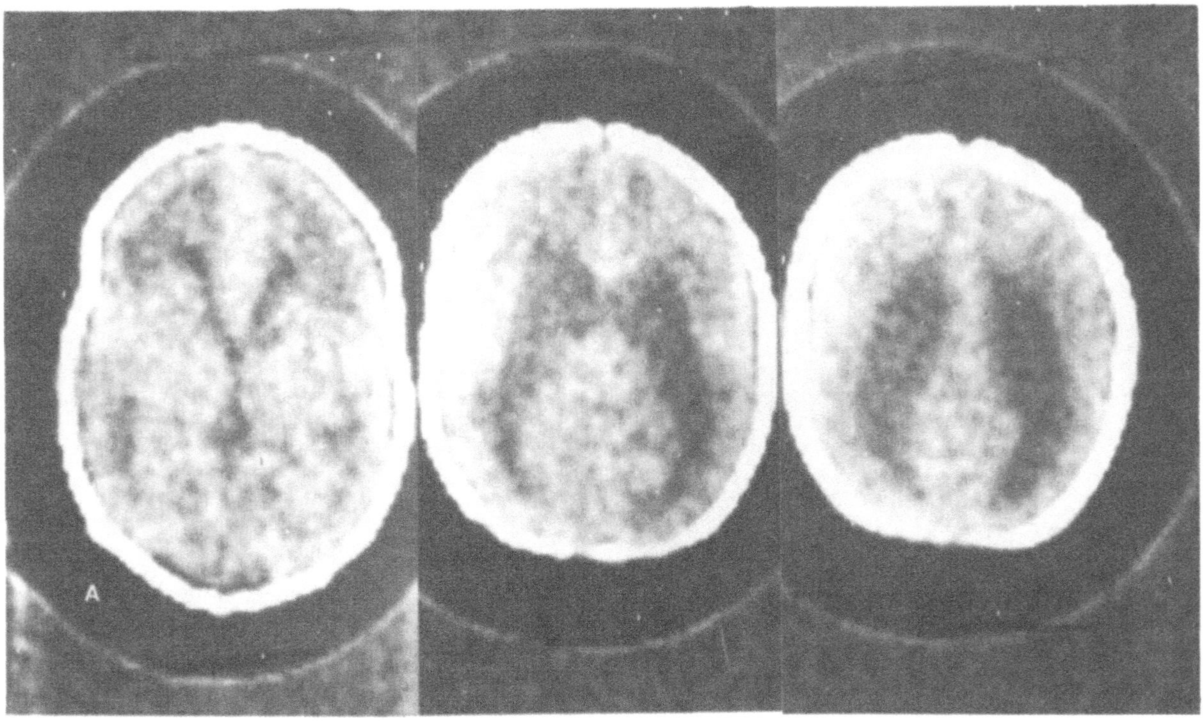

Figure 14. Semilobar holoprosencephaly.

A. CT scan. The interhemispheric fissure is not recognizable indicating continuity of the cerebral hemispheres. The lateral ventricles are malformed. The third ventricle is identifiable.

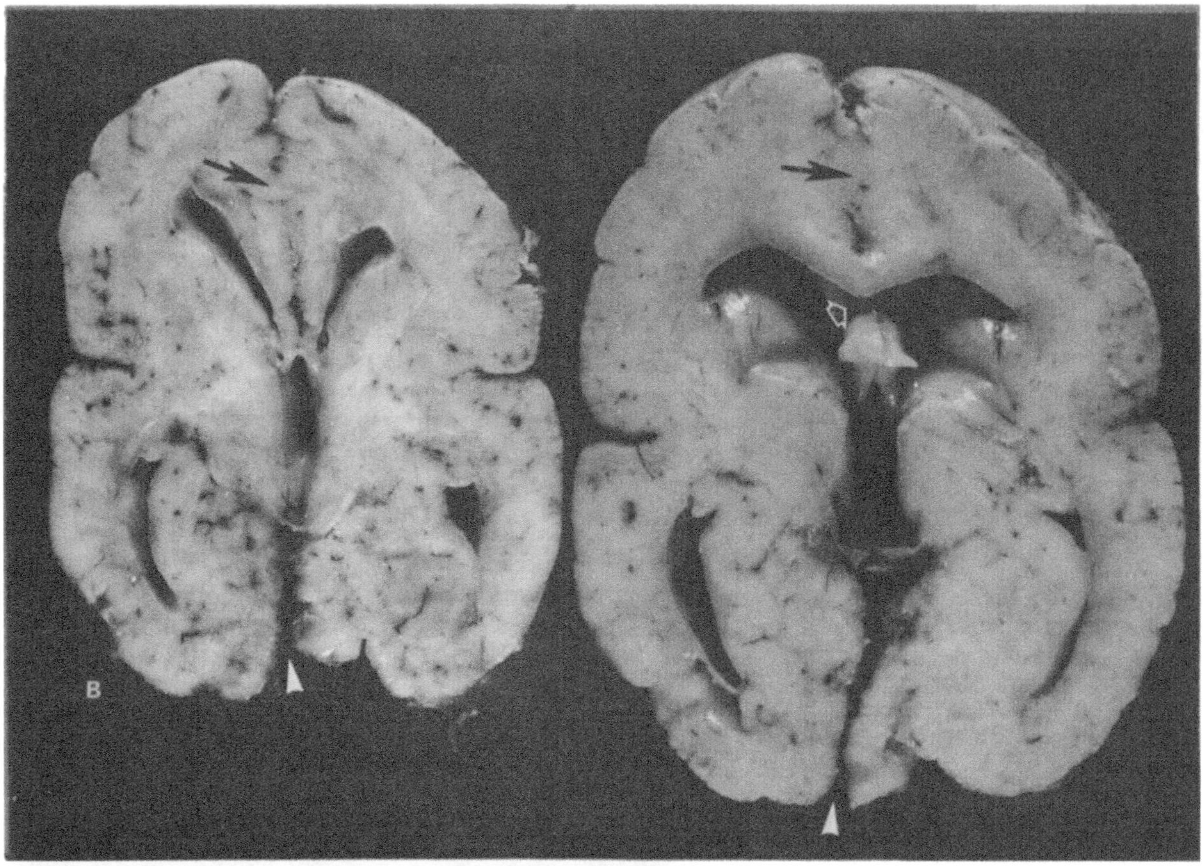

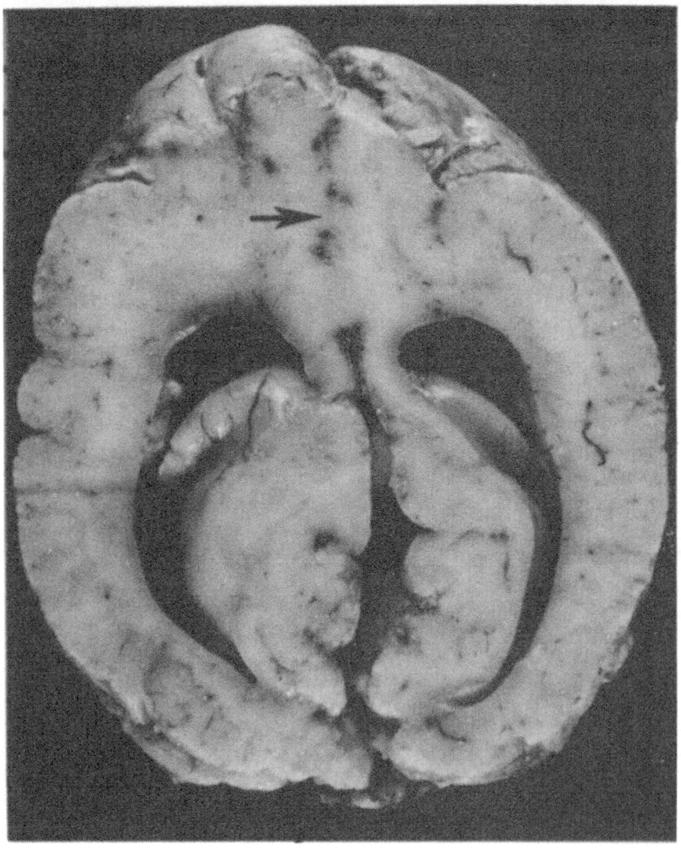

Figure 14. Continued

B. Pathologic specimen. Note the continuity of the cerebral lobes anteriorly (**arrows**) across the poorly formed interhemispheric fissure. This fissure is present posteriorly (**arrowheads**). The lateral ventricles are dysmorphogenic and on one section there is continuity (**open arrows**) between the two sides. The gyri are abnormally wide (pachygyria). The whole brain is variably malformed. There appears to be dysgenesis of the posterior part of the corpus callosum, as well.

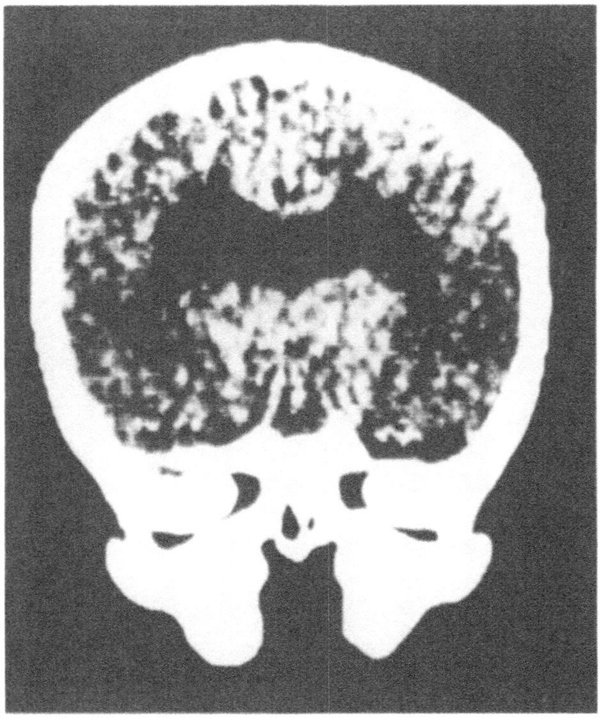

Figure 15. Semilobar holoprosencephaly. Coronal CT. Note nonseparation of the lateral ventricles. [Courtesy D C Harwood-Nash, M.D..]

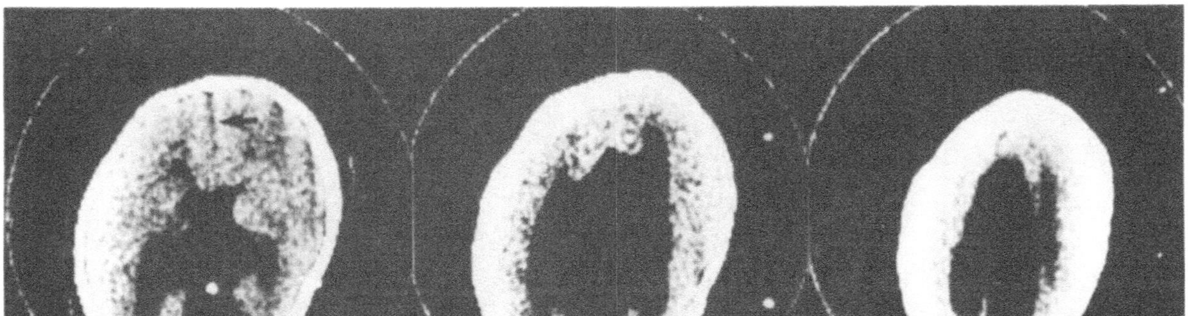

Figure 16. Lobar holopresencephaly in a 1½-year-old girl. Her face was normal except for a rather wide flat nose. The interhemispheric fissure (**arrow**) is present and the interventricular foramina are wider apart. The dorsal sac (**arrowhead**) is eccentric. The broader interventricular foramina and separation of the lateral ventricles might suggest dysgenesis of corpus callosum, the "dorsal sac" then representing the midline arachnoid cyst seen in dysgenesis of corpus callosum. However, the angiographic and ventriculographic findings in this case favored a lobar type of holoprosencephaly rather than dysgenesis of corpus callosum. This case illustrates the difficulty one can encounter in correctly diagnosing these malformations on CT criteria alone. [From (3) with permission.]

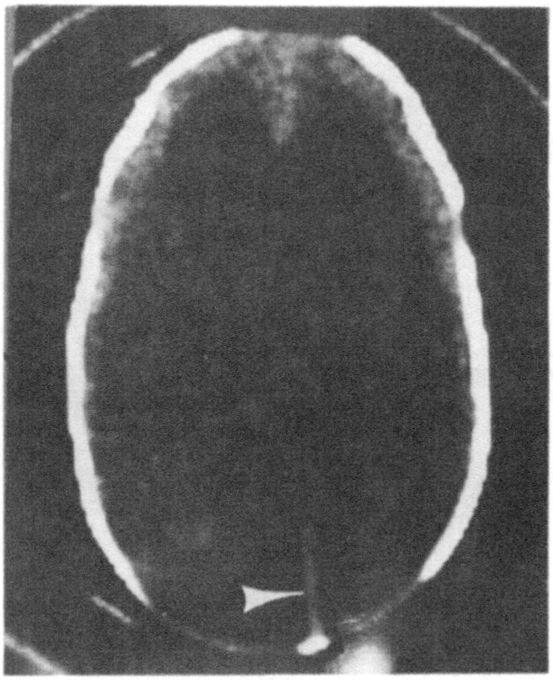

Figure 17. Obstructive hydrocephalus. Note that the fronto-parietal cortical rim and falx **(arrowhead)** are recognizable.

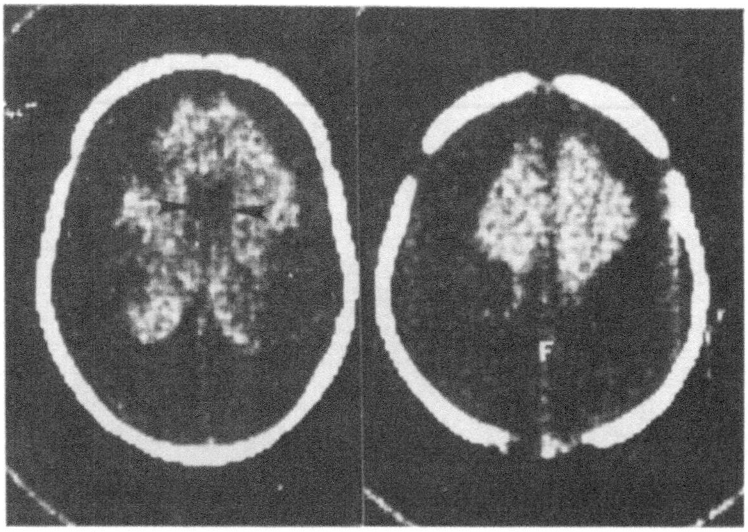

Figure 18. Bilateral massive chronic subdural hematoma in a young child. The cerebral hemispheres have been pushed in from all sides. Sutures are abnormally separated. **Arrowheads** = lateral ventricles. **F** = Falx.

In **multicystic encephalomalacia and polyporencephaly**, the dystrophic cerebral tissue and small cystic areas can become isodense with CSF and therefore may mimic the CT appearance of holoprosencephaly (Fig. 19). However, careful appraisal of the CT scan usually will reveal the ependyma-lined, somewhat dilated ventricular system. On contrast CT scan, the choroid plexi and the ependyma can be identified with ease, thus facilitating the diagnosis. Also, the falx in the IHF becomes easily recognizable, thereby excluding alobar holoprosencephaly.

In the case of **interhemispheric arachnoid cyst associated with dysgenesis of the corpus callosum**, the lateral ventricles, falx and IHF can be identified. The separated interventricular foramina, choroid plexi (espeically on contrast CT scan), and upwardly herniated, dilated third ventricle also help in reaching the correct diagnosis.

In **septo-optic dysplasia**, the flattening of the frontal horns and absence of the septum pellucidum can raise the possibility of lobal holoprosencephaly. However, presence of hypoplastic optic nerves, small optic canals and large chiasmatic cistern seen on thin-section CT scanning should help in reaching the correct diagnosis. Decreased levels of growth hormone with abnormal, visually evoked cortical responses also suggest septo-optic dysplasia.

Major clinical and CT scan features of conditions that should be considered in the differential diagnosis of holoprosencephaly complex are shown in Table I.

SEPTO-OPTIC DYSPLASIA (de MORSIER SYNDROME) (20-25)

History, Definition and Gross Morphology

Septo-optic dysplasia originally was described by de Morsier (20) in 1956. It consists of: 1) primary hypoplasia of the optic nerves; 2) absence of the septum pellucidum; and 3) pituitary dysfunction, especially deficiency of the growth hormone.

The malformation is considered a very mild form of holoprosencephaly complex, probably resulting from an abnormal induction of the prechordal mesoderm. It occurs at about the fourth to sixth week of gestation.

Clinically, these patients are blind and show searching nystagmus. Though it has been reported mainly in the young, it has been recorded in older patients, as well. de Morsier's patient was 84 years old. Dwarfism is related to growth hormone deficiency. Diabetes insipidus may follow hypothalmic dysfunction. The visually evoked responses are abnormal.

CT SCAN FINDINGS

CT scan findings faithfully mirror the pathologic findings and consist of (Fig. 20) 1) hypoplasia of the optic nerves; with thin-section CT scanning, smallness of the optic canals also may be seen; 2) absence of the septum pelludidum; 3) flat roofs of the lateral ventricles on the coronal CT scan. On the axial views, the anterior borders of the lateral ventricles are flat rather than V-shaped; and 4) enlarged suprasellar (chiasmatic) cistern due to chiasmal and hypothalamic dysgenesis.

HYDRENCEPHALY (HYDRANENCEPHALY) (26-34)

Definition and History

Hydrencephaly was described originally by Cruveilhier in 1835 (26). It was Spielmeyer (27), however, who used the term "hydranencephaly" to describe the condition. This malformation is characterized by a normal (usually) or enlarged calvarial cavity (only exceptionally is there micrencephaly) containing thin-walled sac/s filled with CSF in place of the normal cerebral tissue (Fig. 21); the brain tissue is reduced markedly in substance. In fact, the term hydranencephaly is a misnomer since it implies a combination of hydrocephalus and anencephaly. The calvarium does not exist in anencephaly since its growth depends on enlargement of the intracranial contents. Since the skull is well developed in hydrencephaly, obviously anencephaly is not a feature of this disorder. Further, hydrocephalus is rare in this condition. Accordingly, **hydrencephaly** (fluid in the brain) is a preferable term.

Pathogenesis and Gross Pathology

Controversy surrounds the pathogenesis of this malformation. The view that occlusion of the supraclinoid portion of the internal carotid arteries (ICA) occurs in a great majority of cases is not true. Such arterial occlusion is present only in a small percentage of cases. Also, if occlusion of ICA was indeed the cause, abundant collateralization from the ophthalmic and posterior communicating arteries would be expected. However, such collateralization has not been demonstrated consistently in cases of angiographically documented occlusion of ICA. Accordingly, vascular occlusion in cases of hydrencephaly is sufficiently rare that it should be documented pathologically or angiographically before being accepted as the etiologic agent in any given case.

Hypoplasia of the cerebral vessels may be a secondary process due to marked dissolution of the cerebral tissue. The concensus is that this condition results from destruction of the cerebral tissue, which originally had formed to a certain extent. This theory is supported by the presence of normal midline facial structures indicating that telencephalon had developed normally and then undergone a secondary destructive process (see Holoprosencephaly, Chapter 4). This type of destruction usually occurs between 3 months of gestation and term, although destructive changes in the neonate and in the infant occasionally result in a somewhat similar type of cerebral damage. Thus, hydrencephaly may be considered the end result of a destructive process, be it necrotizing encephalitis, vascular injury, trauma, or infection (e.g., rubella, toxoplasmosis). In its broader spectrum, hydrencephaly may be considered to include cases of multiple cystic encephalomalaria, as well.

According to some authors, hydrencephaly can represent a very advanced stage of hydrocephalus. This view certainly merits attention in those patients who have a large head. It is difficult to understand the underlying cause of excessive fluid accumulation unless one considers that necrotic debris may clog the pacchionion granulations resulting in impaired CSF absorption. Pathologically, there are differences between the lining of hydrocephalic ventricles and the fluid-filled sacs in hydrencephaly. In hydrencephaly, the wall of the membranous sac consists of leptomeninges, which are lined internally by a layer of glial tissue that has no ependyma. This is in contrast to hydrocephalus in which cerebral cortex is present to a greater extent and subcortical white matter and ependyma also can be recognized at least in some places.

Whereas a major portion of the cerebral hemisphere is reduced to a membrane, cerebral tissue in the temporal and inferior part of the frontal lobes and in the corpus striatum usually is present in hydrencephaly. The supratentorial compartment transilluminates, implying that the cerebral cortex is less than 1 cm thick. The brain stem is small due to decreased mass of the corticospinal tracts.

CT SCAN FINDINGS

The CT scan findings essentially consist of a CSF-filled supratentorial compartment that also contains basal ganglia (Figs. 22, 23, 24). Rudimentary neural tissue at the frontal lobe/s and/or part of the temporal lobe/s may be recognized (Fig. 25). The CSF-containing sac bears no semblance of separate lateral ventricles. The falx is present. The posterior fossa structures show normal configuration although brain stem is small.

When difficulty is encountered in differentiating hydrocephalus from hydrencephaly, the following features favor hydrocephalus: 1) presence of thin frontal cortical rim; 2) identification of each lateral ventricle as such; and 3) macrocephaly. Absence of any recordable electrical activity on EEG indicates hydrencephaly.

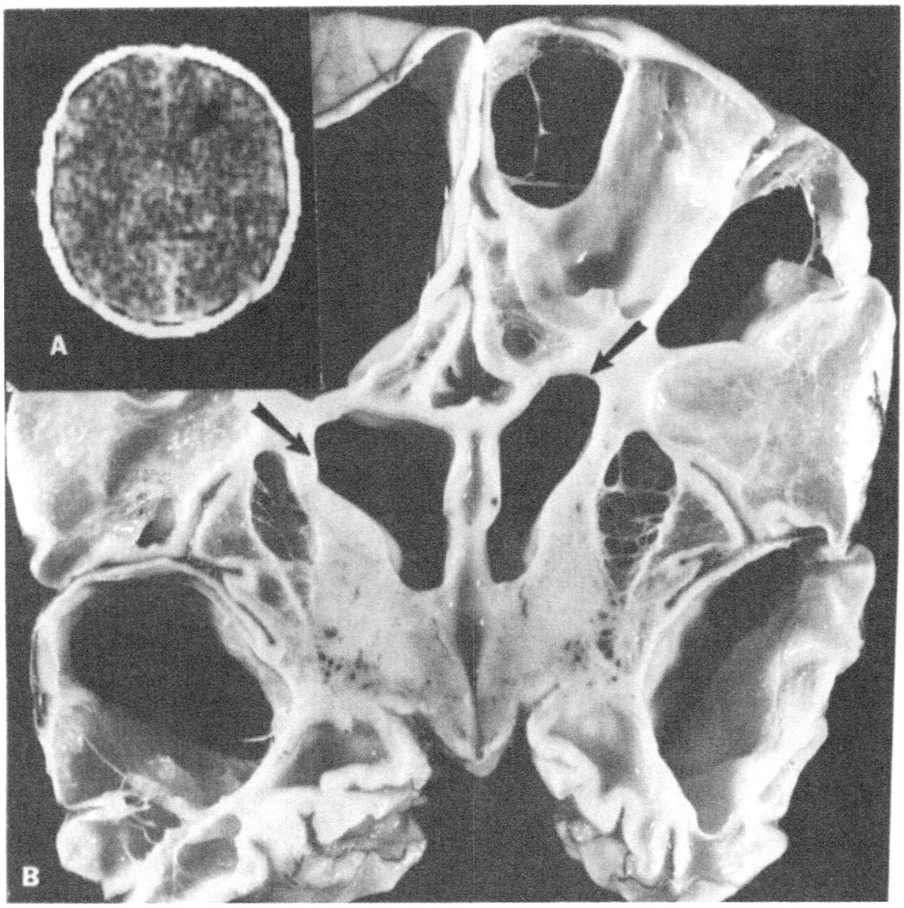

Figure 19. Polyporencephaly in a newborn with anoxia.

A. CT scan. The entire brain is hypodense. The ventricular system **(arrow)** is difficult to recognize as its density is almost the same as that of the ventricular CSF.

B. Pathologic specimen, coronal section. There are multiple areas of porencelphay, some showing septations. Lateral ventricles **(arrows)** are dilated.

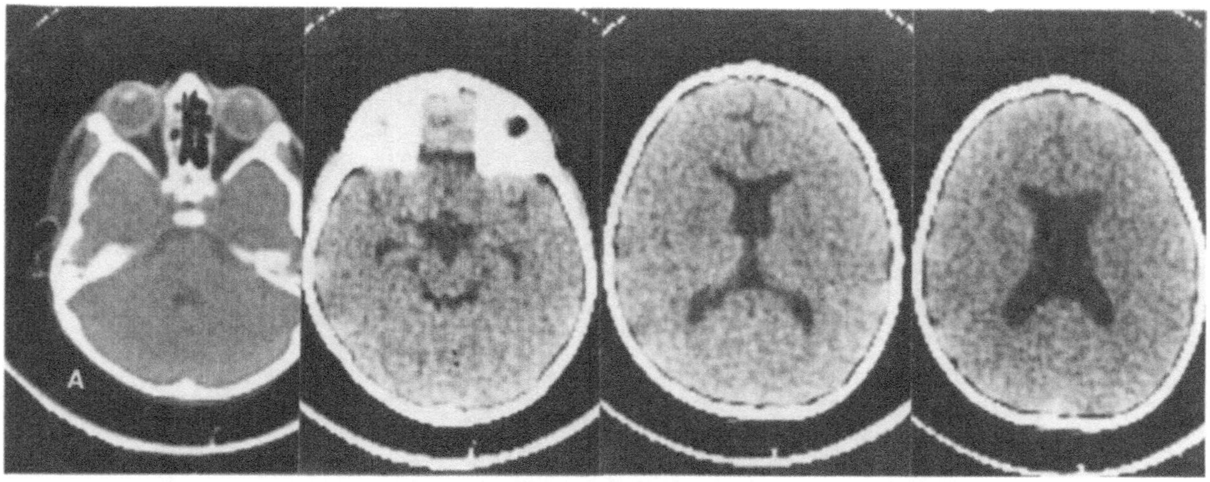

Figure 20. Septo-optic dysplasia in a 1-year-old child.

A. Axial CT scan. There is hypoplasia of the optic nerves, capacious suprasellar cistern, absence of septum pellucidum and flatness of the anterior aspects of the lateral ventricles.

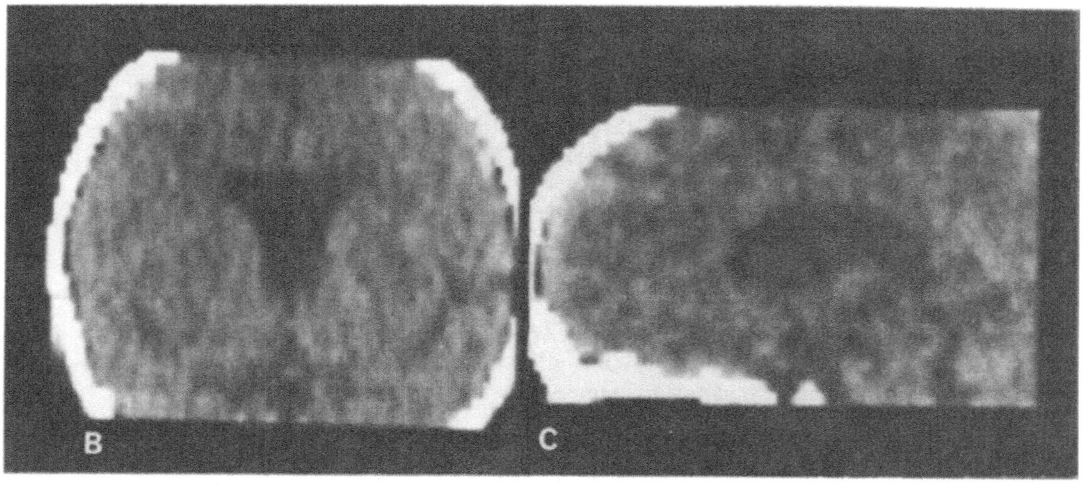

B. Reformatted coronal CT. There is absence of septum pellucidum and flatness of the superior aspects of the lateral ventricles. The suprasellar cistern is generous.

C. Reformatted sagittal CT. Again note prominent suprasellar cistern.

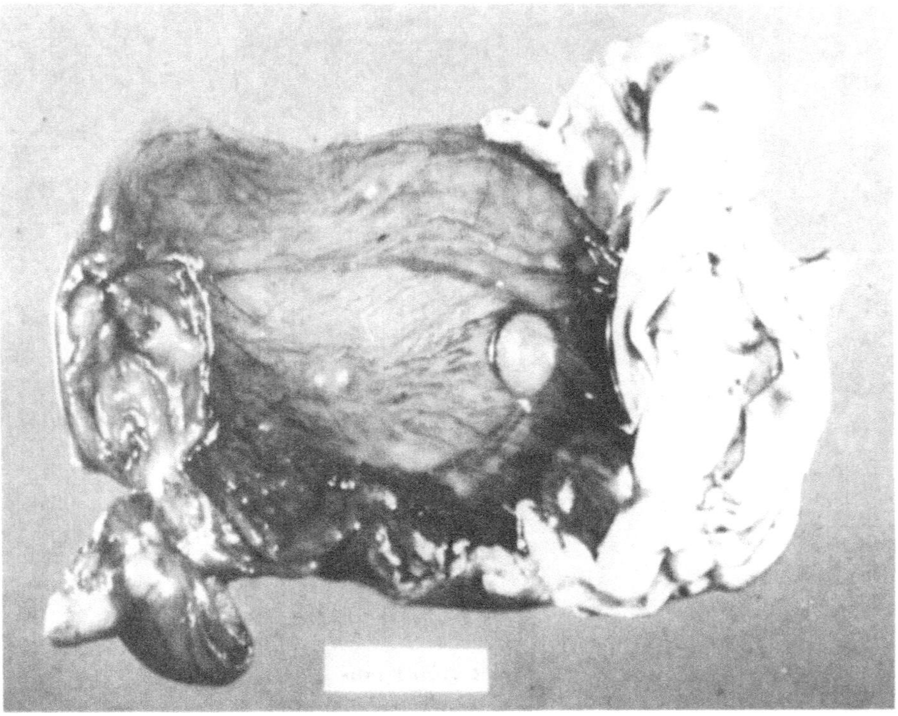

Figure 21. Pathologic specimen of hydrencephaly. The neural tissue has been reduced to a membranous sac. [Courtesy W.F. McCormick, M.D.]

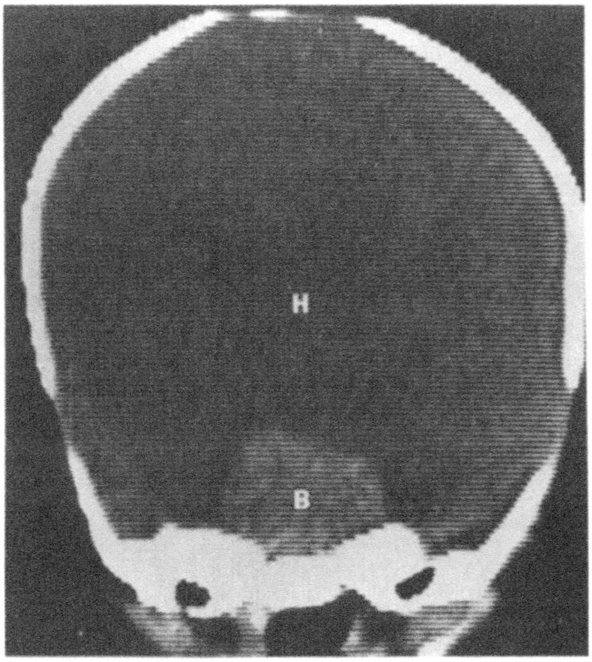

Figure 22. Hydrencephaly (H) as seen on the coronal CT scan. The cerebral tissue is present only at the skull base (B). (From Johnson ML and Rumback CM: *Rad Clin N. America 18:*117-131, 1980, with permission.)

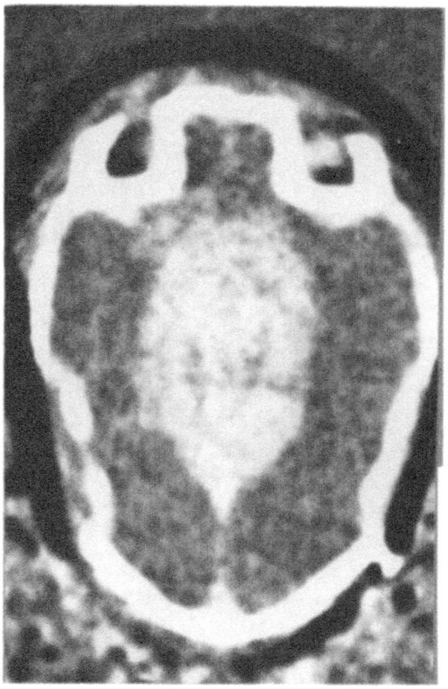

Figure 23. Hydrencephaly. CT scan at level of basal ganglia. Only the midline neural tissue (basal ganglia) is present; the rest of the cerebral hemispheres are transformed into a CSF-containing sac. The posterior fossa structures are normal. [From: *Computed Tomography, 2*:221-235, 1978, with permission.]

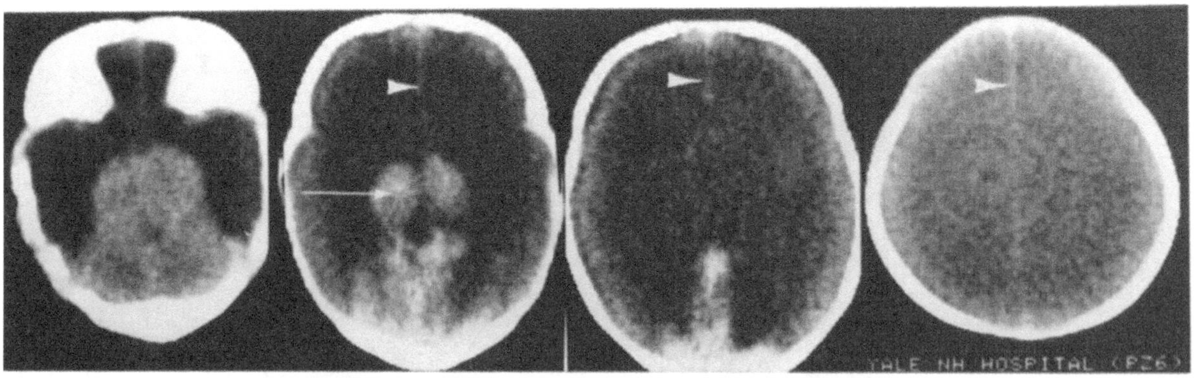

Figure 24. Hydrencephaly in a two-week-old infant. Large size of the head in this case suggests hydrencephaly as a manifestation of the extreme form of hydrocephalus in which hardly any recognizable cerebral hemispheric tissue remains. Preservation of the basal ganglia (**arrow**) and of the posterior fossa structures indicates that in this anomaly the phylogenetically older structures tend to escape the insult; the neopallium suffers the most damage. **Arrowhead** = Falx.

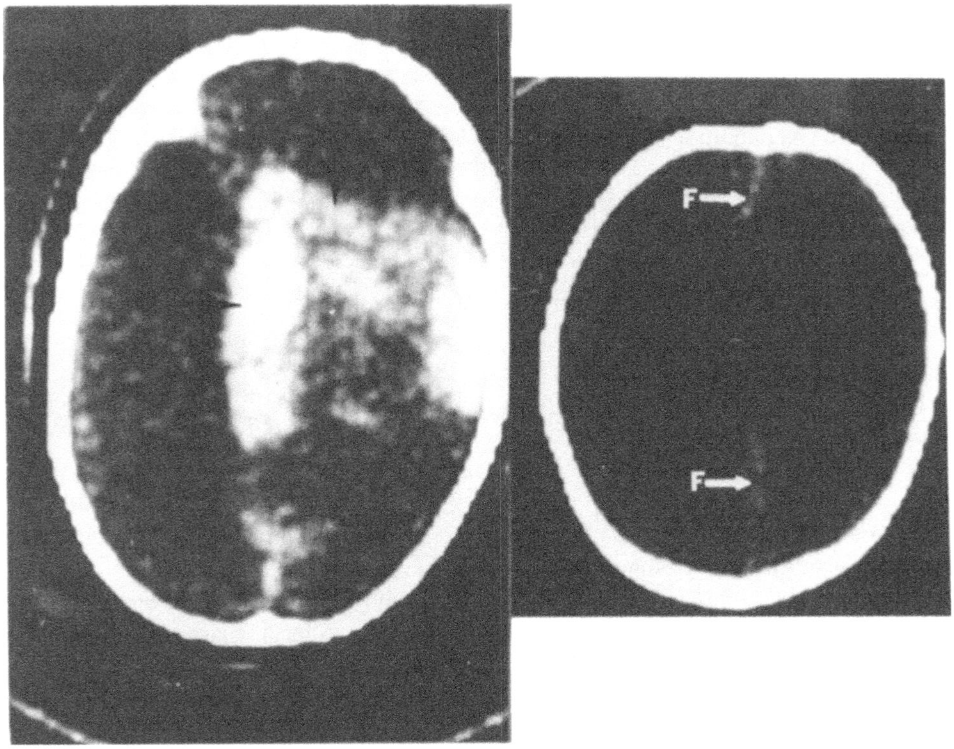

Figure 25. A two-year-old child with hydrencephaly. The neural tissue is present only in the midline and to one side (**arrows**) and at the inferior aspects of the cranial cavity. The rest of the cranial cavity is filled with CSF-containing sacs. Presence of falx (F) excludes alobar holoprosencephaly.

REFERENCES

1. DeMyer W: Holoprosencephaly (Cyclopia-arhinencephaly). In: *Handbook of Clinical Neurology.* Congenital Malformations of the Brain and Skull, Part I. Vol. 30. Eds. Vinken PJ and Bruyn GW: North-Holland Publishing Company, Amsterdam, New York, Oxford, 1977, p 431-478.
2. Probst FP: *The Prosencephalies.* Springer-Verlag, Berlin, Heidelberg, 1979.
3. Osaka K, Matsumoto S: Holoprosencephaly in neurosurgical practice. *J. Neurosurgery, 48:*787-803, 1978.
4. Zingesser LH, Schecter MM, Medina A: Angiographic and pneumoencephalographic features of holoprosencephaly. *Am. J. Reontgenology, 97:*561-574, 1966.
5. DeMyer W, Zeman W: Alobar holopresencephaly (arhinencephaly) with median cleft lip and palate: Clinical electroencephalographic and Nosologic considerations. *Confin Neurol, 23:* 1-36, 1963.
6. Johnston MD, Bhakdinaronk A, Reid YC: An expanded role of the neural crest in oral and pharyngeal development. In: *Oral Sensation and Perception.* 4th Symp. Maryland, National Institutes of Health: 37-52, 1973.
7. DeMyer W: Median facial malformations and their implications for brain malformations. *Birth Defects Orig. Art Series, 11*(7): 155-181, 1975.
8. DeMyer W, Zeman W, Palmer CG: The face predicts the brain: diagnostic significance of median facial anomalies for holoprosencephaly (Arhinencephaly). *Pediatrics, 34:*256-263, 1964.
9. Kurlander GH, DeMyer W, Campbell JA, Taybi H: Roentgenology of holoprosencephaly (Arhinencephaly). *Acta Radiol (Diag), 5:*25-40, 1966.
10. Jellinger K, Gross H, Kaltenback, Grisold W: Holoprosencephaly and agenesis of the corpus callosum:

frequency of associated malformations. *Acta Neuropathol, 55:*1-10, 1981.
11. Hutchison JW, Stovring J, Turner PT: Occipital encephalocele with holoprosencephaly and aqueduct stenosis. *Surg Neurol, 12:*331-335, 1979.
12. Hayashi T, Takasi S, Kuramoto S: A case of holoprosencephaly: with possible association of Dandy-Walker cyst. *Brain Dev, 3:*97-101, 1981.
13. Dallaire L, Fraser FC, Wiglesworth FW: Familial holoprosencephaly. *Birth Defects, 7:*136-142, 1971.
14. Agbata IA, Kovi J, Parshad R, Kovi E. Holoprosencephaly and Trisomy 13 in cyclopia. *JAMA, 241:* 1109, 1979.
15. Burck U, Hayek HW, Zeidler U: Holoprosencephaly in monozygotic twins – clinical and computer tomographic findings. *Am J. Med Genet, 9:*13-17, 1981.
16. Byrd SE, Harwood-Nash DC, Fitz CR, Rogovitz DM: Computed tomography evaluation of holoprosencephaly in infants and children. *J of Computer Assisted Tomography, 1:*456-463, 1977.
17. Manelfe C, Sevely A: Neuroradiological study of holoprosencephalies. *J Neuroradiol, 9:*15-45, 1982.
18. Hayashi T, Yoshida M, Kuramoto S, Takeya S, Hashimoto T: Radiological features of holoprosencephaly. *Surg Neurol, 12:*261-265, 1979.
19. Derakshan J, Sabouri-Deylami-M, Lofti J. Holoprosencephaly. Computerized tomographic and pneumographic findings with anatomic correlation. *Arch Neurol, 37:*55-57, 1980.

Septo-Optic Dysplasia

20. de Morsier G: Agenesie du septum lucidum avec malformation du tractus optique (la dysplasie septo-optique). *Schweiz Arch Neurol Psychiatrie, 77:*267, 1956.
21. Hoyt WF, Kaplan JL, Grombach MM, *et al.*: Septo-optic dysplasia and pituitary dwarfism. *Lancet, 1:* 893-894, 1970.
22. Krause-Brucker W, Gardner DW: Optic nerve hypoplasia associated with absent septum pellucidum and hypopituitarism. *J Ophthalmol, 89:* 113-120, 1980.
23. Manelfe C, Rochiccile P: CT of septo-optic dysplasia. *Am J Roentgenol, 113:*1156-1160, 1979.
24. Ellenberger C, Runyan TE: Holoprosencephaly with hypoplasia of the optic nerves, dwarfism, and agenesis of the septum pellucidium. *Am J Ophthalmol, 70:*960, 1970.
25. O'Dwyer JA, Newton TH, Hoyt WF: Radiologic features of septo-optic dysplasia: de Morsier Syndrome. *AJNR, 1:*443-447, 1980.

Hydrencephaly

26. Crome L, Sylvester P: Hydranencephaly. *Arch Dis Child, 33:*235, 1958.
27. Spielmeyer W: Ein hydranencephales Zwillingspaar. *Arch Psychiat Nervenkr, 39:*807, 1905.
28. Dublin AR, French BN: Diagnostic image evaluation of hydranencephaly and pictorially similar entities, with emphasis on computed tomography. *Radiology, 137:*81-91, 1980.
29. Hamby WB, Krauss RF, Beswick WF: Hydranencephaly: Clinical diagnosis. Presentation of seven patients. *Pediatrics, 6:*371-383, 1950.
30. Myers RE: Brain pathology following fetal vascular occlusion: an experimental study. *Invest Ophthal, 8:*41-50, 1969.
31. Osborn BI, Silverstein AM: Animal model for human disease: Hydranencephaly, porencephaly, congenital cysts, retinal dysplasa, C.N.S. malformation. *Am J Path, 67:*221-241, 1972.
32. Osborn BI, Silverstein AM, Prendergast RA, Johnson RT, Parshall CJ: experimental viral induced congenital encephalopathies. I. Pathology of hydranencephaly and porencephaly caused by blue-tongue vaccine virus. *Lab Invest, 25:*197-205, 1971a.
33. Osborn BI, Johnson RT, Silverstein AM, Prendergast RA, Jochim MM, Levy SE: Experimental virus induced congenital encephalopathies. II. The pathogenesis of blue-tongue vaccine virus infection in fetal lambs. *Lab Invest, 25:*206-210, 1971b.
34. Sutton LN, Bruce DA, Schut L: Hydranencephaly versus maximal hydrocephalus: An important clinical distinction. *Neurosurgery, 6:*35-38, 1980.

5

Arnold-Chiari Malformation

DEFINITION AND PATHOLOGY (1-13)

Arnold-Chiari malformation is commonly recognized by its primary features of ponto-cerebellar dysgenesis. However, other brain anomalies form equally important components of this disorder. The ponto-cerebellar dysgenesis is characterized by failure of the pontine flexure to develop and by caudal herniation through the foramen magnum of the inferior cerebellum and other posterior fossa structures (fourth ventricle, medulla oblongata).

The pathogenesis of this disorder is poorly understood and no single theory explains the entire spectrum of the malformation. One of the various theories offered to explain caudal dislocation of the posterior fossa contents is that it results from traction exerted by the myelomeningocele (9), an almost constant feature of the Arnold-Chiari malformation Type II. This has been shown to be incorrect as the nerve roots pursue a normal course five vertebral levels cephalad to the site of myelomeningocele (1); if this theory were correct, all the nerve roots should be angled cephalad in this anomaly. A second theory (originally proposed by Chiari himself in 1895 and pursued by Gardner (6)) postulates that continued impermeability of the roof of the developing fourth ventricle results in persistent embryonic encephalo-hydromyelia causing caudal midbrain herniation. This explanation appears attractive conceptually, but absence of hydrocephalus in some cases and patency of foramen of Magendi at birth in most cases of Arnold-Chiari malformation would suggest that this theory is not applicable in every instance. Patten (1, 11) proposed that a primary overgrowth of the neural tissue, starting at the fourth week of gestation, results in transforaminal herniation of the posterior fossa contents. A concomitant hypoplasia of the occipital bone per se might further contribute to the dysmorphology of this malformation at the posterior fossa level. Large massa intermedia and large caudate nuclei, prominent anterior commissure and occasional megalencephaly seen in this disorder seem to support the concept of neural tissue overgrowth. The neural tissue overgrowth may be a manifestation of defective regression in size of certain parts of the neural tissue, an important stage in normal development of the central nervous system. Kelch *et al.* (14) have suggested that Arnold-Chiari Type I may be an acquired lesion due to excessive CSF absorption along spinal absorptive pathways as seen in lumboperitoneal shunt placement for hydrocephalus. That is, increased rate of CSF absorption along spinal nerve roots may lead to a relative decreased pressure at skull base causing tranforaminal herniation of cerebellar tonsils.

An interesting and seemingly plausible hypothesis was advanced by Cameron (3). According to him, escape of CSF into the amniotic cavity from the invariably associated myelocele or myelomeningocele results in unbalancing of the amniotic and intraventricular pressures. The resultant greater amniotic volume and pressure squeezes the pliable calvarial cavity (the calvarium begins to ossify by about seventh month of gestation) such that the intracranial contents are forced through the foramen magnum. This effect naturally is borne mainly by structures located close to the foramen magnum-brain stem, fourth ventricle and inferior cerebellum. It thus explains their caudal herniation which is the main morphological feature of Arnold-Chiari malformation Type II. This squeezing effect might explain fusion of thalami and thickening of the massa intermedia (due to apposing of third ventricle walls) and maldevelopment of falx and interdigitations of neural tissue in IHF (again due to coming together of the medial aspects of cerebral hemispheres). The pressing of midbrain can explain aqueductal narrowing. The forcing of CSF into the central canal can explain hydrosyringomyelia.

The time of occurrence of the malformation is at about 100 mm stage (near the third month of gestation) (3).

Of the associated anomalies, an obstructive aqueductal lesion is frequently present. Other anomalies consist of syringohydromyelia, craniolacunia (Luckenschadel), dysgenesis of the corpus callosum, polymicrogyria, platybasia and basilar invagination.

CRANIOLACUNIA is characterized by oval to circular lucencies in the skull (because of disordered ossification of membranous bone) separated by ridges of normal appearing bone. Poor sutural ossification can give an erroneous appearance of their splitting. This condition is almost exclusively seen in craniospinal dysraphic states (encephalomeningocele, myelomeningocele). It probably represents a mesencymal alteration in combination with neural dysgenesis. It rarely persists after six to nine months of age.

For descriptive purposes, Arnold-Chiari malformation has been classified into three types:

> TYPE I is charactarized by displacement of the cerebellar tonsils and of inferior cerebellum (mainly inferior vermis) into the upper cervical canal; the medulla oblongata and fourth ventricle are not displaced downward. It is usually seen in older children and adults.
>
> TYPE II includes the features in Type I plus caudal displacement of the elongated lower pons and medulla oblongata; the fourth ventricle also is caudally displaced and elongated. The medulla oblongata buckles up at its junction with the spinal cord. A myelomeningocele almost invariably accompanies this malformation. Type II is the most common and is seen in infants and young children.
>
> TYPE III consists of displacement of the medulla oblongata, the fourth ventricle and almost all of the cerebellum into an occipital and high cervical encephalomeningocele.

Hydrocephalus in Arnold-Chiari malformation usually cannot be explained by a single cause; a multitude of factors probably operate in various combinations (15). These include: a) aqueductal obstructive lesion (usually stenosis); b) compression of the subarachnoid spaces at the foramen magnum and at the tentorial incisura; c) obstruction of the outlet foramina of the fourth ventricle; and d) compression of the pliable venous sinuses of the posterior fossa leading to increased venous pressure and consequent impairment of CSF absorption (16). It also is quite likely that ventriculomegally may, in part, be a manifestation of cerebral dysgenesis (telencephalopathy), especially when the temporal horns are not proportionately enlarged. Hydrocephalus, compensatory hydromyelia (dilation of the central canal of the spinal cord) and developmental scoliosis have an interesting relationship in patients with Arnold-Chiari malformation and myelomeningocele (8). It is believed that if an anatomic cause (e.g., segmentation anomaly of the spine) of scoliosis is absent in patients with myelomeningocele, the disorder may be explained on the basis of hydromyelia. This hypothesis seems to be borne out by the reduction in size of the enlarged spinal cord shadow on myelography after ventricular shunting concomitant with arrest or improvement in scoliosis deformity and improvement in extremity weakness and spasticity.

CLINICAL SYMPTOMATOLOGY

In the pediatric age group, the major neurologic defect is related to hydrocephalus. Cerebellar dysfunction and brain stem compression further add to the neurologic impairment, and respiratory distress due to medullary compression is not an uncommon presentation (17). Medullary vascular lesions – hemorrhage and necrosis – seen in pathologic specimens are believed a consequence of stretched arteries due to brain stem descent (17, 18).

CT SCAN FINDINGS (19-25)

CT findings primarily reflect the following pathologic characteristics of Arnold-Chiari malformation Type II:

1) Hydrocephalus.
2) Caudal dislocation of the cerebellar tonsils, fourth ventricle and brain stem.
3) Hypoplasia of the falx and tentorium.
4) Overgrowth of certain parts of the brain resulting in deformity of the adjacent ventricular system. Telencephalopathy manifests itself by an alteration in shape of the lateral ventricles.
5) Crowding of the posterior fossa contents resulting in secondary adaptive changes of the bone and compression of the subarachnoid spaces.

The CT scan findings shown in Table I are of Arnold-Chiari malformation Type II.

TABLE I
SUMMARY OF CT SCAN FINDINGS OF ARNOLD-CHIARI MALFORMATION TYPE II*

A. VENTRICLES AND CISTERNS

- Smallness and poor visualization of the caudally displaced fourth ventricle.

TABLE I (continued)

- Indentation on the third ventricle caused by the large massa intermedia (75%).
- Asymmetric dilation of the lateral ventricles. The occipital horns are disproportionately larger than the frontal horns. On coronal images, there is medial pointing of the frontal horns of the lateral ventricles at the interventricular foramen level. On axial images, the frontal horns may be normal, pointed (beaked) or slightly bulbous at the end.
- Absence of the septum pellucidum (50%).
- Prominence of the interhemispheric fissure and of adjacent sulci with interdigitations of the gyri, seen after ventricular shunting.
- Compression of the posterior fossa subarachnoid spaces. The cisterna magna is seldom seen in these patients.

B. SKULL AND DURA

- Craniolacunia (85%) (Fig. 1).
- Flattening or scalloping of the posterior aspects of the petrous pyramids (90%).
- Partial absence and/or fenestration of the falx (usually in the fronto-parietal region) (50-100%).
- Tentorial hypoplasia and wide and elongated tentorial incisura (in almost all cases).
- Small posterior fossa and large foramen magnum.

C. MIDBRAIN AND CEREBELLUM

- Tectal (mesencephalic) beaking (89%).
- Towering cerebellum (76% of post-shunted cases).
- Sharp anterior cerebellar margins.
- Excessive overlapping by cerebellum of the mid to upper brainstem. Such overlapping of pons can result in masses at the cerebello pontine angles (CPA) (93%).
- Posterior fossa pseudotumors.

*NOTE: The figures in parentheses represent percent incidence of that anomaly seen on CT and are primarily derived from Naidich *et al.*, 1980.

A. VENTRICULAR SYSTEM

Lateral Ventricles

Usually, the occipital horns are disproportionately larger than the frontal horns (Fig. 2). This finding probably is explained on the basis of dysgenesis of forceps major of the corpus callosum, thalamus, optic radiations, and calcarine cortex. The normal development of these structures determines the size of the occipital horns.

The frontal horns may be of normal shape, show a variable degree of pointing (beaking) or be slightly bulbous at the extreme end on the axial images. The beaking is usually more pronounced on the medial aspects. This change in shape very likely is determined by the size of the caudate nucleus. Medial pointing of the frontal horns on coronal images is similarily explained (Fig. 3). The frontal horns may assume a somewhat flat or cup-shaped pattern (instead of normal V-shape). Part of the explanation of lateral ventricular dysmorphology probably lies in defective development of the telencephalon such that the lateral ventricles do not assume their characteristic appearance.

Some asymmetry in size of the lateral ventricles is usually apparent in the non-shunted state; however, this asymmetry becomes more pronounced after shunting. The lateral ventricle ipsilateral to the shunt commonly becomes smaller than its counterpart (Figs. 11,19). This may be related to partial transmission of the endoventricular choroid plexus pulse wave along the shunt tubing such that reduced pulse wave is available for ventricular distention (26).

Irregularity of borders of lateral ventricles (usually at their lateral aspects) is not uncommon. This irregularity in the non-shunted state is quite likely a manifestation of gray matter heterotoia (a defect of peripheral migration of the neuronal cell population). In the shunted state, such an irregularity is difficult to distinguish from that caused by ependymitis.

Third Ventricle

The third ventricle is not prominently enlarged probably due to the tethering effect of the enlarged massa intermedia (Fig. 4). The large massa intermedia lies closer to the interventricular foramina than normally. The third ventricle walls are parallel or biconcave. Occasionally, diverticuli at the front and/or hind end are present when this ventricle exhibits an unusual distention. These diverticuli add CSF density to the suprasellar and quadrigeminal cisterns.

Fourth Ventricle

The fourth ventricle is small, elongated and caudally displaced (Figs. 5, 6, 7). Since displacement may be difficult to recognize on axial images, sagittal views are ideal for evaluation of caudal dislocation of the fourth ventricle and of the cerebellar tonsils.

B. DURA AND ITS COMPARTMENTS

Hypoplasia of the falx and tentorium is an important pathologic characteristic of Arnold-Chiari malformation. The falx hypoplasia (representing telencephalopathy) is best appreciated on the contrast CT scan wherein the falx is seen as a partially interrupted and/or thinly enhanced linear structure (Figs. 7,8). The falx aplasia or hypoplasia is most pronounced in the anterior and/or the middle third. In all cases, the posterior part is the most developed. At points where the falx is fenestrated or absent, the pial surfaces of gyri of the neighboring cerebral hemisphere may appose and thus obliterate the interhemispheric fissure. The hypoplastic tentorium is manifested by a wide and elongated tentorial incisura which is inserted on the occipital bone lower than normal (Figs. 8,9,11). The tentorial leaves, instead of normally converging posteriorly (to assume a V-shape) (Fig. 10), pursue a somewhat parallel or laterally convex course on contigous slices, and join each other more posteriorly than normal. Wide tentorial incisura can be appreciated far more clearly on the contrast CT scan as the dural leaves show prominent enhancement.

Occasionally, when the tentorial incisura is exceptionally wide, elongated and low, the CSF space along its borders appears as a wide arc between the cerebellar hemispheres and the occipital lobes. This appearance should not be misconstrued as a collar of edema around a mass lesion (Fig. 11). Similarly, slight increase in density of the cerebellar tissue, as it lies within the wide tentorial incisura surrounded by CSF density, can mimic a mass lesion (pseudotumor) (22) (Fig. 12). Such mimicry may become more pronounced on the contrast CT scan.

It should be noted that the tentorial incisura may be excessively wide normally. Unless other corroborative CT scan findings of Arnold-Chiari malformation exist, the isolated presence of wide tentorial incisura should not be considered a sign of this disorder.

C. CHANGES AT THE ABNORMALLY WIDE TENTORIAL INCISURA

1. Tectal (Mesencephalic) Beaking

This is a manifestation of partial or complete fusion of colliculi of the quadrigeminal plate (Figs. 2,5, 9,13,14). The normal groove between the colliculi is not recognizable except in the mild form of the malformation. The aqueduct is seen poorly or not at all; when seen it is flattened from sides. The mesencephalic beaking primarily represents developmental arrest (that is, impaired elimination of a certain population of cells) since the human fetus of 14-50 mm length shows a similar caudal projection of the quadrigeminal plate. Collicular compression from sides by the upwardly herniated overgrown cerebellum partly explains the mesencephalic beaking. The dorsal projection of the beaked mesencephalon over cerebellum is akin to the dorsal projection of the medullary tissue over the upper cervical cord. The mesencephalic beaking is a very reliable sign of this malformation and is invariably present.

2. Overgrowth of the Cerebellar Hemispheres

Such an overgrowth involves mainly the central and the superior areas of the cerebellum. The ascent of the overgrown cerebellum causes elevation of the temporo-occipital lobes, the atria and the occipital horns resulting in the creation of prominent CSF space around it in the midline – the so-called pericerebellar cistern (Figs. 8,11,15). This pericerebellar cistern becomes especially noticeable after shunting when further ascent of the overgrown cerebellum (upward transtentorial herniation) occurs. At a lower and anterior level, the overgrown cerebellum may result in rounded masses at the cerebello-pontine angle cisterns as it overlaps the pons (Figs. 12,15,16).

D. ADAPTIVE POSTERIOR FOSSA CHANGES DUE TO TIGHT PACKING OF ITS CONTENTS

Smallness of the posterior fossa and hypertrophy of the cerebellum result in secondary adaptive changes in the posterior fossa. These include: 1) scalloping (posterior concavity) of the petrous bones and the clivus (Fig. 17); 2) truncation of the medial ends of the internal auditory canals; and 3) compression of the infratentorial subarachnoid spaces. The cisterna magna is poorly developed or not developed at all in these cases.

E. CHANGES AT AND BELOW THE LARGE FORAMEN MAGNUM (Fig. 18)

The classic radiographic demonstration of tonsillar and/or fourth ventricular descent below the foramen magnum seen on air studies or at myelography is difficult to ascertain on axial images. At metrizamide CT cisternography, the caudally displaced cerebellar tonsils can be demonstrated (Fig. 19), but due to volume averaging and angulation of the beam, it is difficult to be sure whether the visualized cerebellar tonsils are normal or abnormally displaced caudally. Sagittal CT scans are ideal for studying this perspective.

F. INTERHEMISPHERIC FISSURE (IHF) AND ADJACENT SUBARACHNOID SPACES

In the unshunted state of this disorder, the IHF and subarachnoid spaces at the tentorial incisura are variably compressed due to hydrocephalus and ascent of the overgrown cerebellum. After shunting, these subarachnoid spaces become prominent, espceially IHF

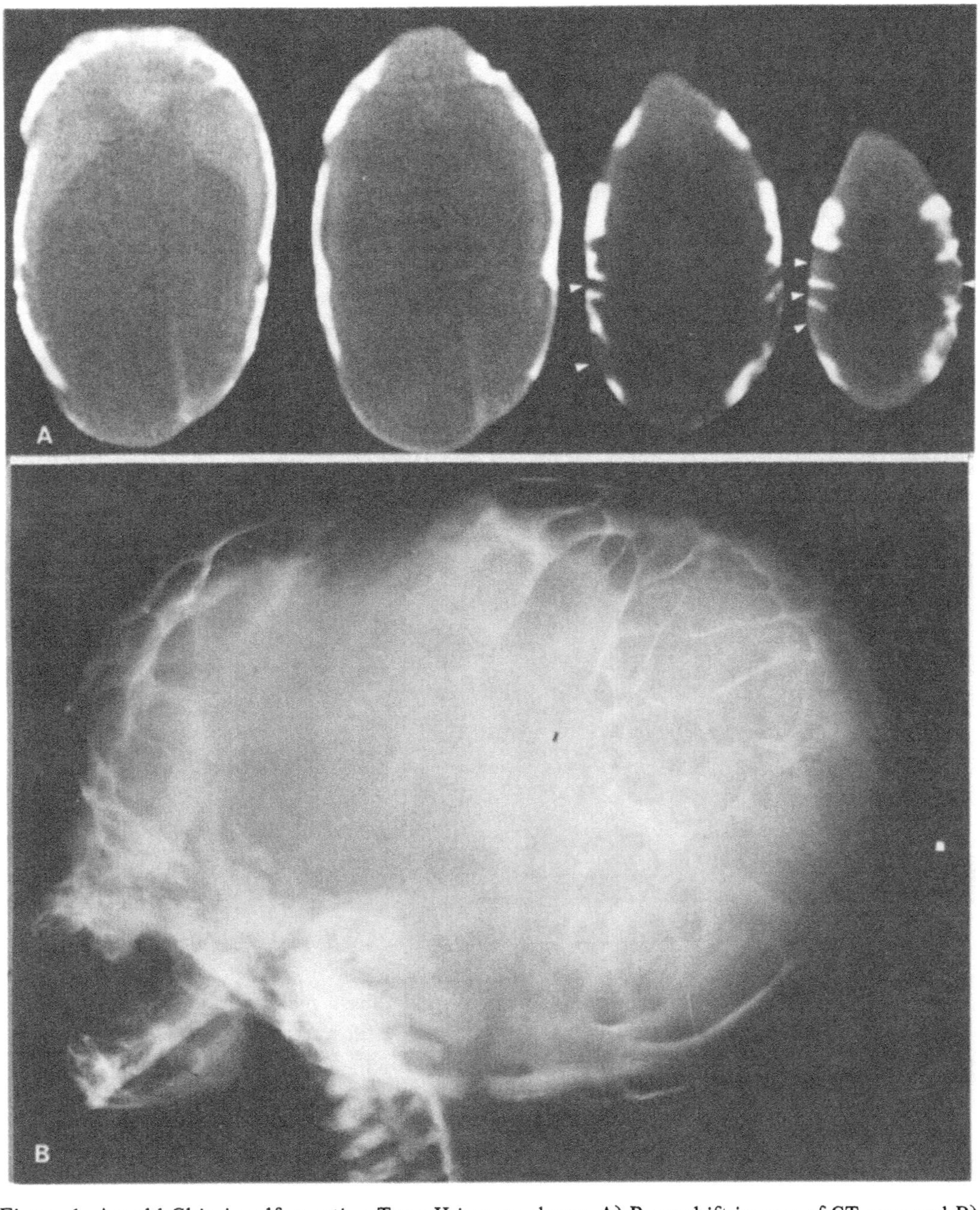

Figure 1. Arnold-Chiari malformation Type II in a newborn. A) Bone shift images of CT scan and B) lateral skull film. Note craniolacunia involving the entire calvarial thickness at many places (**arrowheads**). Usually it involves the inner table and the superior aspect of the skull.

(Fig. 20). Such a prominent IHF interposed between the lateral ventricles should not be mistaken to suggest the concomitant presence of dysgenesis of corpus callosum. To diagnose dysgenesis of corpus callosum, the IHF must be traceable to the anterior wall of the third ventricle on contiguous CT slices at level of the frontal horns and third ventricle. (See chapter on Dysgenesis of Corpus Callosum.)

It should be noted that many of the CT findings described above can be present singly or in combination without the concomitant presence of Arnold-Chiari malformation.

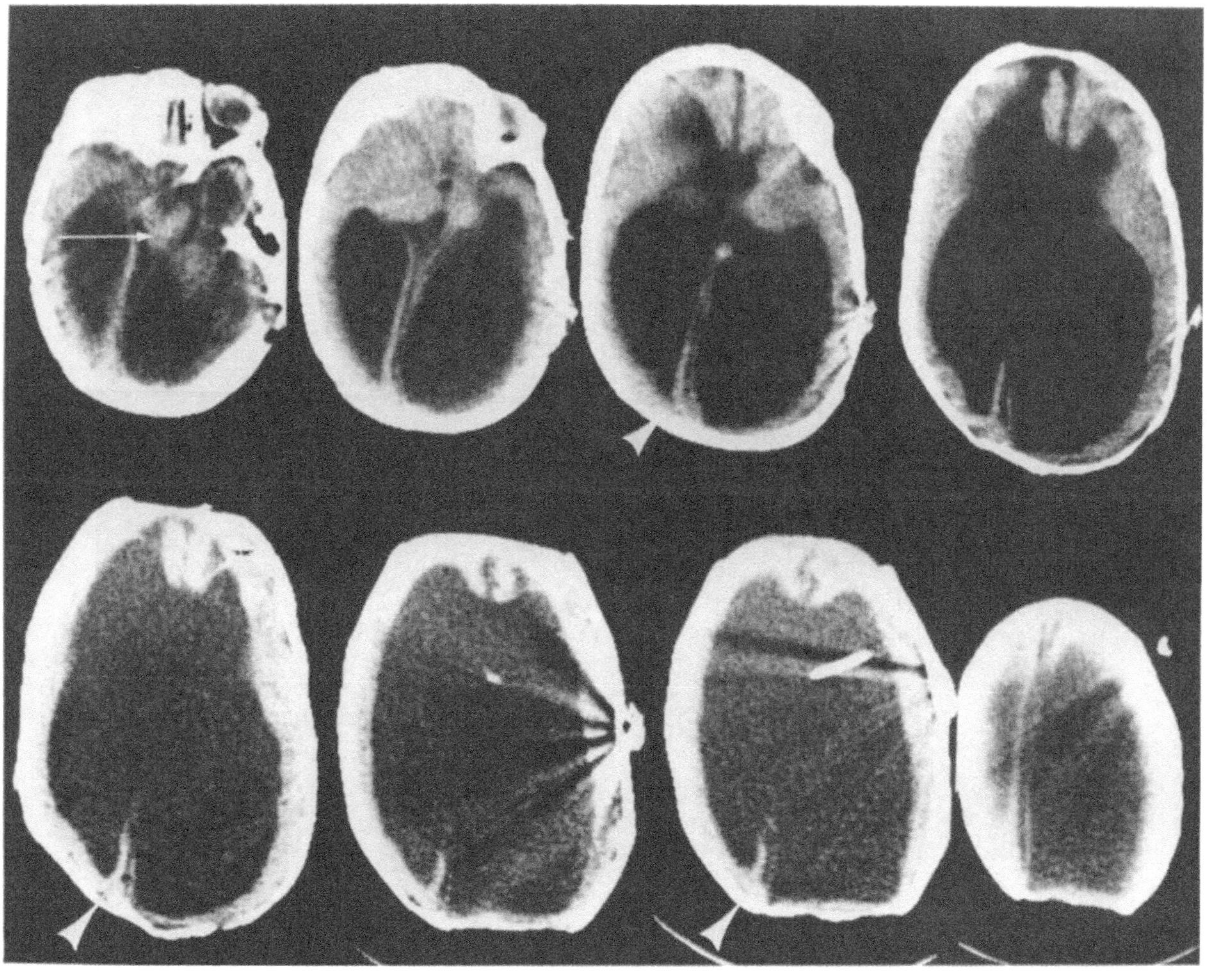

Figure 2. An infant with Arnold-Chiari malformation Type II. This case shows that in the presence of marked ventriculomegaly many of the features of Arnold-Chiari malformation Type II can be masked. However, mesencephalic beaking **(arrow)** usually is a helpful clue to the presence of the malformation in such a situation. Also note that eccentric placement of the falx **(arrowheads)** indicates that this malformation occurs at about, or before, 3 months of gestation.

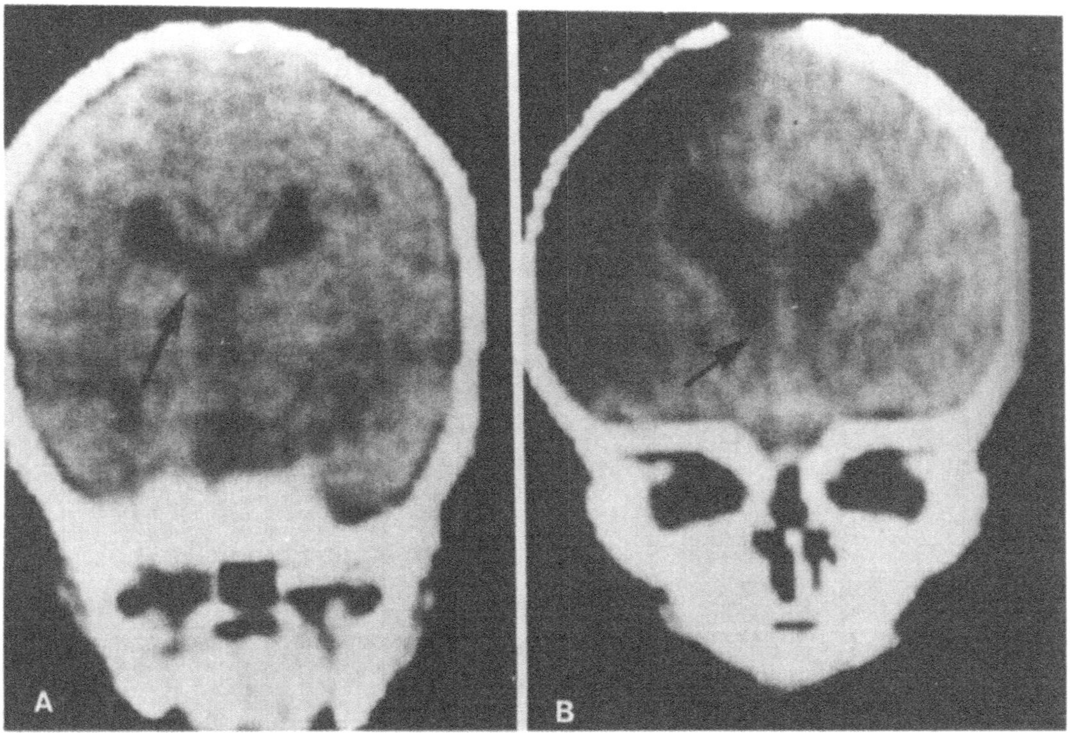

Figure 3. Arnold-Chiari malformation Type II. Separate cases. Coronal CT scans. Note pointing of the floor of the lateral ventricles (**arrows**). (From Naidich *et al. Radiology, 134:*657, 1980, with permission.)

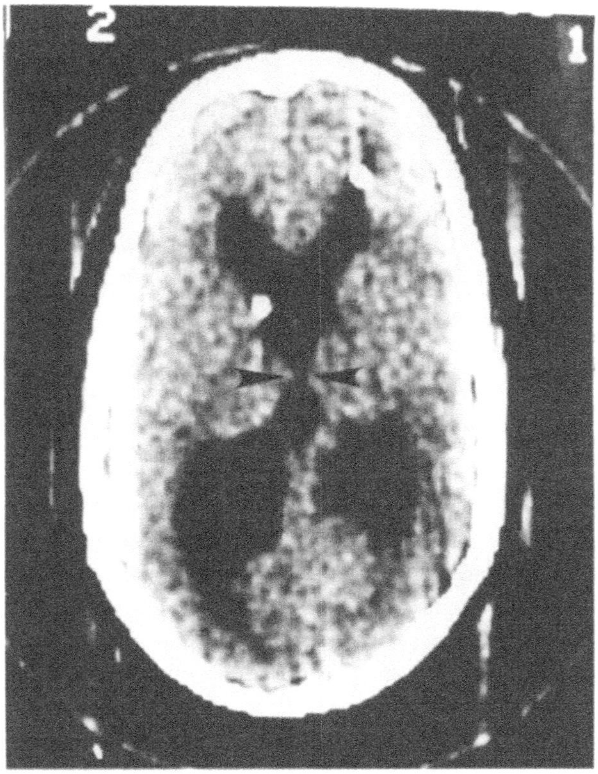

Figure 4. Arnold-Chiari malformation Type II. CT scan at third ventricle level. Waist-like deformity of the third ventricle is caused by large massa intermedia (**arrowheads**). Note disproportionate dilatation of the occipital horns.

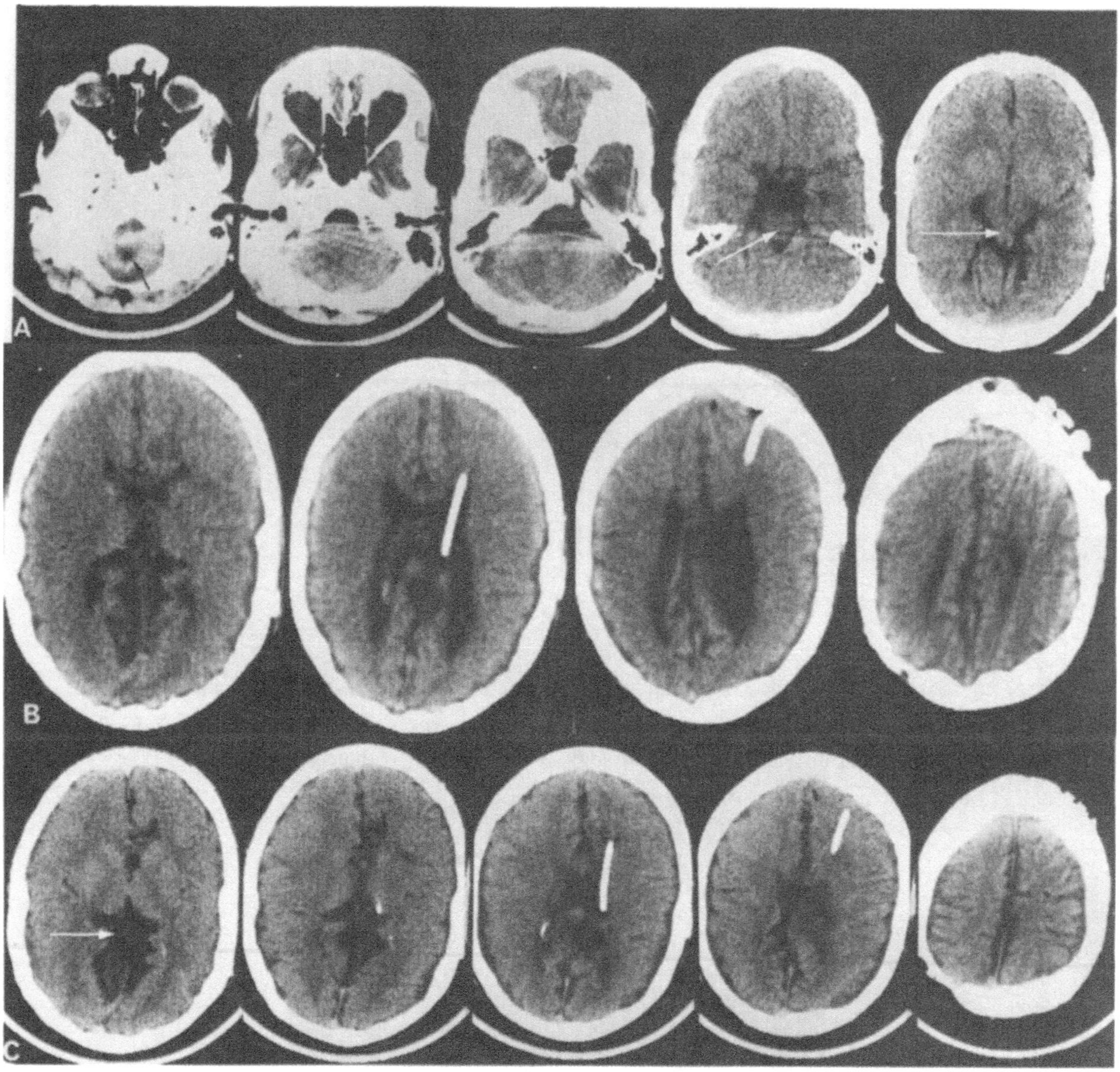

Figure 5. Arnold-Chiari malformation Type II. A) The fourth ventricle is caudally displaced (**black arrow**); it should be present on the CT slice shown in the middle of the row. There is mesencephalic beaking (**white arrows**) as well. B) and C) CT scans after shunting. In C), the lateral ventricles have become far smaller. There is prominence of the interhemispheric fissure as well as of the superfical cortical sulci. The prominent subarachnoid spaces (**arrow**) at the tentorial incisura represent confluence of cistern velum interposition and retropulvinar, posterior pericallosal and superior vermian cisterns. It can assume a diamond-shaped configuration. This finding is frequently seen following shunting. See text for explanation.

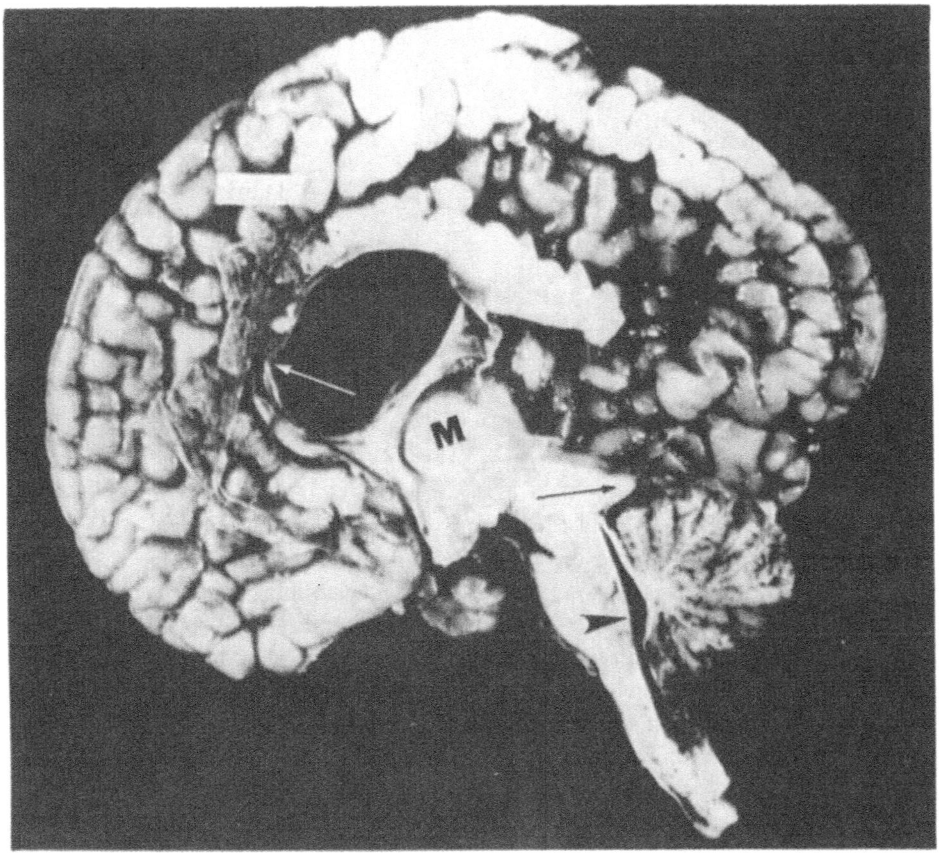

Figure 6. Pathologic specimen of the Arnold-Chiari malformation Type II. There is a large massa intermedia (**M**), tectal beaking (**black arrows**) and caudal displacement of the flattened and elongated fourth ventricle (**arrowheads**). There is dysgenesis of the anterior part of the corpus callosum (**white arrow**) and polymicrogyria, as well. (Courtesy McClure Wilson, M.D.)

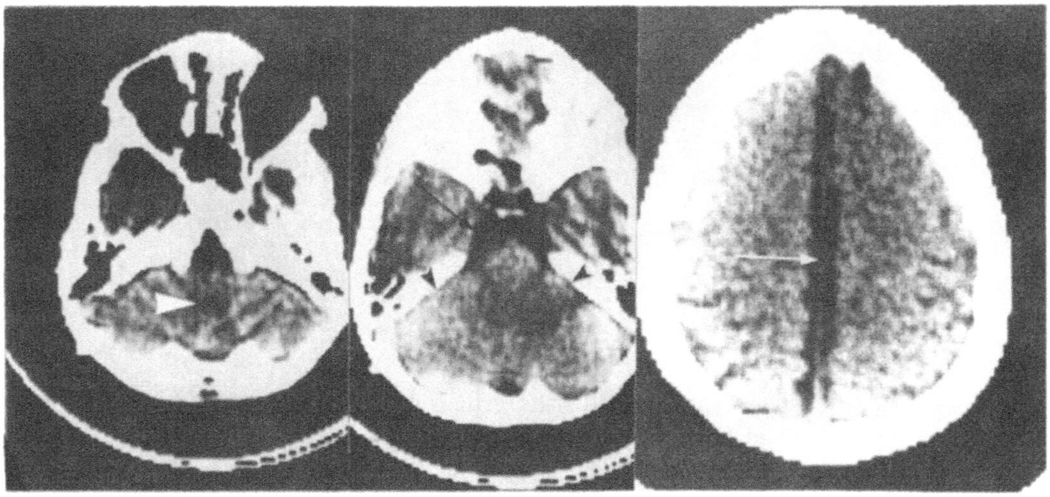

Figure 7. Arnold-Chiari malformation Type II. Non-contrast CT. Note the following: 1) petrous scalloping (**black arrowheads**), 2) low-placed fourth ventricle (**white arrowhead**), [it should have been visible at the slice level shown in the middle], and 3) hypoplastic falx (**white arrow**).

The prepontine cistern (**black arrow**) in the middle CT slice is prominent. Suprasellar, prepontine and lateral pontine cisterns are often prominent in this malformation.

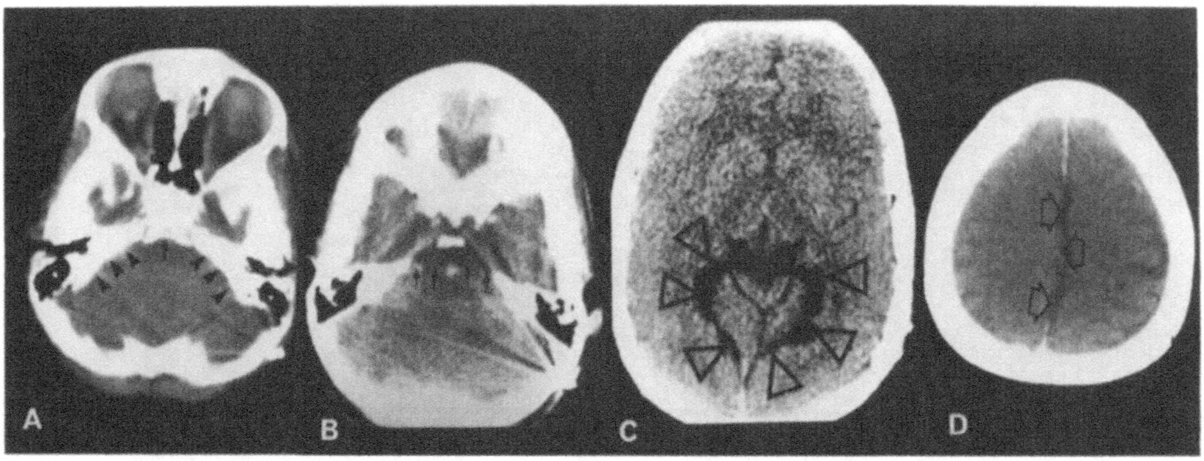

Figure 8. Arnold-Chiari malformation Type II. Contrast CT scan. Note the following: 1) petrous (**arrowheads**) and clivus (**arrow**) scalloping in (A) forming an arc; 2) prominent prepontine cistern (**arrows**) in (B); 3) pericerebellar cistern (**arrowheads**) around the anterior and superior cerebellum at level of the wide tentorial incisura in (C); and 4) hypoplastic falx (**arrows**) in (D). (Courtesy Solomon Batnitzky, M.D.)

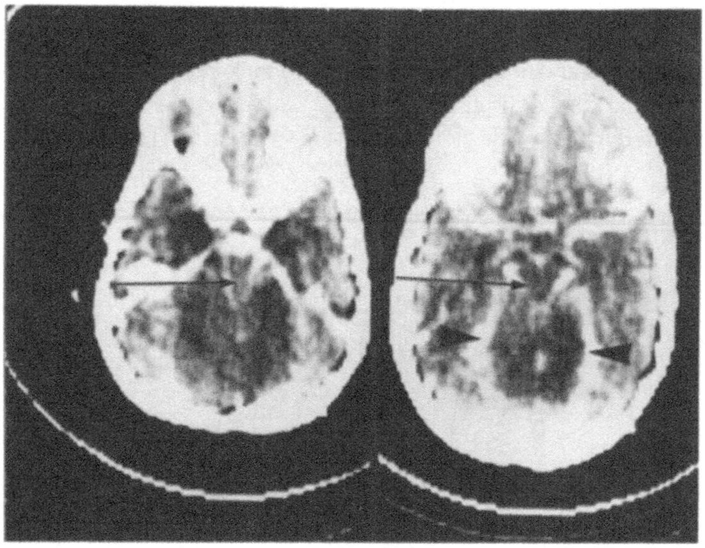

Figure 9. Arnold-Chiari malformation Type II in a three-year-old boy. The patient had meningitis as well which resulted in good visualization of the subarachnoid spaces on the contrast CT scan because of the presence of exudate in them. Note mesencephalic beaking (**arrows**) and wide tentorial incisura (**arrowheads** are at tentorial edges). The tentorium is low placed. The wide tentorial incisura must be visible on all contiguous slices.

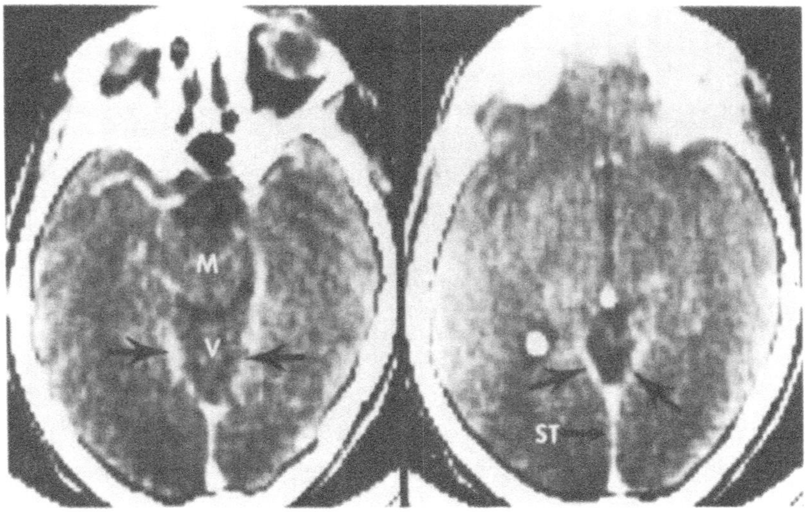

Figure 10. Normal contrast CT scan at mesencephalon (M) and tentorial incisura (**arrows**) level. Note the normal shape of mesencephalon and posterior convergence of the tentorial lea . ST = straight sinus. V = vermis.

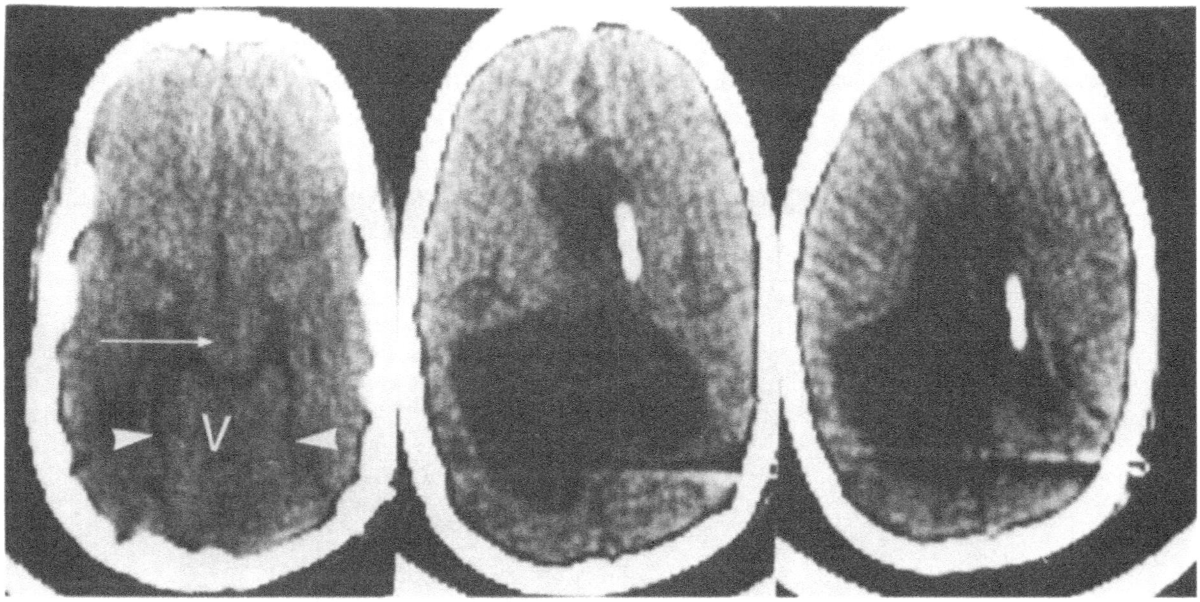

Figure 11. Arnold-Chiari malformation Type II. Disproportionate enlargement of the occipital horns and apposition of their medial borders should not be mistaken for a cyst. The vermis (V) in this wide and elongated tentorial incisura (**arrowheads** are at the CSF along the tentorial edges-pericerebellar cistern) should not be misinterpreted as a mass lesion. Note mild mesencephalic beaking (**arrow**). Observe that the shunt containing lateral ventricle is smaller than its companion.

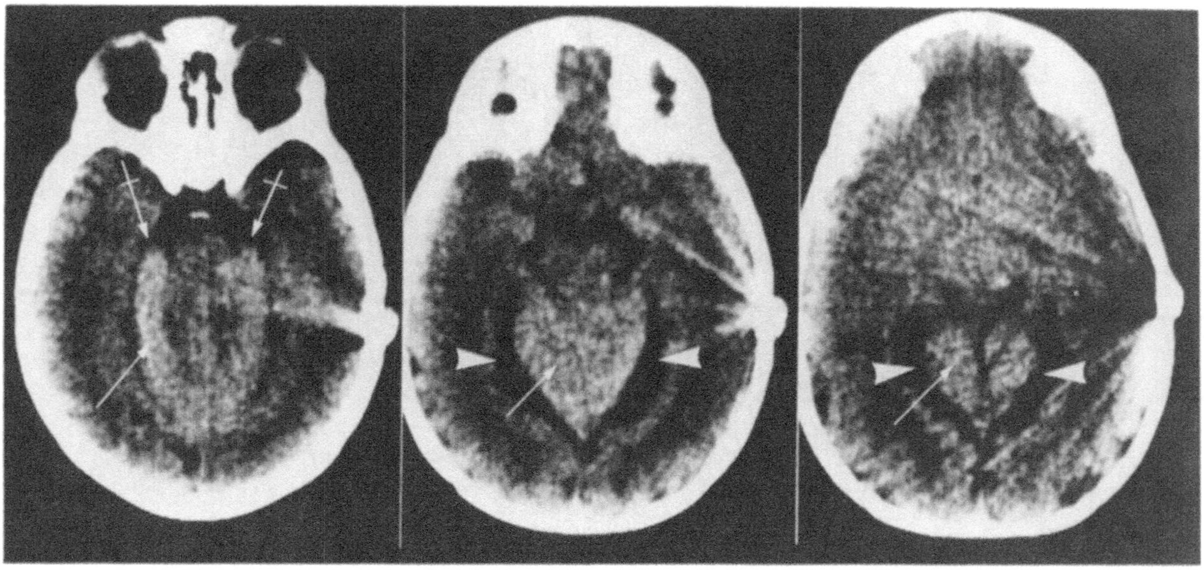

Figure 12. Arnold-Chiari malformation Type II. The cerebellum, for some unknown reason, can sometimes assume a very dense appearance (**arrows**) and be highly echogenic. This appearance should not be mistaken for a hemorrhage or a neoplasm. The part of the cerebellum that surrounds the brainstem simulates a mass lesion (pseudotumor) at the cerebellopontine angles (**crossed arrows**). The prominent pericerebellar cistern (**arrowheads**) is well-shown.

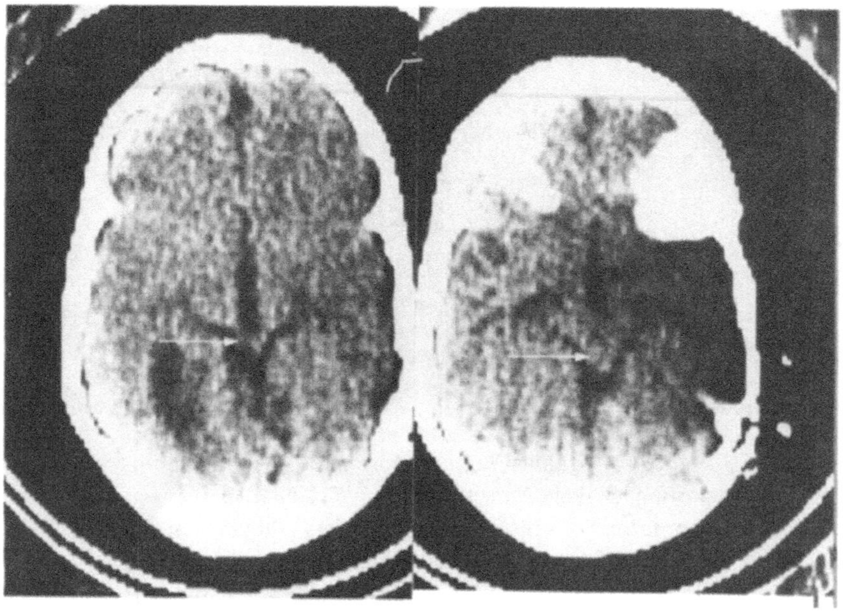

Figure 13. Arnold-Chiari malformation Type II. There is prominent mesencephalic beaking (**arrows**).

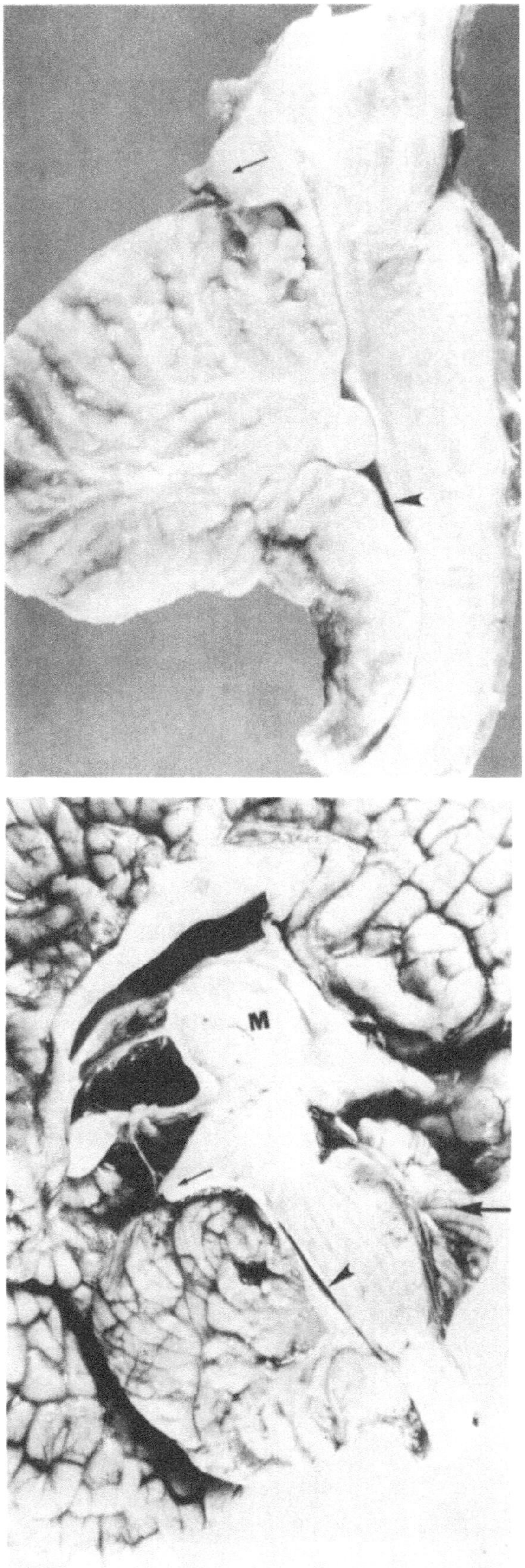

Figure 14. Pathologic specimens of Arnold-Chiari malformation Type II. Two separate cases. Note varied configuration of the mesencephalic beaking (**thin arrows**). The beaked mesencephalon excessively overlies the adjoining cerebellum which can become invaginated. The fourth ventricle is elongated, flattened and caudally displaced (**arrowheads**). Massa intermedia (M) is quite prominent. In the illustration on the right, the cerebellum has extended forward on the side of pons to be located anterior to it (**thick arrow**). This part of the forwardly placed cerebellum appears as a cerebellopontine angle mass on CT.

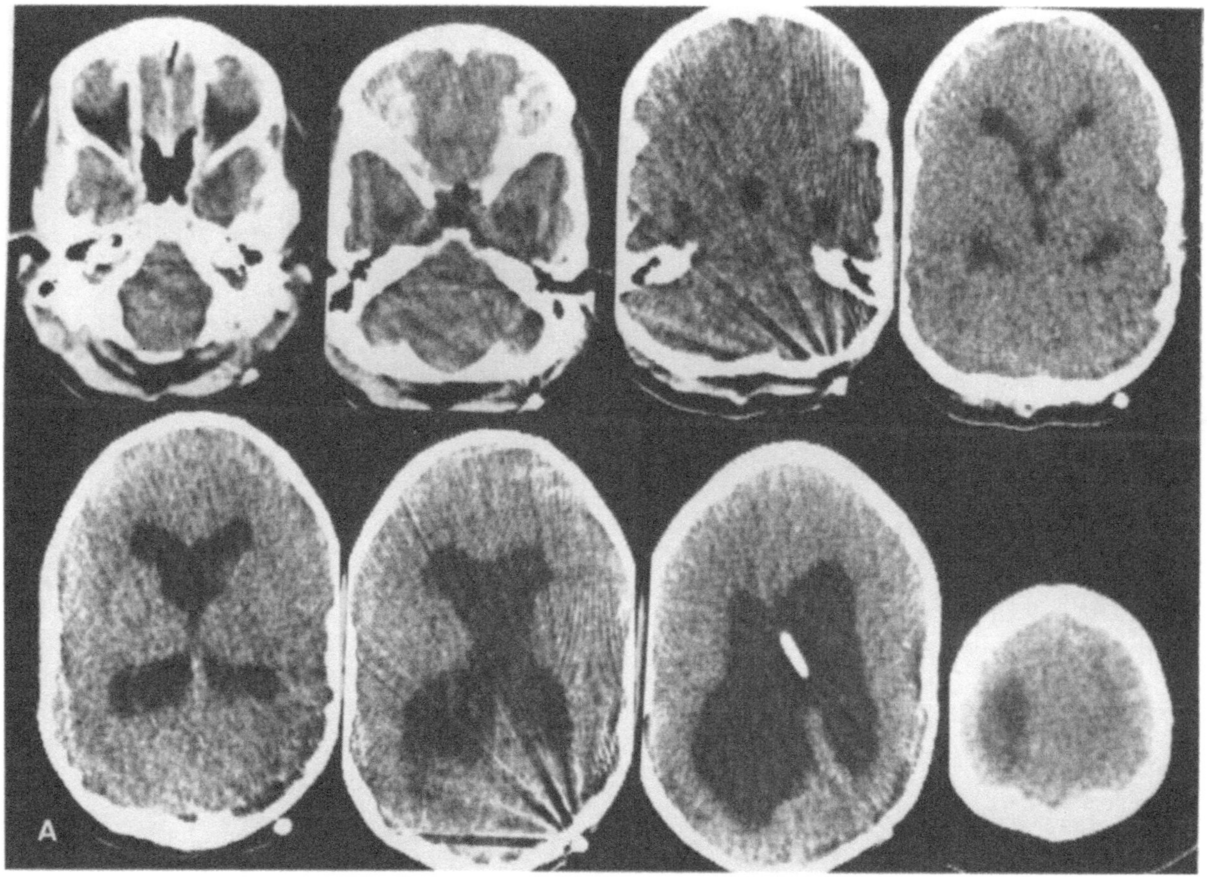

Figure 15. Arnold-Chiari malformation Type II. The overgrown cerebellum overlaps the pons and can present as soft tissue masses at cerebellopontine angles (**white arrows** in [A,B]). This case also shows that the morphologic features of this malformation become far more readily recognizable after the lateral ventricles become smaller following their shunting. A) large ventricles, B) collapsed ventricles.

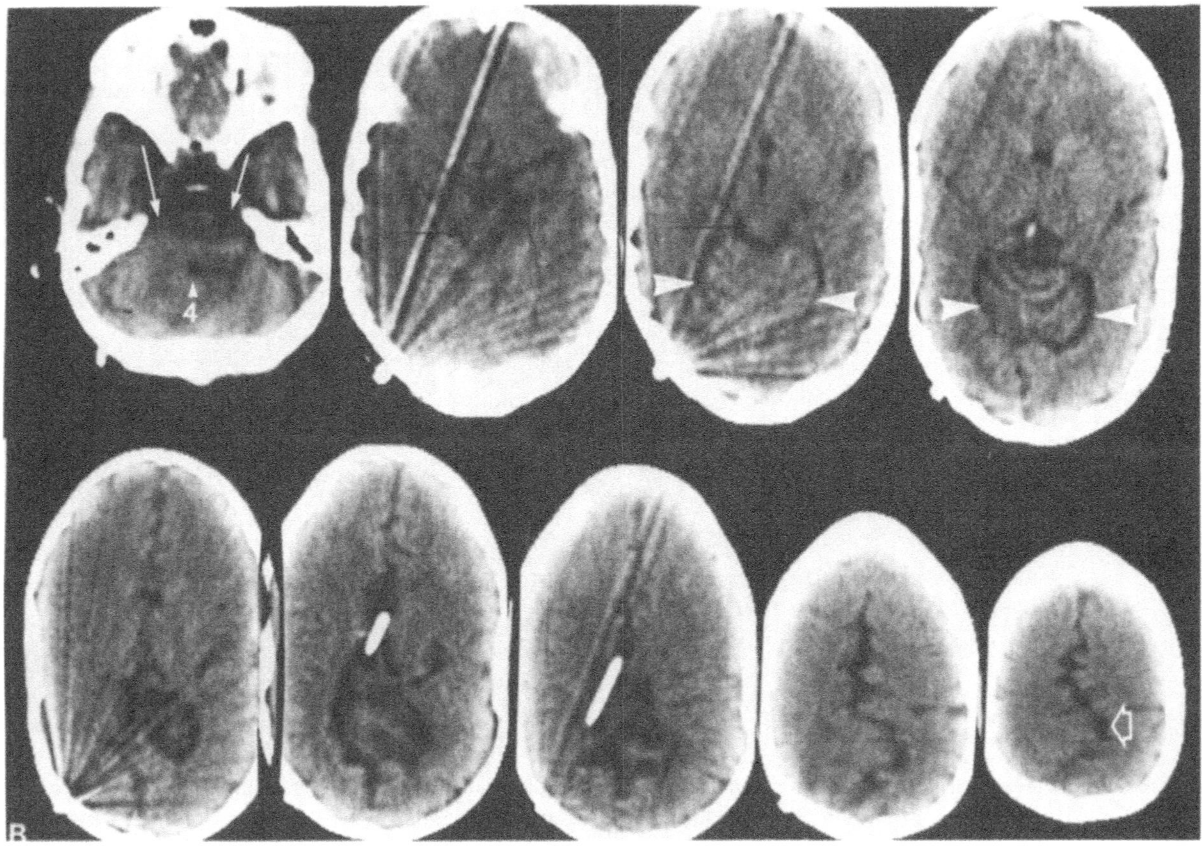

Figure 15. Continued

On the CT scan shown in (B), note the following which were not identifiable in (A): 1) prominence of the interhemispheric fissure with interdigitating pattern of the gyri; 2) wide tentorial incisura (**arrowheads**) containing the superior cerebellum with its pericerebellar cistern; and 3) mesencephalic beaking (**black arrows**). The posterior part of the interhemispheric fissure (**open arrow**) is buckled to the side because of its expansion from underneath by the higher placed and overgrown cerebellum. The fourth ventricle (4) in (B) is almost normally placed because it has ascended concurrent with ascending transtentorial herniation following ventricular shunting. Note petrous scalloping in (A).

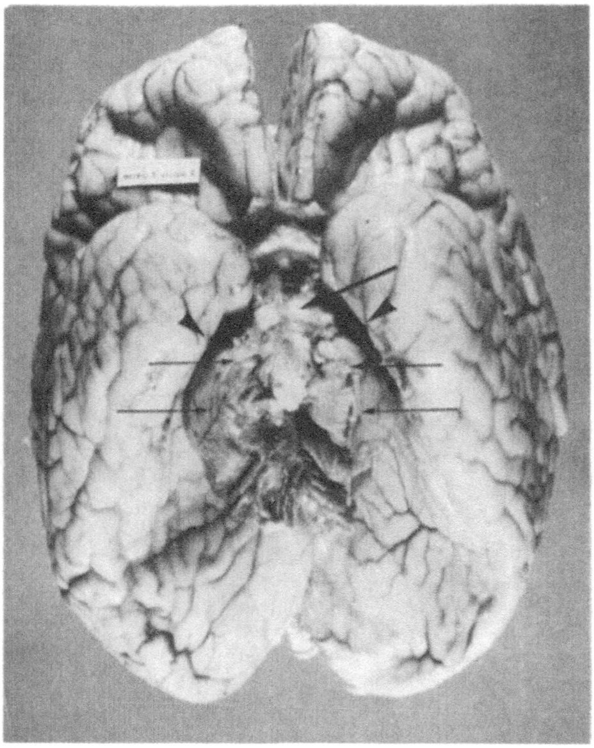

Figure 16. Arnold–Chiari malformation Type II. Base view of the pathologic specimen. The overgrown cerebellum **(thin arrows)** overlaps the brainstem **(thick arrow)** and lies between it and the medial temporal lobes **(arrowheads).** Note the associated polymicrogyria. (Courtest W.F.'McCormick, M.D.)

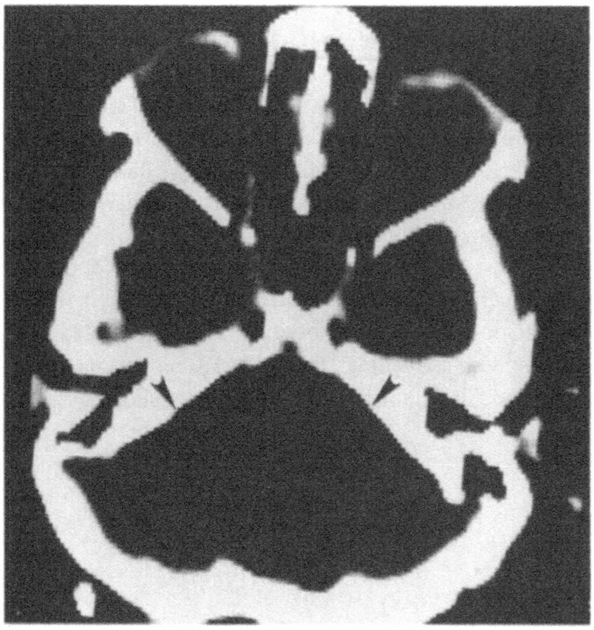

Figure 17. Petrous scalloping **(arrowheads).** If occurs at level between the petrous ridges and above the jugular tubercles. The internal auditory canals in such cases are shortened and eroded from pressure of the tightly packed posterior fossa structures. Petrous scalloping becomes more pronounced with growth of the cerebellum.

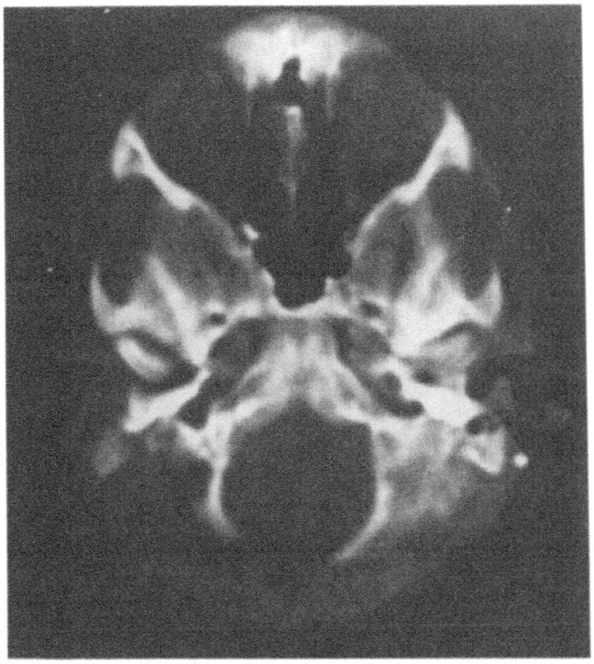

Figure 18. Arnold-Chiari malformation Type II. Note the large foramen magnum.

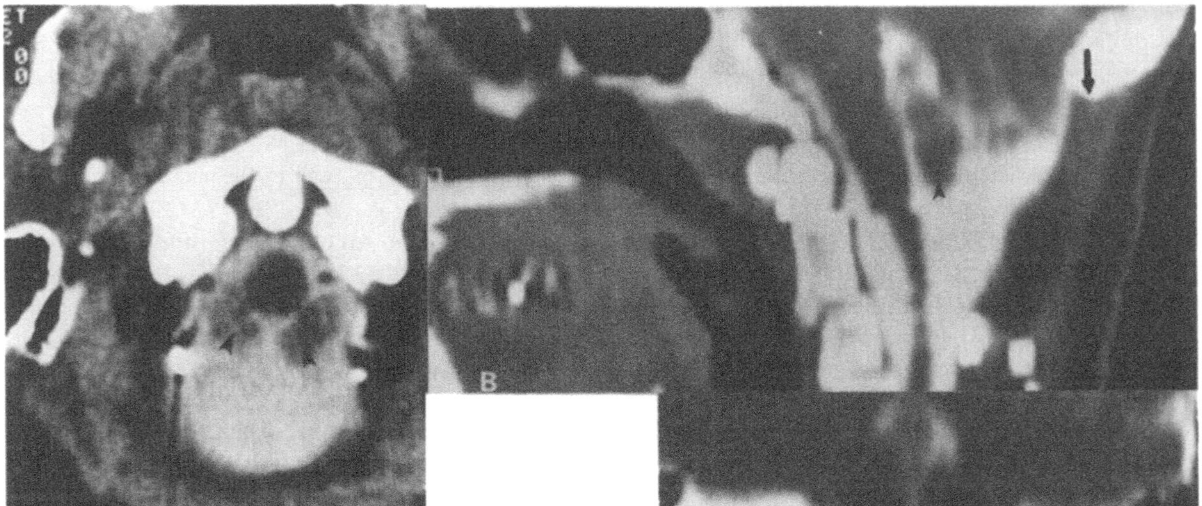

Figure 19. A 14-year-old female with Arnold-Chiari malformation Type I. Metrizamide CT scan. A) Axial CT at C_1 level, B) reformatted saggital and C) reformatted coronal CT at and about foramen magnum level. The cerebellar tonsils **(arrowheads)** are below the foramen magnum **(arrows)**. The fourth ventricle was normal in shape and location.

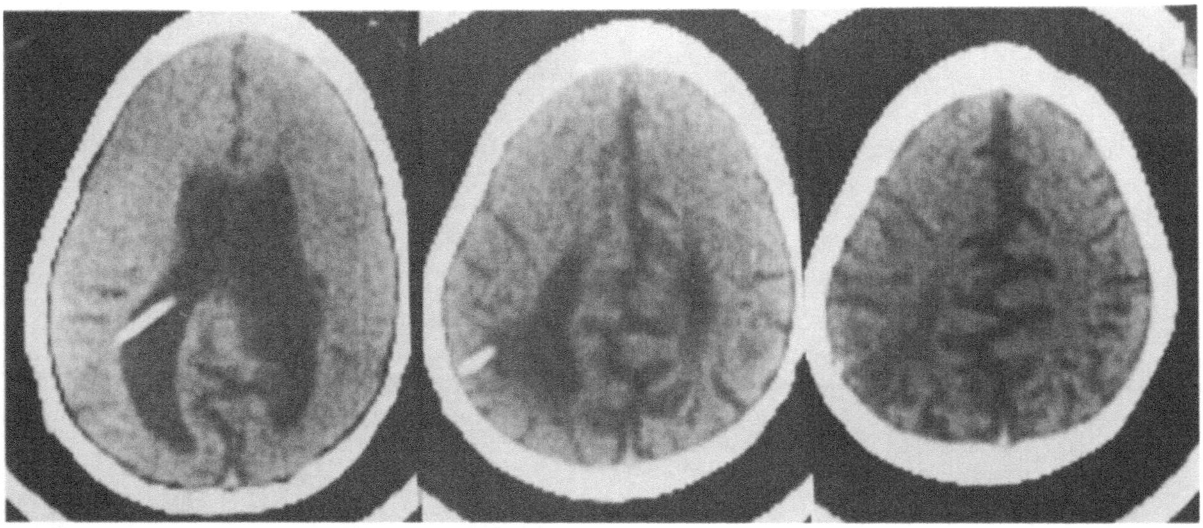

Figure 20. Arnold-Chiari malformation Type II. There is marked prominence of the interhemispheric fissure following ventricular shunting. Also observe that there is interdigitating pattern of the gyri at the interhemispheric fissure. The shunt containing lateral ventricle is smaller than its companion.

REFERENCES

1. Barry A, Patten BM, Stewart BI: Possible factors in development of Arnold-Chiari malformation. *J Neurosurg, 14:*285-301, 1957.
2. Bamberger BC: The Chiari II malformation: Arnold Chiari of the literature. *J Neuroradiol, 9:*47-70, 1982.
3. Cameron AH: The Arnold-Chiari and other neuroanatomical malformations associated with spina bifida. *J Path Bact, 73:*195-211, 1957.
4. Daniel PM, Strich SJ: Some observations on the congenital deformity of the central nervous system known as the Arnold-Chiari malformation. *J Neuropath Exp Neurol, 17:*255-266, 1958.
5. Feigin I: Arnold-Chiari malformation with associated analogous malformation of the midbrain. *Neurology, 6:*22-31, 1956.
6. Gardner WJ: Anatomical features common to Arnold-Chiari malformation and Dandy-Walker malformation suggest common origin. *Clev Clin Quart, 26:*206, 1959.
7. Gooding CA, Carter A, Hoare RD: New ventriculographic aspects of the Arnold-Chiari malformation. *Radiology, 89:*626-632, 1967.
8. Hall P, Lindseth R, Campbell R, *et al.*: Scoliosis and hydrocephalus in myelocele patients. The effects of ventricular shunting. *J Neurosurg, 50:* 174-178, 1979.
9. Lichtenstein BW: Atresia and stenosis of the aqueduct of sylvius with comments on Arnold-Chiari complex. *J Neuropath Exp Neurol, 18:*3, 1958.
10. Masters CL: Pathogenesis of the Arnold-Chiari malformation: the significance of hydrocephalus and aqueduct stenosis. *J Neuropath Exp Neurol, 37:*56-74, 1978.
11. Patten BM: Overgrowth of the neural tube in young human embryos. *Anat Rec, 113:*381-393, 1952.
12. Peach B: The Arnold-Chiari malformation. *Arch Neurol, 12:*527-535, 1965.
13. Van Hoytema GJ, vandenBerg R: Embryological studies of the posterior fossa in connection with Arnold-Chiari malformation. *Dev Med Child Neurol supp, 11:*61-87, 1966.
14. Welch K, Shillito J, Strand R *et al.*: Chiari I malformation – an acquired disorder. *J Neurosurg, 55:* 604-609, 1981.
15. Yamada H, Nakamura S, Tanaka Y, Tajima M and Kageyama N: Ventriculography and cisternography with water soluble contrast media in infants with myelomeningocele. *Radiology, 143:*75-83, 1982.
16. Mueller SM, Reinertson JE: Reversal of emissary vein blood flow in achondroplastic dwarfs. *Neurology, 30:*769-772, 1980.
17. Papasozomenos S, Roessmann V: Respiratory distress and Arnold-Chiari malformation. *Neurology, 31:*97-100, 1981.
18. DeReuck J, Vandere Ecken H: The arterial angio-

architecture of the Arnold-Chiari malformation. *Arch Biol, 88:*61-65, 1977.

19. Naidich TP, Pudlowski RM, Naidich JB, *et al.*: Computed tomographic signs of the Chiari II malformation. Part I: Skull and dural partitions. *Radiology, 134:*65-71, 1980.
20. Naidich TP, Pudlowski RM, Naidich JB: Computed tomographic signs of Chiari II malformation. II: Midbrain and cerebellum. *Radiology, 134:*391-398, 1980.
21. Naidich TP, Pudlowski RM, Naidich JB: Computed tomographic signs of the Chiari II malformation. III: Ventricles and cisterns. *Radiology, 134:*657-663, 1980.
22. Zimmerman RD, Breckbill D, Dennis MW, Davis DO: Cranial CT findings in patients with meningocele. *Am J Roentgenol, 132:*623-629, 1979.
23. Di-Lorenzo N, Bozzao L, Antonelli M, Fortuna A: Arnold-Chiari malformation detected by unenhanced multiplanar CT scan. *Surg Neurol, 16:*340-345, 1981.
24. Weisberg L, Shraberg D, Meriwether RP, Robertson H, Goodman G: Computed tomographic findings in the Arnold-Chiari type I malformation. *Comput Tomogr, 5:*1-9, 1981.
25. Forbes WS, Isherwood I: Computed tomography in syringomyelia and the associated Arnold-Chiari type I malformation. *Neuroradiology, 15:*73-78, 1978.
26. Linder M, Diehl JT, Sklar FM: Significance of post shunt ventricular asymmetries. *J Neurosurg, 55:* 183-186, 1981.

6

Dandy-Walker Malformation

DEFINITION

This developmental anomaly ususally consists of: 1) hydrocephalus; 2) maldevelopment of the vermis; 3) dilatation of the fourth ventricle; 4) large posterior fossa; and 5) elevation of transverse sinuses, confluence of sinuses, and tentorium (1).

According to Hart *et al.* (2), this anomaly should consist of a triad of: a) hydrocephalus; b) vermian dysgenesis (ranging from aplasia to mere hypoplasia); and c) large posterior fossa cyst communicating with an enlarged fourth ventricle (Figs. 1,2).

HISTORY (1)

Whereas it is generally believed that this disorder was first described by Sutton in 1887 (2), Costa da Costa *et al.* in 1973 (3) attributed the first description of this entity to Virchow in 1863, and to Tusari in 1891. Be that as it may, it was after the publications of Dandy and Blackfan in 1914 (4) and Dandy in 1921 (5) that this clinical and pathologic entity was clearly recognized as such. They suggested congenital atresia of the outlet foramina of the fourth ventricle as the underlying cause of this disorder. Taggert and Walker in 1942 (6) further elucidated this entity and supported the concept of Dandy and Blackfan. Benda in 1954 (7) objected to the concept of foraminal obstruction as being too simplistic an explanation of this disorder.

PATHOGENESIS (1-16)

That obstruction of the outlet foramina is *the* cause of the Dandy-Walker malformation is an oversimplification and probably a misrepresentation of the embryologic facts. Such an outlet foraminal obstruction is not present in all cases. There is a variable degree of patency of one, two or all of the outlet foramina in almost all cases. During the pneumoencephalography era, it was not uncommon to fill the posterior fossa cyst with air by injecting it in the lumbar subarachnoid space.

The acceptable embryologic basis of the malformation will be the one that embraces: a) elevated torcular; b) large posterior fossa; c) chronology of vermian morphogenesis and patency of outlet foramina of the fourth ventricle; and d) production of CSF in the entire ventricular system and its escape from the fourth ventricle. Enlargement of the posterior fossa and elevation of the torcular in all cases indicate that this malformation occurs before 12 weeks of gestation since the torcular attains its normal location by that time. The fact that there is seldom concurrent myelomeningocele in this disorder suggests that it occurs after four to five weeks, the point at which neural tube normally closes. From this, one can deduce that the anomaly occurs within five to twelve weeks of gestation. This timing is earlier than the generally accepted (16) 16 to 20 weeks when the outlet foramina of the fourth ventricle normally become patent, the cerebellum having attained its normal configuration by 16 weeks. Before that time, the CSF, which the ventricular choroid plexus begins to produce at 6 weeks, escapes from the fourth ventricle through its permeable roof. In other words, the failure of the outlet foramina of the fourth ventricle to become patent at 16 to 20 weeks cannot explain a malformation that seems to originate before 12 weeks.

If outlet foraminal obstruction is not the cause, then how else can one explain this disorder? Some workers have suggested (2,14) that vermian dysgenesis occurs and leads to secondary fourth ventricular distension. This hypothesis alone cannot explain the exceedingly disproportionate enlargement of the fourth ventricle and the occurrence of the cyst, let alone the enlargement of the posterior fossa. In any dysgenetic process, the secondary enlargement of the neighboring ventricular and/or subarachnoid spaces should not result in concomitant enlargement of the adjacent cranial cavity. If one now invokes the impaired permeability of the fourth ventricle roof (12,14) as a plausible cause, then it is possible to explain the fourth ventricle distension and its secondary effect on the morphogenesis of the vermis. That is, the distended fourth ventricle disturbs midline fusion of the vermis and its proper development.

Whereas the pathogenesis of Dandy-Walker malformation seems far from being clearly established, I believe the best embryologic explanation is the impaired permeability of the fourth ventricle membranous roof and vermian dysgenesis.

Histologically, the cyst wall contains arachnoid membrane and an ependymal layer; irregularly scattered cerebellar tissue may be found in the cyst wall. Associated CNS malformations – dysgenesis of corpus callosum, syringo-hydromyelia, gray matter heterotopia, polymicrogyria – are present in more than 50 per cent of cases (2). The most common is dysgenesis of corpus callosum. Concurrent systemic anomalies (e.g., cleft palate, polydactyly, Klippel-Feil Syndrome) have been reported in as many as 25 per cent of patients (2).

ETIOLOGY

Genetic, chemical or multiple factors may play a part in its causation, but the exact etiology is uncertain. The occurrence of a wide variability in the degree of vermian dys(hypo-)genesis, hydrocephalus, and associated anomalies (17) suggests variable expression of the damaging influence(s).

CLINICAL SYMPTOMATOLOGY (17,18)

The symptoms are mainly those of hydrocephalus and cerebellar dysfunction. There is no sex predilection, and about 60% of the cases occur before three years of age, although it can occur in adults. The familial occurrence of Dandy-Walker malformation has been described (19,20).

CT SCAN FINDINGS

In a typical case, the characteristic findings include a large fourth ventricle that communicates dorsally with the cyst, which is of variable size (Figs. 3,4,5). In an atypical case this malformation may involve mainly the inferior part of the fourth ventricle at inferior medullary velum level (21) (Fig. 6). The vermis is totally or partially absent. The cerebellar hemispheres are always present but may be slightly smaller. The posterior fossa is larger in volume and the torcular elevated. The higher placed tentorium is best appreciated on the coronal CT (Figs. 7,8). Hydrocephalus, of variable degree, is almost always present; only in an exceptional case is the ventricular system mildly dilated or not dilated at all (Fig. 9).

DIFFERENTIAL DIAGNOSIS

The following conditions need to be considered in the differential diagnosis:

1) Posterior fossa extra-axial arachnoid cyst
2) Large cisterna magna
3) Massive enlargement of the fourth ventricle in communicating hydrocephalus and the so-called isolated (trapped) fourth ventricle
4) Ponto cerebellar atrophy
5) Fourth ventricular arachnoid cyst

In the case of POSTERIOR FOSSA EXTRA-AXIAL ARACHNOID CYST (22-25), the cyst does not blend with the fourth ventricle. Instead, the fourth ventricle is compressed (Fig. 10). The notch (Fig. 11) between the forwardly displaced cerebellar hemispheres should not be misinterpreted as the fourth ventricle. When recognizable, the fourth ventricle has a pointed rather than the flat anterior aspect as seen in Dandy-Walker malformation. In doubtful cases, instillation of metrizamide into one of the lateral ventricles (metrizamide ventriculography) will show passage of the contrast medium into the compressed and forwardly dislocated fourth ventricle (Fig. 12). These cysts may be trabeculated (Fig. 13). The lateral ventricles usually are enlarged. The occipital bones may be thinned from cyst compression. These patients usually reveal signs of posterior fossa compression.

SOMEWHAT LARGE CISTERNA MAGNA (25-27) is not an uncommon finding at all ages (26). Shape and size (Figs. 14,15,16) are variable, ranging from 2 x 2 to 6 x 4 cm. (26) A 0.4 per cent incidence has been reported in consecutive CT scans performed for various reasons (26). The main feature that distinguishes this entity from posterior fossa extra-axial cyst is the absence of compression of the fourth ventricle and lack of ventricular enlargement. The disorder may reveal arachnoidal septations and peripheral enhancement not exhibited by extra-axial cyst. Contrast enhancement may be related to associated anomalous venous pattern or surrounding dural membrane.

Typically, such cases do not manifest signs of posterior fossa compression. Large cisterna magna is a reflection of developmental cerebellar hypoplasia or, less likely, atrophy eluding clinical recognition.

In an extremely exceptional case, one may have to carefully exclude lesions such as cystic astrocytoma, cystic hemangioblastoma, and an epidermoid, which may mimic it.

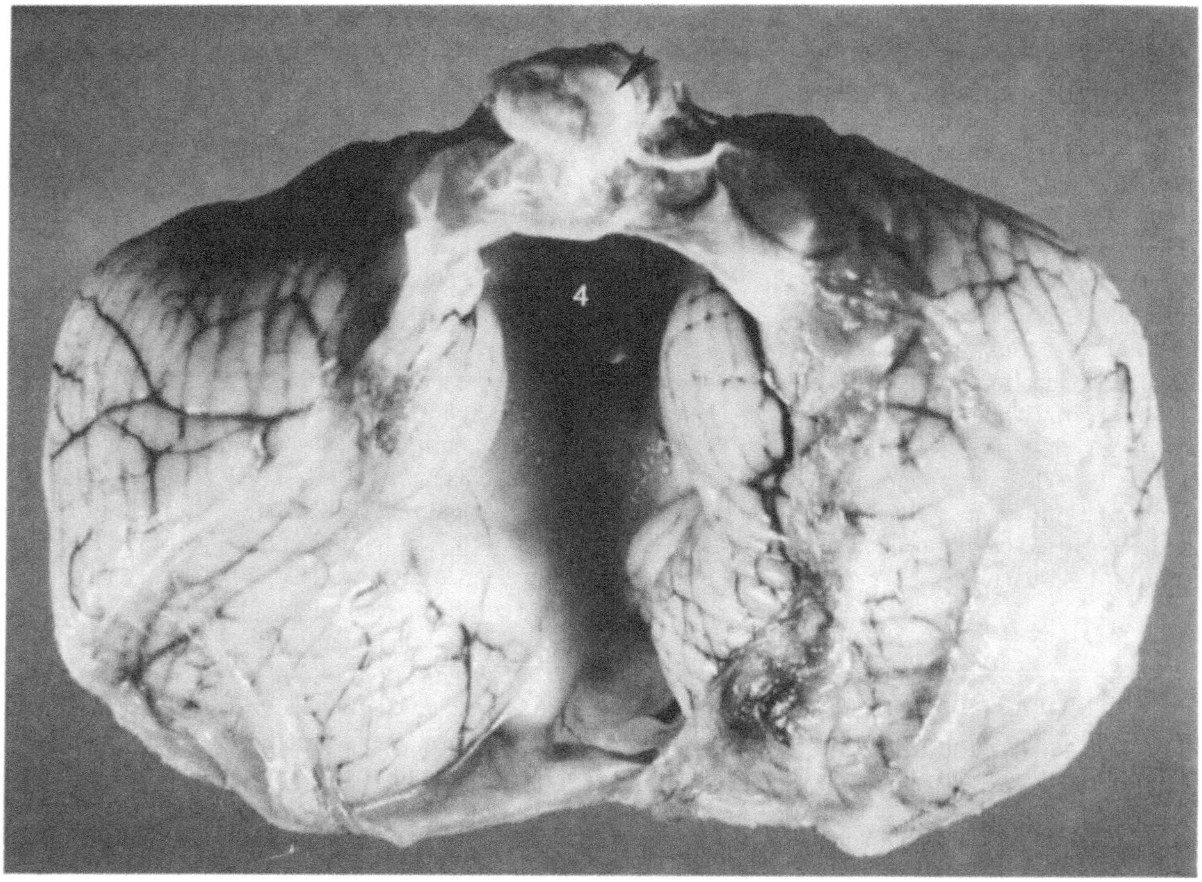

Figure 1. Pathologic specimen of Dandy-Walker malformation. Note dorsad continuation of the dilated fourth ventricle (4) into the cyst that has thin membrane (collapsed in this specimen). There is no vermis. The cerebellar hemispheres are present. Observe flat anterior aspect of the fourth ventricle. **Arrowhead** = Brainstem.

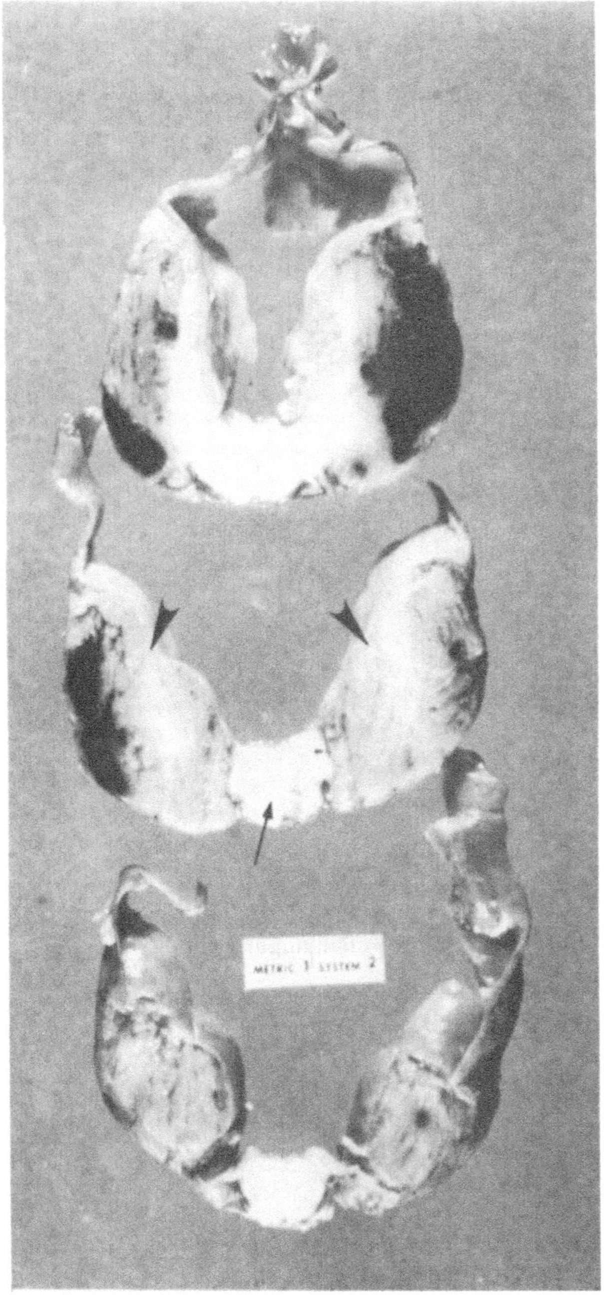

Figure 2. Pathologic specimen of Dandy-Walker malformation. In addition to vermian agenesis, there is hypoplasia of the cerebellar hemispheres **(arrowheads)** probably due to pressure atrophy from the distended fourth ventricle and the cyst. **Arrow** = Brainstem.

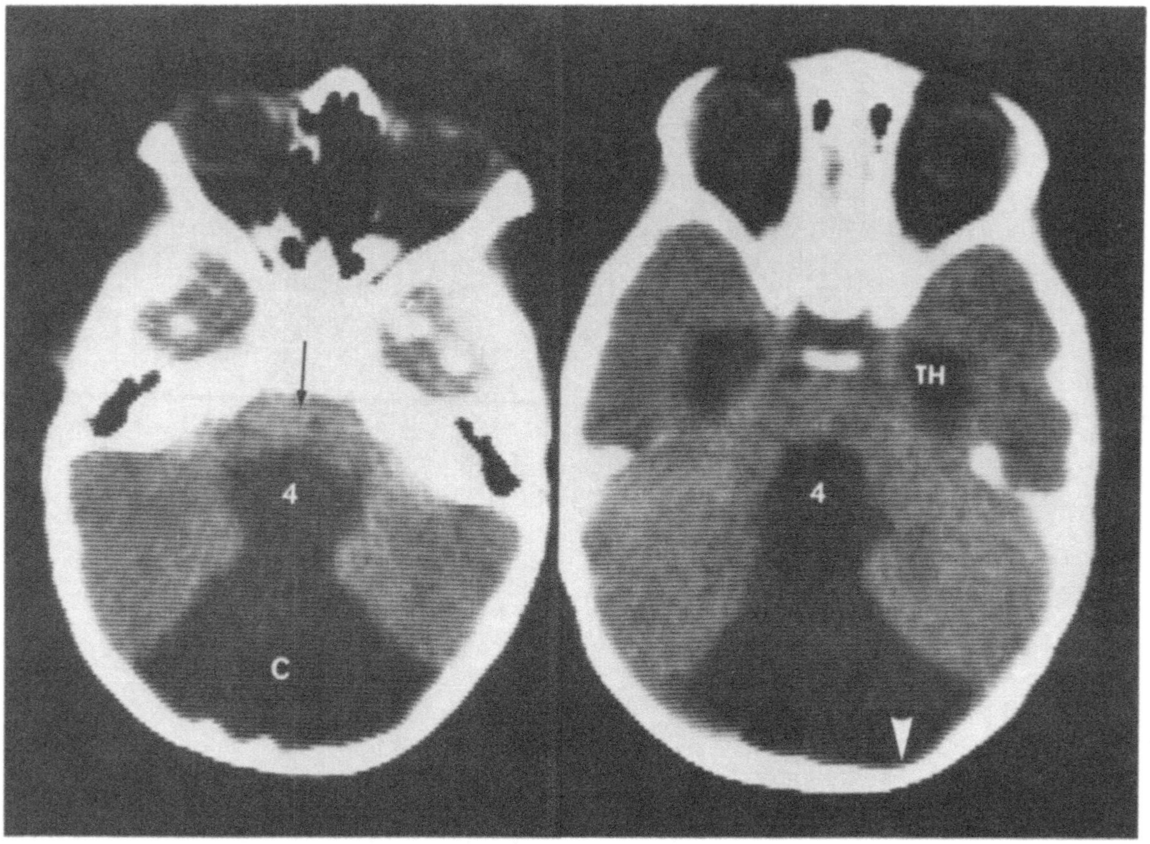

Figure 3. Typical CT scan findings of Dandy-Walker malformation. The anterior aspect of the fourth ventricle (4) is flat. It continues into the cyst (C) and no intervening vermian tissue is present. Note localized bone thinning (**arrowhead**). TH = Dilated temporal horn, as part of generalized hydrocephalus. **Arrow** = Brainstem (courtesy of Dr. Guinto).

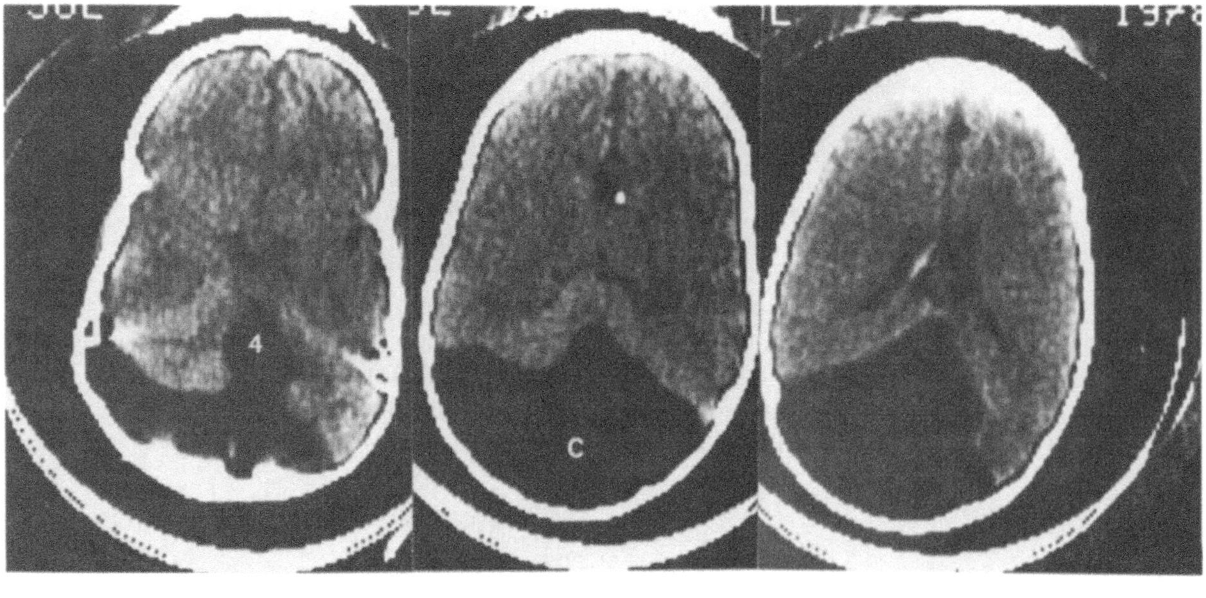

Figure 4. Dandy-Walker malformation. The asymmetric cyst (C) is huge and extends into the supratentorial compartment. 4 = fourth ventricle.

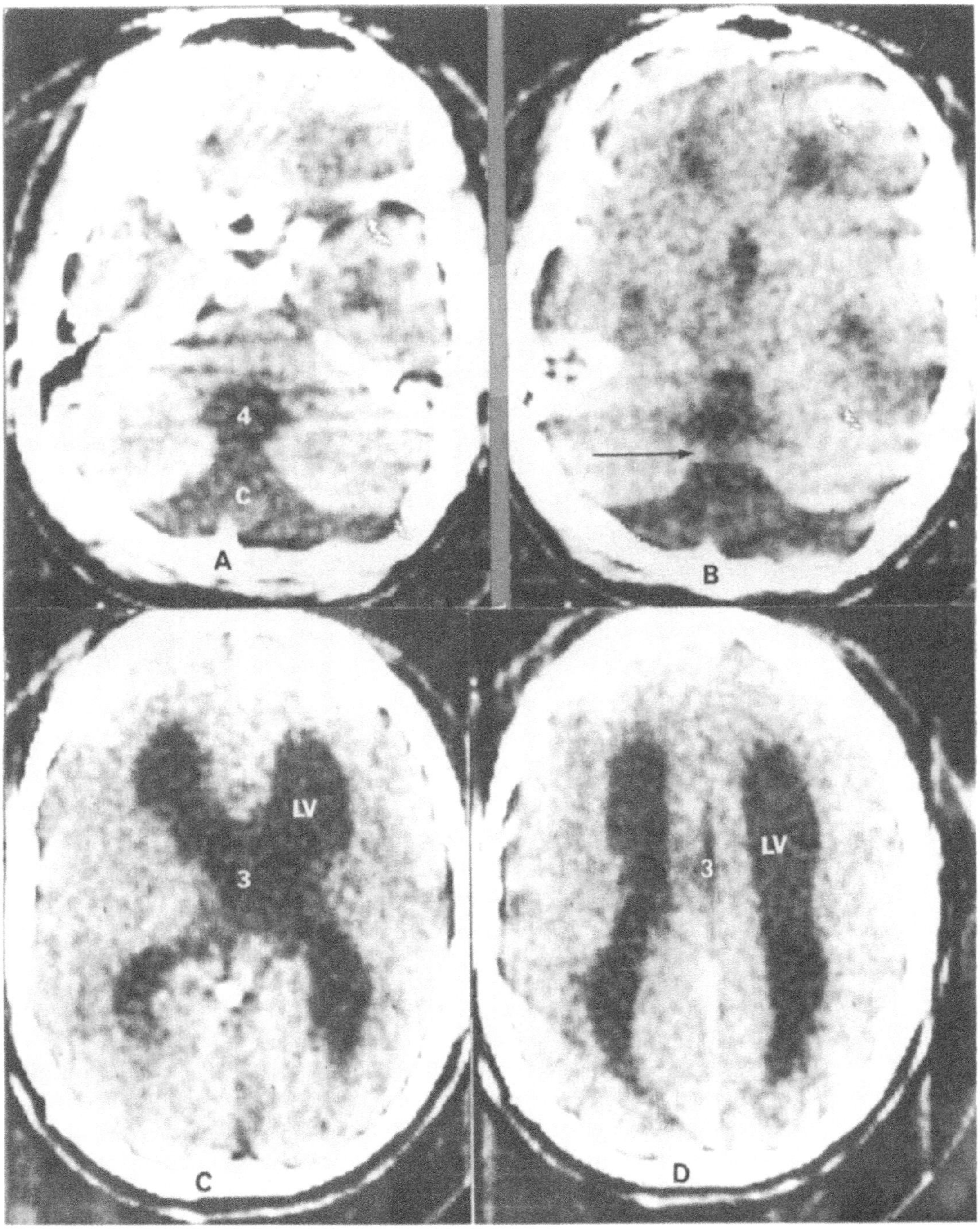

Figure 5. Dandy-Walker malformation and associated dysgenesis of corpus callosum. The fourth ventricle (4) merges posteriorly into the cyst (C). A rudiment of vermian tissue (**arrow**) is present behind the fourth ventricle in (B). Dysgenesis of corpus callosum is represented by separation of the lateral ventricles (LV) and interposition of the dilated third ventricle (3) between them.
This 26-year-old mad had seizures, psychomotor retardation, dyslexia and ataxia since childhood. Clinical diagnosis was "chronic schizophrenia, undifferentiated."

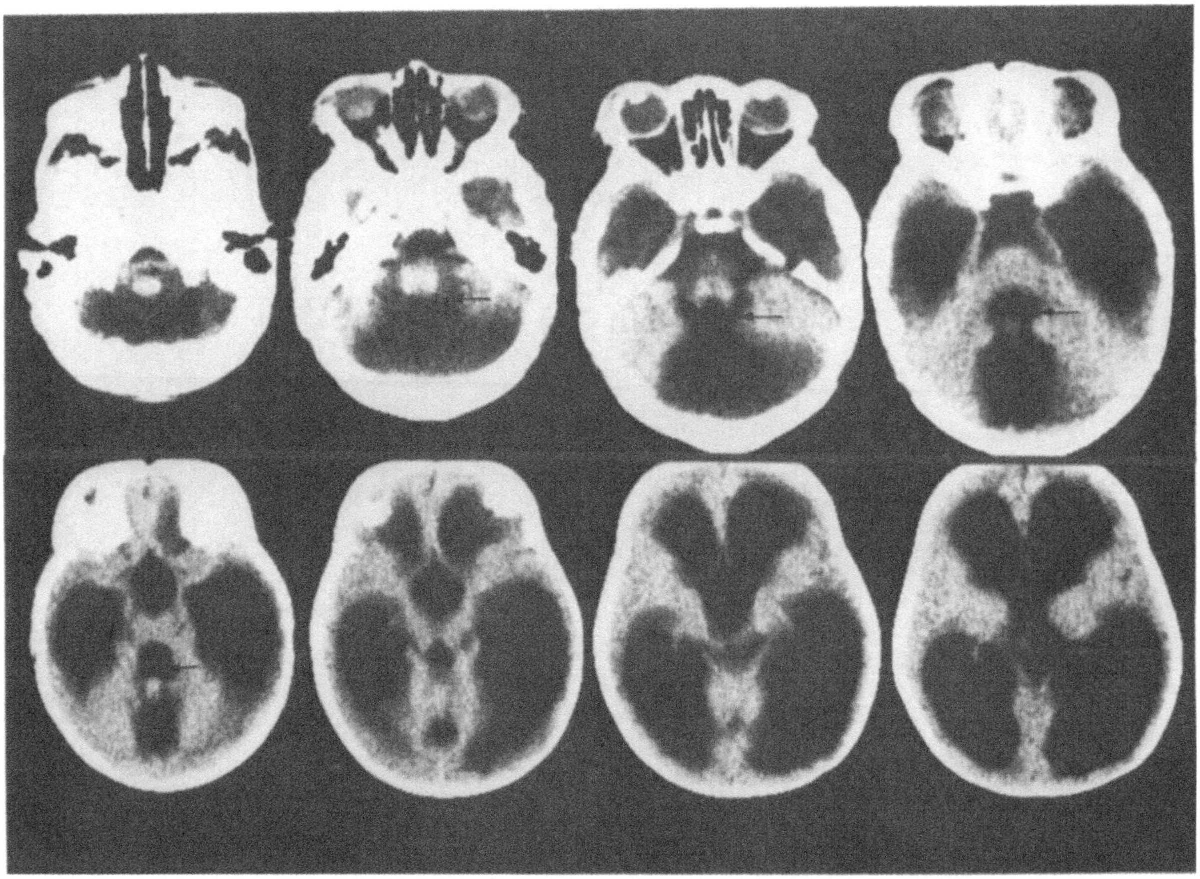

Figure 6. Probable Dandy-Walker malformation in a 3-month-old. This is somewhat an atypical form involving mainly the inferior part of the fourth ventricle (**arrows**) at the inferior medullary velum level. The mid to upper part of the fourth ventricle is only slightly dilated and it maintains almost the normal shape. The presence of enlarged subarachnoid spaces around the brainstem makes one wonder if the CT appearance is an exceptional manifestation of the extraventricular obstructive ventriculomegaly (communicating hydrocephalus) with the posterior fossa cystic structure representing a massively enlarged cisterna magna. Notice marked hydrocephalus.

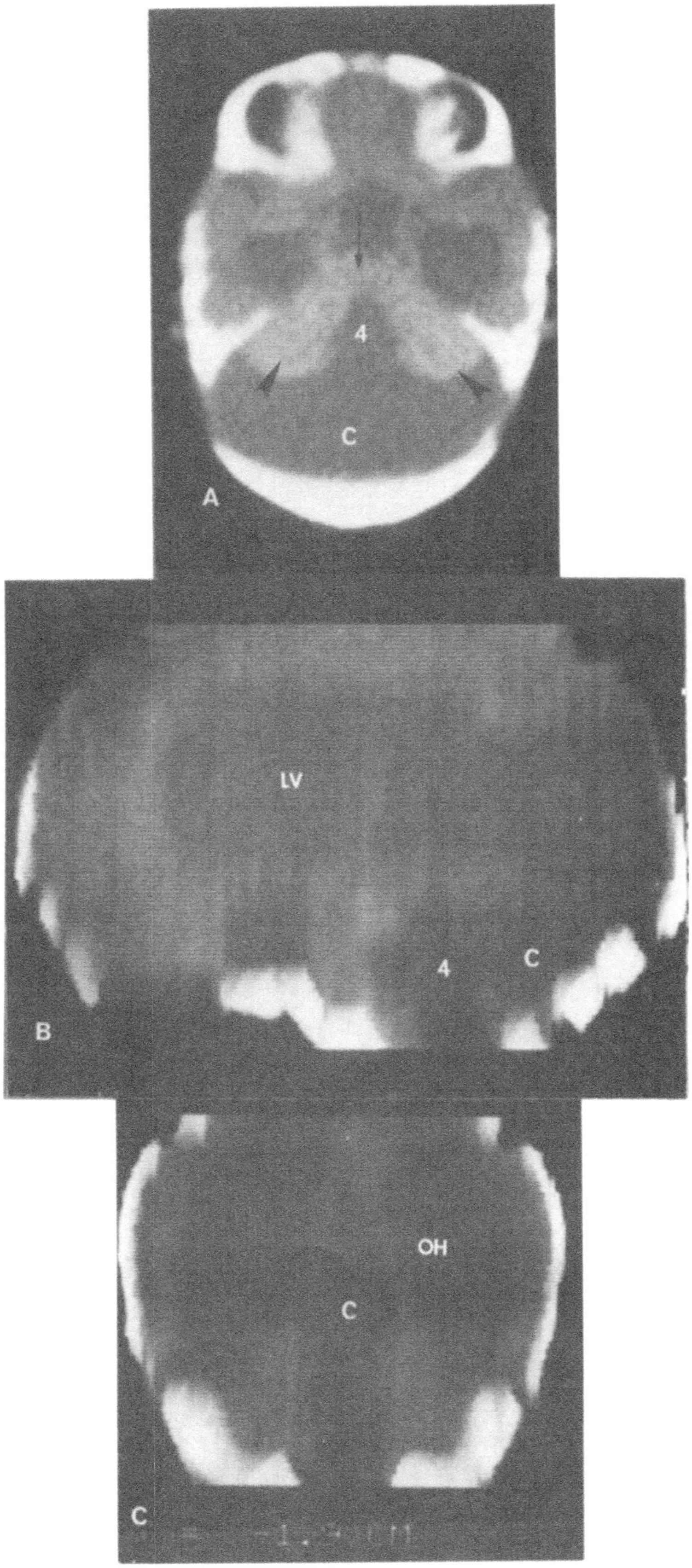

Figure 7. Dandy-Walker malformation. Axial (A) and reformatted sagittal (B) and coronal (C) CT images. The cerebellar hemispheres (**arrowheads**) are hypoplastic. 4 = fourth ventricle, C = cyst, LV = lateral ventricle, OH = occipital horn. **Arrow** = Brainstem. (Courtesy Dr. Guinto.)

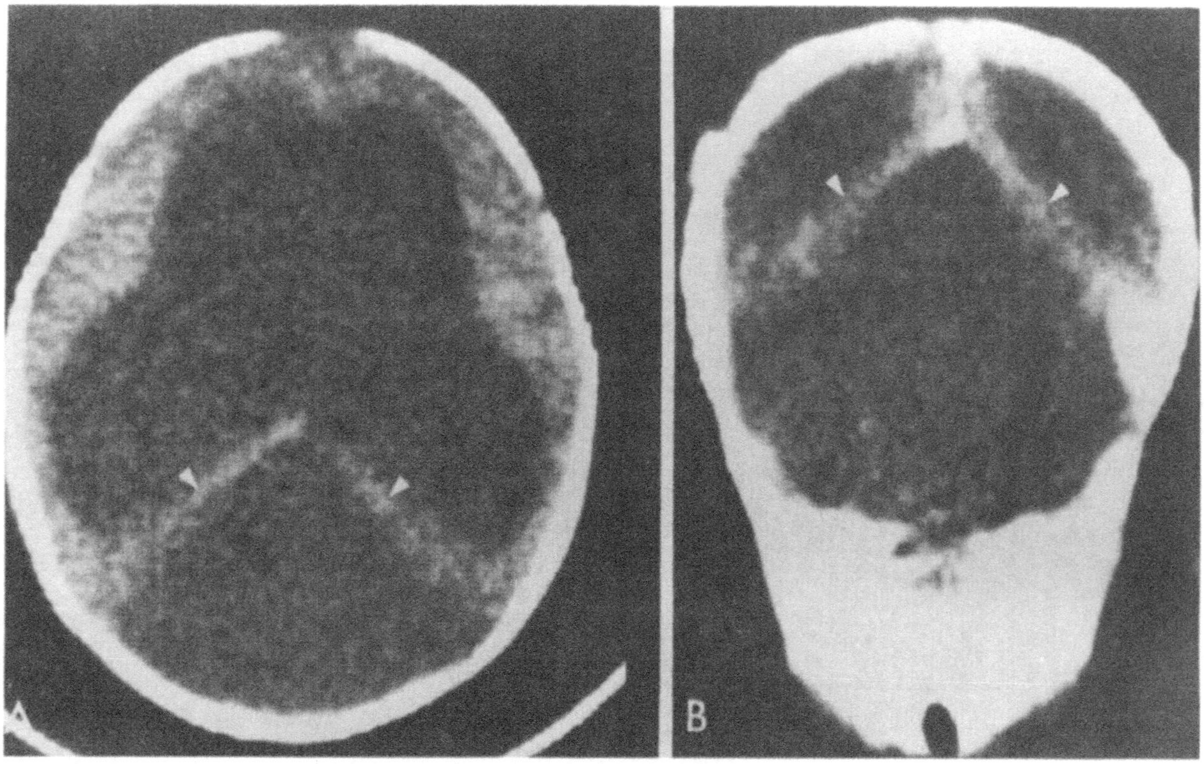

Figure 8. Dandy-Walker malformation in a 2-month-old boy. (A) axial and (B) coronal CT scan. Note high position of the tentorium (**arrowheads**). [From Naidich *et al., Rad. Cl. N. America,* Vol. 20, March 1980 (with permission).]

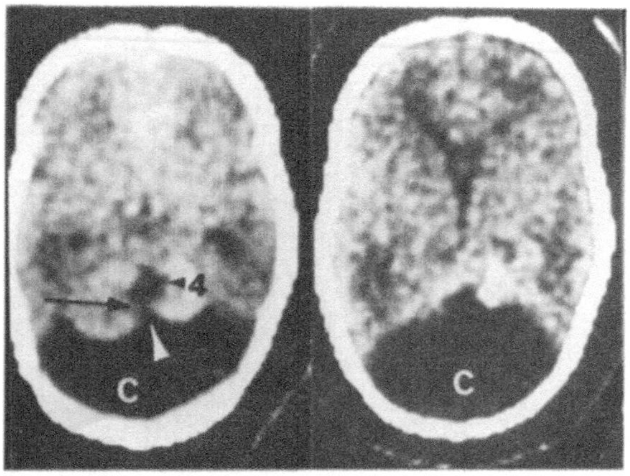

Figure 9. A milder form of Dandy-Walker malformation. The midline notch between the cerebellar hemispheres (**white arrowhead**) is not seen in the severe form. A rudimentary vermian tissue (**arrow**) also is present. The fourth ventricle (4) has a somewhat unusual shape. The lateral ventricles are only minimally if at all dilated. C = cyst.

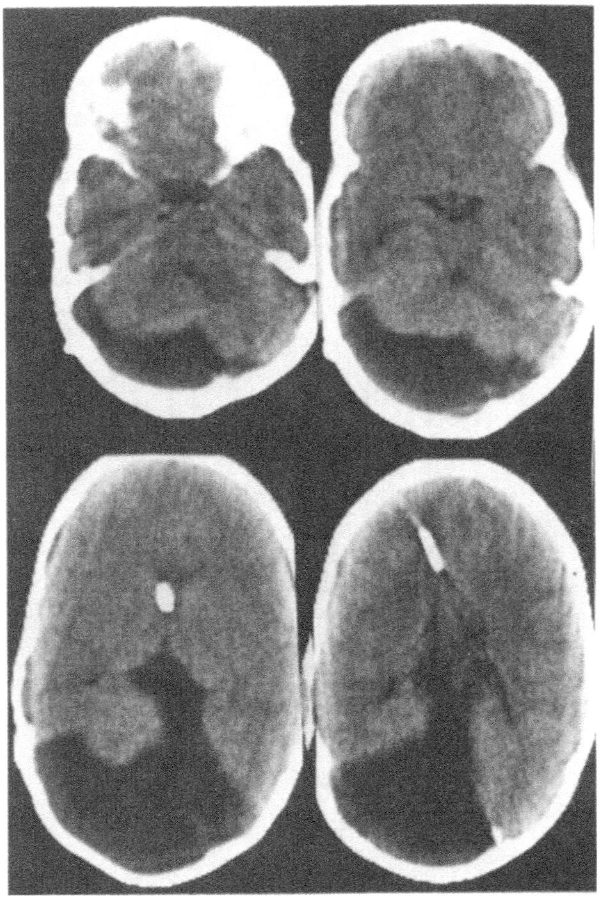

Figure 10. A posterior fossa extra-axial arachnoid cyst in a 4-year-old child. It is asymmetric and has supratentorial component as well. Because of associated hydrocephalus due to compression of the fourth ventricle, ventricular shunting was required.

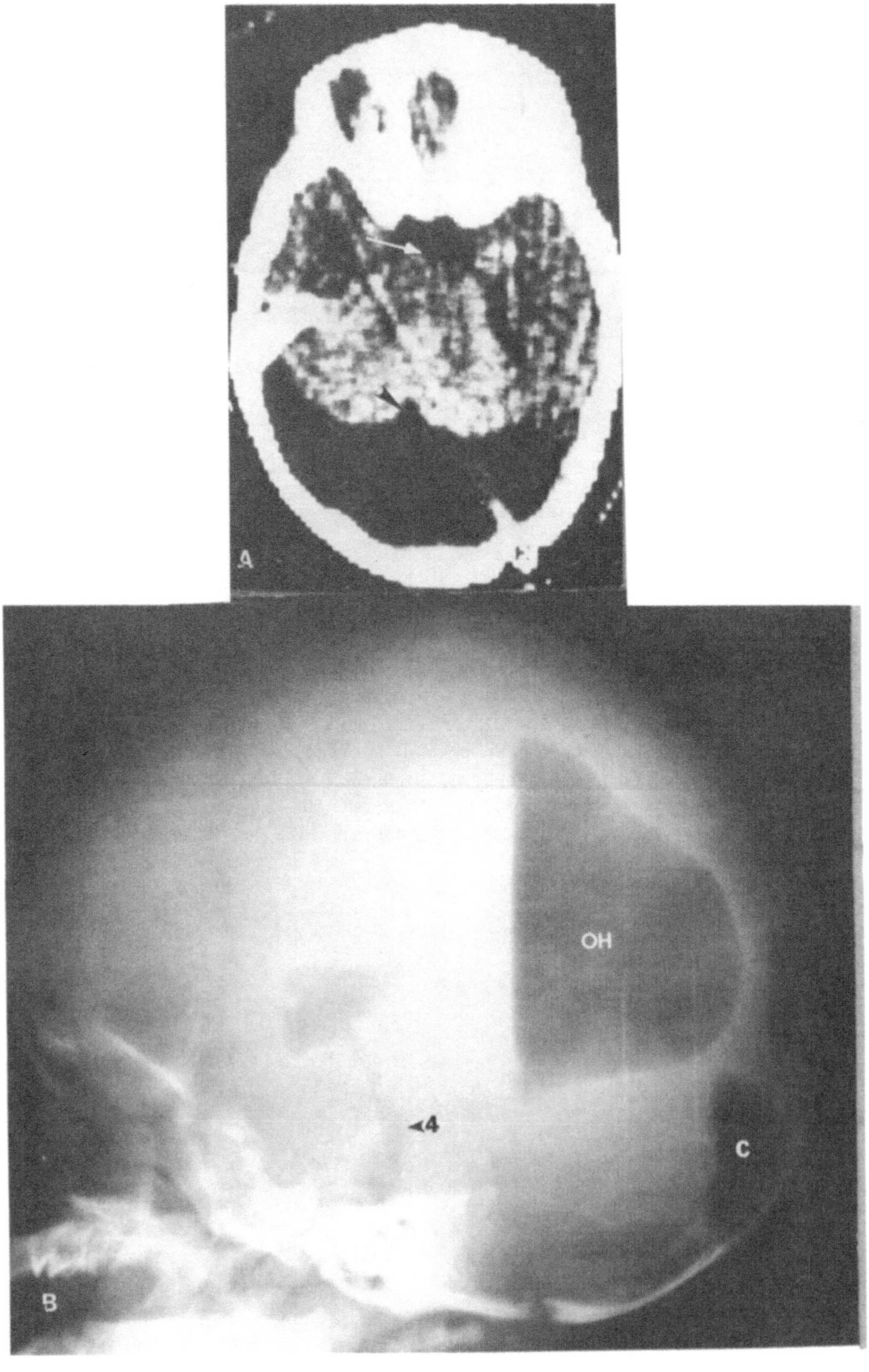
A
OH
◄4
C
B

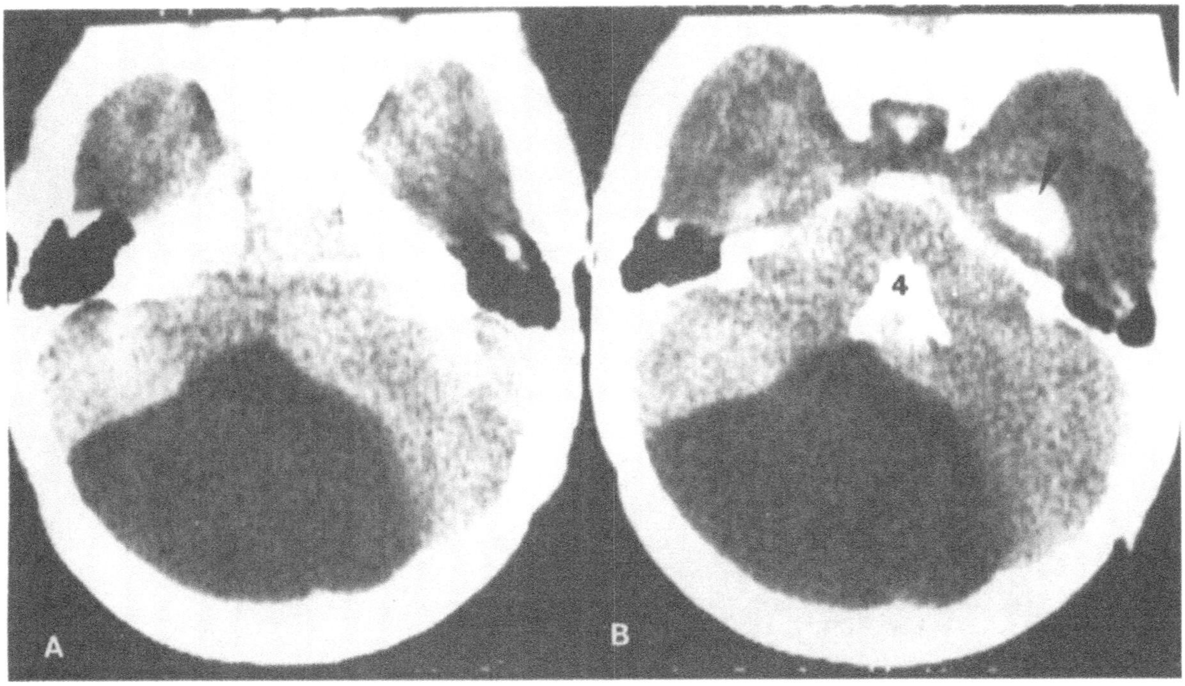

Figure 12. Posterior fossa extra-axial arachnoid cyst.
A. This scan is likely to be confused with Dandy-Walker malformation, the fourth ventricle presumed being continuous with the cyst. However, if one were to measure the size of the apparent brainstem, it would be abnormally large rather than compressed. In such cases, metrizamide CT scanning provides useful information by opacifying the fourth ventricle.
B. Metrizamide CT scan. The compressed fourth ventricle (4) is displaced anteriorly. Note that it has maintained its normal shape. Its postero-lateral recesses are clearly recognizable. This will not happen in Dandy-Walker malformation. Note associated hydrocephalus as suggested by dilated temporal horn **(arrowhead)**. (Courtesy Dr. Marc.)

← Figure 11. Posterior fossa extra-axial arachnoid in an infant.

A. CT scan. The compressed fourth ventricle is not recognizable. The midline notch **(arrowhead)** between the cerebellar hemispheres should not be confused with the fourth ventricle. If it were indeed the fourth ventricle then the brainstem size as measured from its anterior surface **(arrow)** to the presumed fourth ventricle would be enormous. Taking into consideration the minification factor, the pons at this level normally should not measure more than 3 cm.

B. Pneumoencephalogram, lateral view. The fourth ventricle (4) is displaced anteriorly by the partly air-filled cyst (C). OH = Dilated occipital horn.

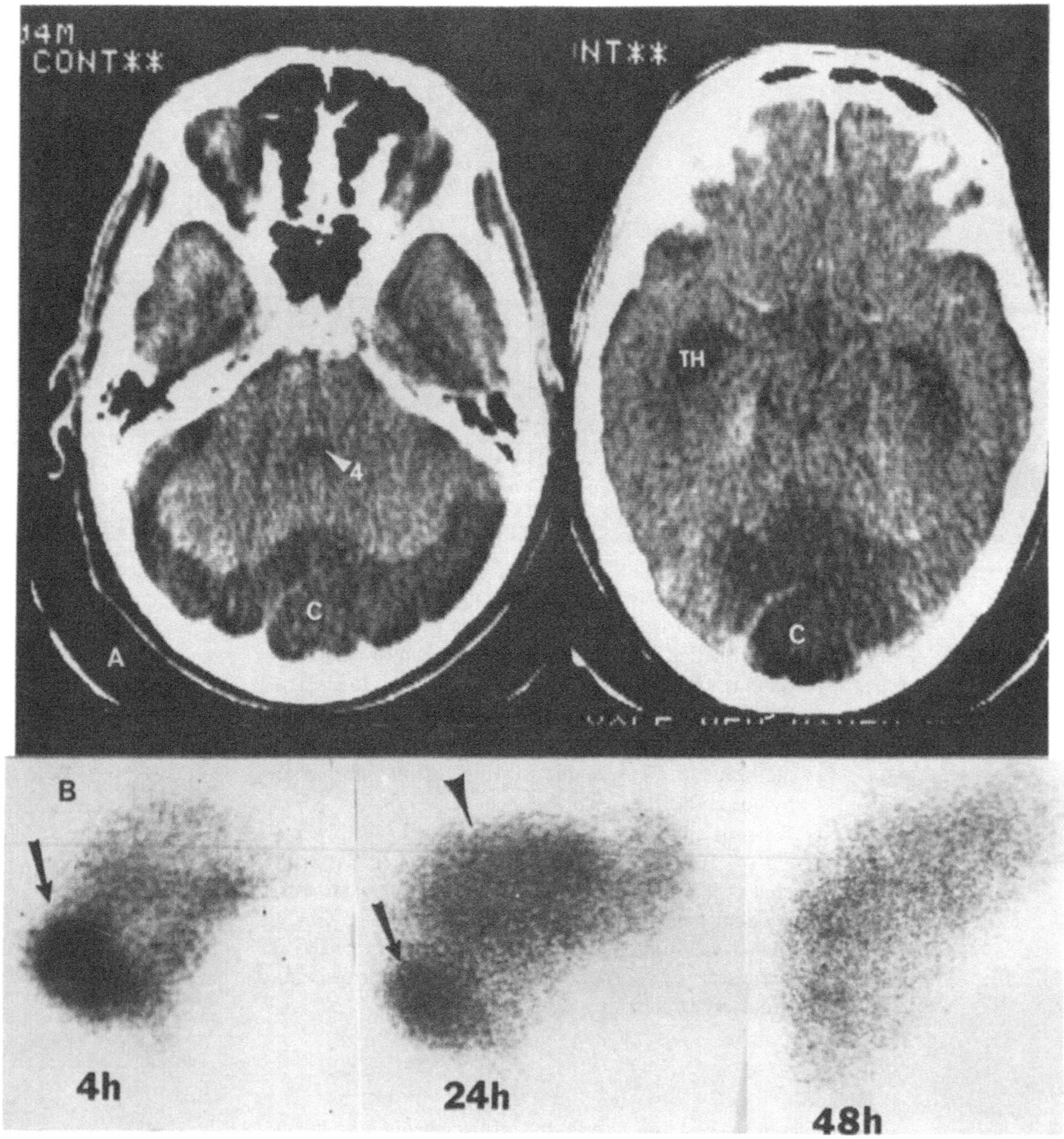

Figure 13. A. CT scan. Partly trabeculated posterior fossa extra-axial arachnoid cyst (C). Fourth ventricle (4) is displaced forward. TH = Dilated temporal horn. B. Isotope cisternogram. Note that the isotope enters the cyst (**arrows**) indicating its communication with the subarachnoid space. Its escape, however, is delayed as evidenced by persistent radioactivity on the 24 hr image. The isotope also enters the dilated lateral ventricles (**arrowhead**) with delayed clearance.
This 76-year-old demented male had presented with subarachnoid hemorrhage.

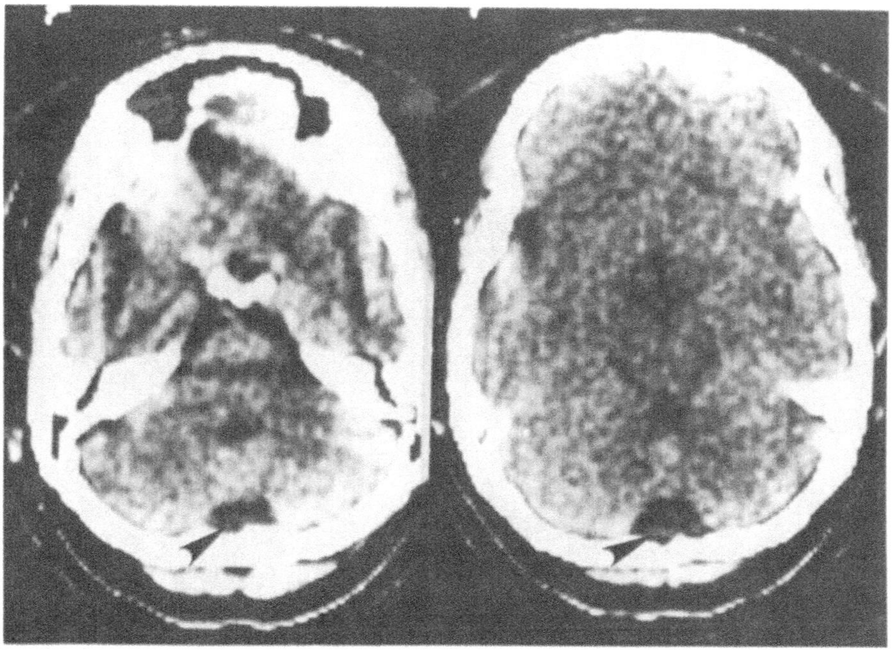

Figure 14. A mildly enlarged cisterna magna (**arrowheads**).

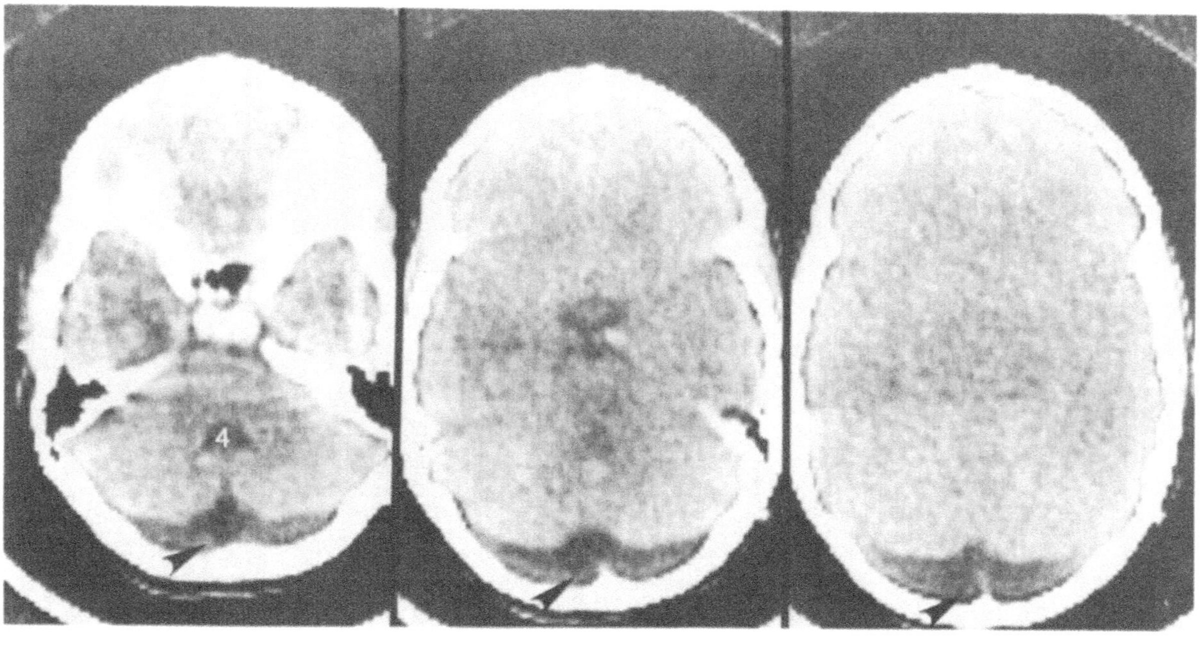

Figure 15. A moderate sized cisterna magna (**arrowheads**). The fourth ventricle (4) is not compressed. There was no hydrocephalus.

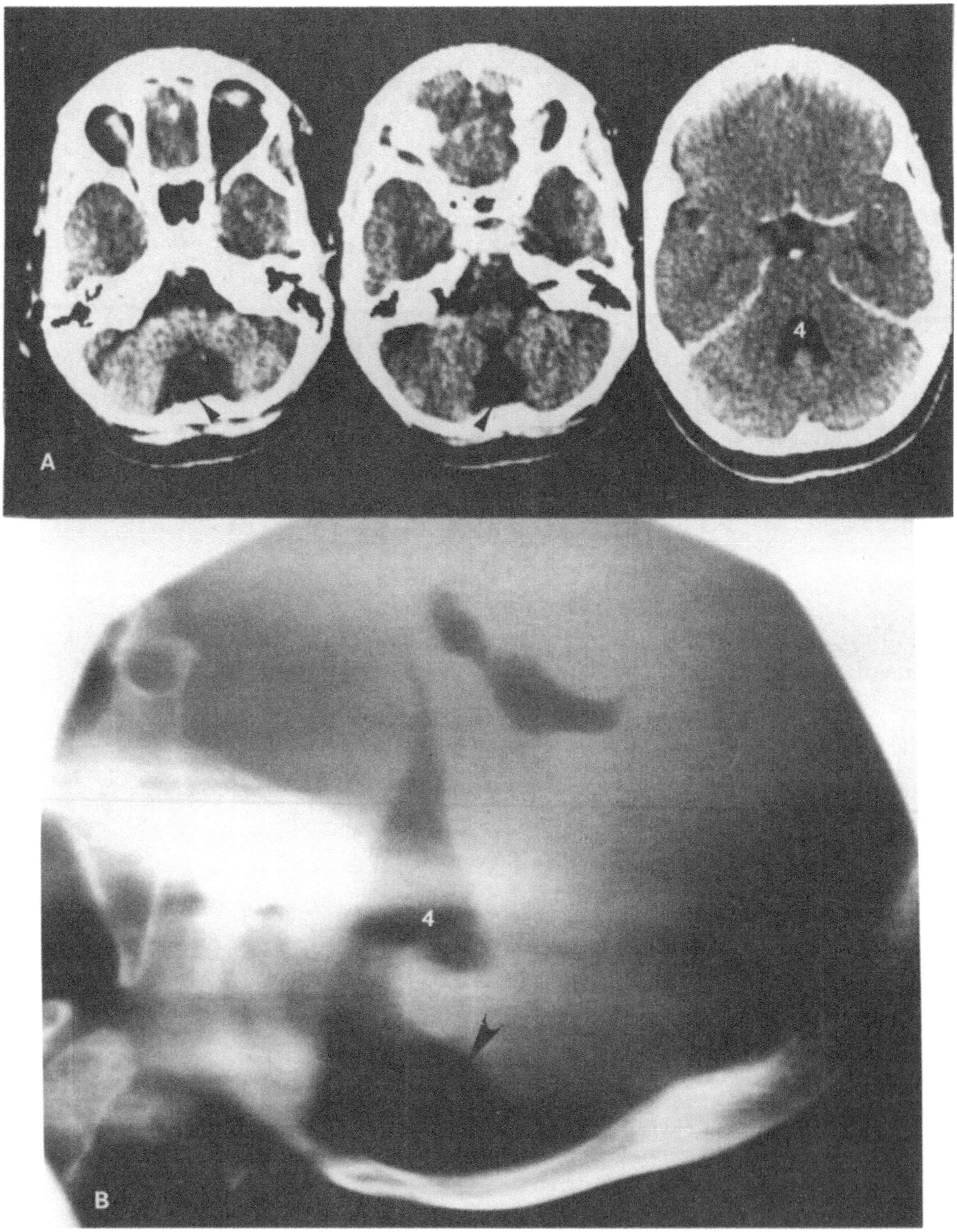

Figure 16. Large cisterna magna.
A. CT scan. Note that the large cisterna magna (**arrowheads**) does not compress the tourth ventricle (4). There was no hydrocephalus.
B. Pneumoencephalogram, lateral view. The large cisterna magna (**arrowhead**) communicates with the fourth ventricle (4) through vallecula and foramen of Magendie.

Occasionally, in COMMUNICATING HYDROCEPHALUS, the fourth ventricle can assume a considerable size, although it maintains its usual shape and vermis is easily recognized (Fig. 17). Commonly, it becomes smaller after shunting the dilated lateral ventricles (Fig. 18). If the fourth ventricle does not shrink after lateral ventricular shunting, one may have to suspect the fourth ventricle having been transformed into the so called TRAPPED OR ISOLATED FOURTH VENTRICLE (28-31). This implies a blockage of the outlet foramina of the fourth ventricle and of the aqueduct, a condition that invariably follows CSF infection. Such an entrapped fourth ventricle (Fig. 19) can cause brain stem compression, which may require alleviation by directly shunting the fourth ventricle.

In PONTO-CEREBELLAR ATROPHY, the fourth ventricle and poster-fossa subarachnoid spaces are enlarged.

FOURTH VENTRICULAR ARACHNOID CYST is an extremely uncommon condition (32). A cyst that has completely obstructed the aqueduct, is almost impossible to distinguish from an entrapped fourth ventricle even in metrizamide ventriculography. However, a partially patent aqueduct may allow the contrast medium to layer around the lesion, thereby disclosing its true identity.

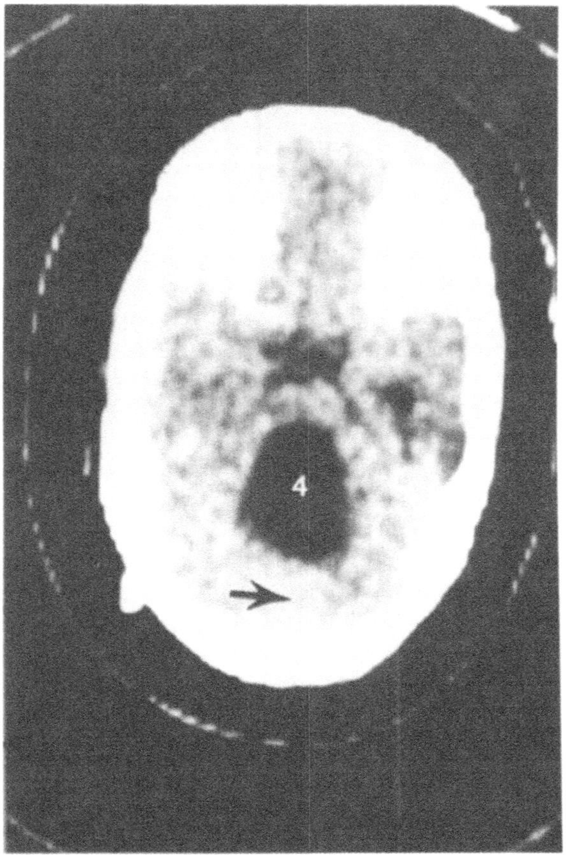

Figure 17. Trapped fourth ventricle (4). The vermis (**arrow**) is present behind it. This 1-month-old child had meningitis.

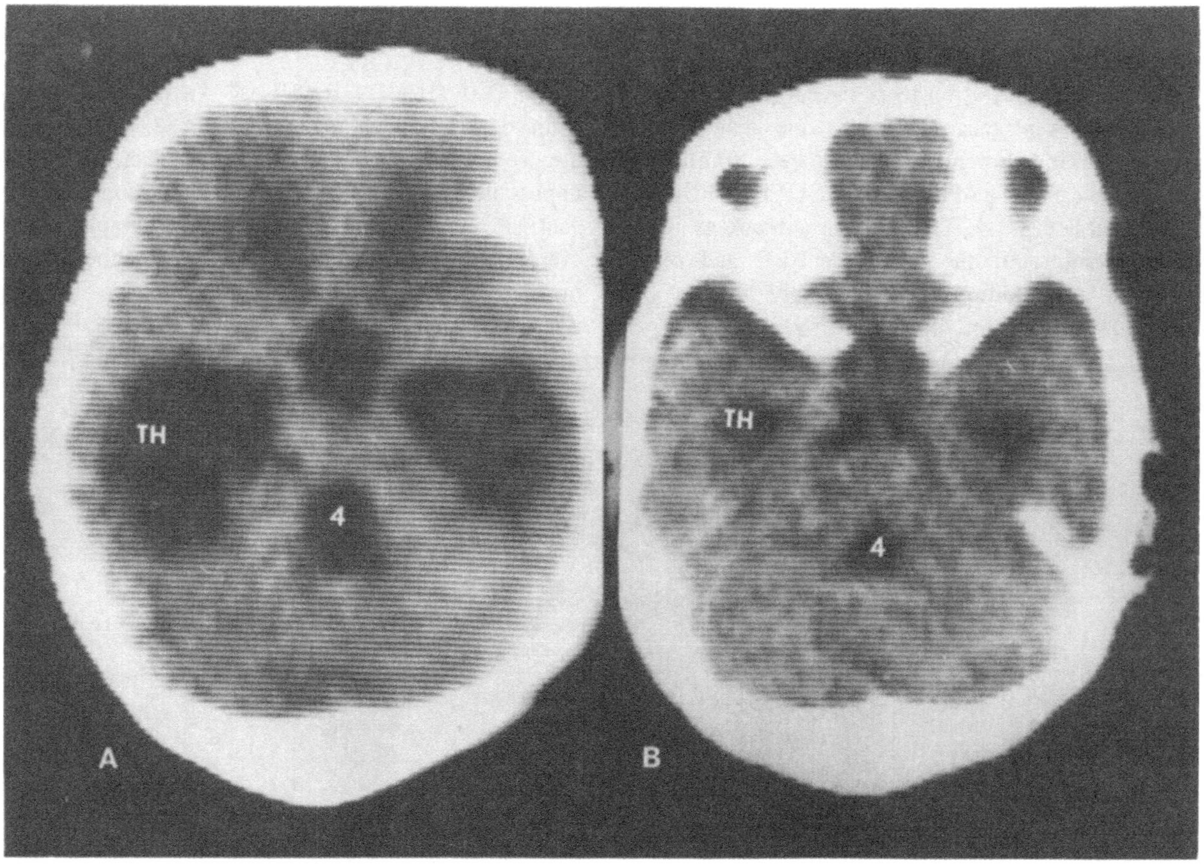

Figure 18. Reduction in size of the fourth ventricle (4) with decrease in size of the lateral ventricles following shunt therapy. A. before shunting, B. following shunting. TH = temporah horns.

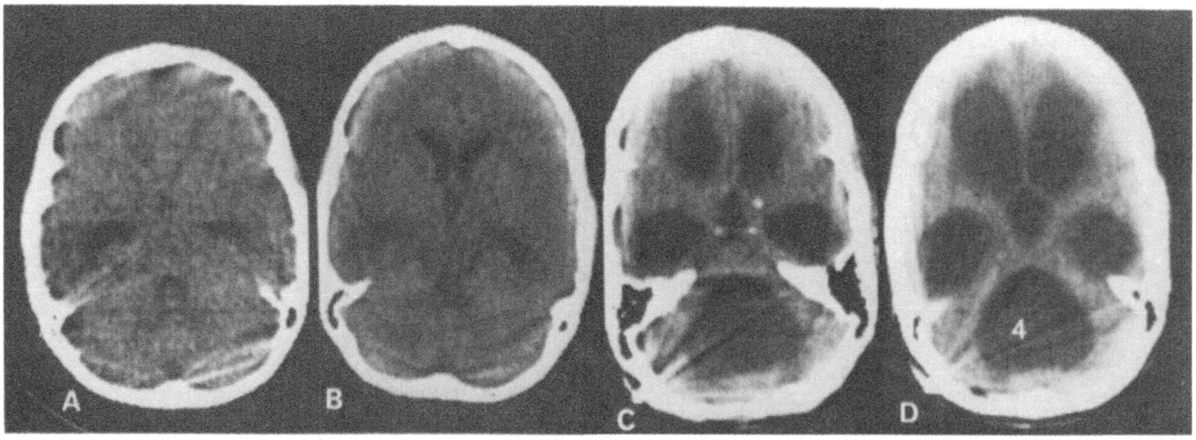

Figure 19. Entrapped fourth ventricle. This 8-year-old child presented with subarachnoid hemorrhage from a ruptured posterior inferior cerebellar artery aneurysm. Note progressive enlargement of entire ventricular system. The fourth ventricle (4) became trapped as seen in (C) and (D). (A) was done on 6/11/81; (B) on 6/16/81; (C) and (D) on 5/29/82.

REFERENCES

1. Brown JR: The Dandy-Walker Syndrome. In: *Handbook of Clinical Neurology. Congenital Malformations of the Brain and Skull.* Part 1, Vol 30. Eds. Vinken PJ, Bruyn GW, North Holland Publishing Co., Amsterdam, New York, Oxford, page 623, 1977.
2. Hart MN, Malamud N, Ellis WG: The Dandy-Walker Syndrome: a clinico-pathological study based on 28 cases. *Neurology, 22:*771-780, 1972.
3. Costa da Costa J, Anicet A, Ferreira Coutinho M: Sindrome De Dandy-Walker. *Arg Neuro Psiquiat (Sau Paulo), 31:*46-52, 1973.
4. Dandy WE, Blackfan KD: Internal hydrocephalus, an experimental, clinical and pathological study. *Am J Dis Chils, 8:*406-482. 1914.
5. Dandy WE: The diagnosis and treatment of hydrocephalus due to occlusion of the foramina of Magendie and Luschka. *Surg Gynecol Obst, 32:* 112-124, 1921.
6. Taggart JK, Walker AE: Congenital atresia of the foramina of Luschka and Magendie. *Arch Neurol Psychiat, 48:*583-612, 1942.
7. Benda CE: The Dandy-Walker syndrome or so-called atresia of foramen Magendie. *J Neuropath Exp Neurol, 13:*12-29, 1954.
8. Walker AE: A case of congenital atresia of the foramina of Luschka and Magendie: surgical cure. *J Neuropath Exp Neurol, 3:*368-373, 1944.
9. Lagger RL: Failure of pyramidal tract decussation in the Dandy-Walker syndrome. Report of two cases. *J Neurosurg, 50:*328-387, 1979.
10. Gardner E, O'Rahilly R, Prolo D: The Dandy-Walker and Arnold-Chiari malformations. Clinical, developmental and teratological consideration. *Arch Neurol, 32:*393-407, 1975.
11. Weed LH: The development of the cerebro-spinal spaces in pig and in man. Vol 5. In: *Carnegie Institution: Contributions to Embryology.* Washington, D.C., Carnegie Institute of Washington (1917).
12. Gardner WJ: *The Dysraphic States, From Syringomyelia to Anencephaly.* Excerpta Medica, Amsterdam, p 201, 1975.
13. D'Agostino AN, Kernohan JW, Brown JR: The Dandy-Walker syndrome. *J Neuropath Exp Neurol, 22:*450-470, 1963.
14. Brodal A, Hauglie-Hanssen E: Congenital hydrocephalus with defective development of the cerebellar vermis (Dandy-Walker syndrome): Clinical and anatomical findings in two cases with particular reference to the so-called atresia of the foramina of Magendie and Luschka. *J Neurol Neurosurg Psychiat, 22:*99-108, 1959.
15. Wolpert SM: Dural sinus configuration: measure of congenital disease. *Radiology, 92:*1511-1516, 1969.
16. Wilson JT: On the nature and mode of origin of the foramen of Magendie. *J Anat, 71:*423-428, 1936-1937.
17. Tal Y, Freigang B, Dunn HG *et al.*: Dandy-Walker syndrome: Analysis of 21 cases. *Dev Med Child Neurol, 22:*189-201, 1980.
18. Sawaya R. McLaurin RI: Dandy-Walker syndrome: Analysis of 23 cases. *J Neurosurg, 55:*89-98, 1981.
19. Jenkyn LR, Roberts DW, Merlis AI, Rozycki AA, Nordgren RE: Dandy-Walker malformation in identical twins. *Neurology (NY), 31:*337-341, 1981.
20. Lehman RM: Dandy-Walker syndrome in consecutive siblings: Familial hindbrain malformation. *Neurosurgery, 8:*717-719, 1981.
21. Masden JC, Dobben GD, Azar-kia B: Dandy-Walker syndrome studied by computed tomography and pneumoencephalogy. *Radiology, 147:*109-114, 1983.
22. Raybaud C: Cystic malformations of the posterior fossa: abnormalities associated with the development of the roof of the fourth ventricle. *J Neuroradiol, 9:*103-133, 1982.
23. Archer CA, Darwish H, Smith K Jr.: Enlarged cisternae magnae and posterior fossa cysts simulating Dandy-Walker syndrome on computed tomography. *Radiology, 127:*681-686, 1978.
24. Carteri A, Gerosa M, Gaini SM, Vallani R: The dysraphic state of the posterior fossa. Clinical review of the Dandy-Walker syndrome and the so-called arachnoid cysts. *J Neurosurg Sci, 23:* 53-59, 1979.
25. Vaquero J, Carrillo R, Cahezudo JM, Nombela L, Bravo G: Arachnoid cysts of the posterior fossa. *Surg Neurol, 16:*117-121, 1981.
26. Adam R, Greenberg JO: The mega cisterna magna. *J Neurosurg, 48:*190-192, 1978.
27. Just NWM, Goldenberg M: Computed tomography of the enlarged cisterna magna. *Radiology, 131:* 385-391, 1979.
28. Giuseppe S, Musgrave MA, Fitz CR, Harwood-Nash D.C.: The isolated fourth ventricle in children: CT and clinical review of 16 cases. *AJR, 135:* 1233-1238, 1980.
29. Hawkins JC III, Hoffman HJ, Humphreys RP: Isolated fourth ventricle as a complication of ventricular shunting. Report of three cases. *J Neurosurg, 49:*910-913, 1978.

30. Foltz EL, Shurtleff DB: Conversion of communicating hydrocephalus to stenosis or occlusion of the aqueduct during ventricular shunt. *J Neurosurg, 24:*520-529, 1966.

31. Zimmerman RA, Bilaniuvk LT, Gallo E: Computed tomography of the trapped fourth ventricle. *AJR, 130:*503-506, 1978.

32. Korosue K, Tamaki N, Fujiwara K, Matsumoto S: Arachnoid cyst of the fourth ventricle manifesting normal pressure hydrocephalus. *Neurosurg, 12:* 108-110, 1983.

7

Hydrocephalus

DEFINITION

Ventricular enlargement (ventriculomegaly) does not automatically imply hydrocephalus. Ventriculomegaly can be caused by tissue loss (atropic ventriculomegaly) or obstruction to cerebrospinal fluid (CSF) pathways (obstructive ventriculomegaly). Hydrocephalus denotes ventriculomegaly that is or has been under increased pressure; such pressure may be constant or intermittent. The destructive effect of hydrocephalus is best conveyed by the concept of force as envisaged by LaPlace's law: F = P x A (F = force, P = pressure, and A = area).

The two basic types of hydrocephalus are intra- and extraventricular obstructive hydrocephalus. In INTRAVENTRICULAR OBSTRUCTIVE HYDROCEPAHLUS, the obstruction lies in the ventricular system, which includes the *exit* foramina of the fourth ventricle. In EXTRAVENTRICULAR OBSTRUCTIVE HYDROCEPHALUS (communicating hydrocephalus), the obstruction is in the non-ventricular subarachnoid pathways.

CONGENITAL HYDROCEPHALUS is defined as ventriculomegaly of undetermined cause occurring in utero. Generally, a self-limiting disease with no identifiable cause, (Fig. 1) BENIGN EXTERNAL HYDROCEPHALUS (1) is characterized by enlargement of the non-ventricular subarachnoid spaces and normal or somewhat enlarged ventricles. Most of the children present with rapid head growth and no serious neurologic dysfunction. This chapter is limited to a discussion of hydrocephalus as seen in the pediatric age group.

CT CRITERIA OF HYDROCEPHALUS

Mild hydrocephalus may escape clinical recognition, and ventriculomegaly can precede rapid head growth following prenatal intracranial hemorrhage (2). Recognition of this circumstance should have prompted establishment of some rigid CT criteria for assessing hydrocephalus. Unfortunately, no such criteria exist. Measurements used in the pneumoencephalography era and as they are applied to the CT scan (3) may be employed; bicaudate and bifrontal ratios (4) may be used (Fig. 2), but these have a wide range of variation. Therefore, we prefer to assess the ventricular size qualitatively. Although this approach to assessing ventricular enlargement in its earlier stages is very tenuous, no disagreement prevails in moderate to severe cases of hydrocephalus. Rounding off and somewhat bulbar configuration of the superolateral angles of the frontal horns is the earliest sign of ventriculomegaly and is very reliable.

SOME PHYSIOLOGIC AND DYNAMIC ASPECTS OF CEREBROSPINAL FLUID PRODUCTION, FLOW AND ABSORPTION (5-13)

CSF is produced primarily by the choroid plexus. Extraventricular sites of CSF production include parenchymal extracellular space with transependymal passage to the ventricle and along nerve roots. Its approximately 0.35 ml per minute secretion rate results in the production of about 500 ml of CSF within a day. The ventricular volume ranges from 15 to 25 ml and subarachnoid space compartment holds roughly 120 ml; thus, CSF turnover is at least three to four times its daily production. Increased hydrostatic pressure within the hydrocephalic ventricles reduces CSF secretion only slightly.

The CSF circulation is unidirectional from the ventricles to the subarachnoid spaces and is believed to be propelled by pulsation of the choroid plexus transmitted to ventricular CSF (endoventricular CSF pulse pressure). Some CSF travels along the spinal subarachnoid spaces; some is thought to be absorbed along spinal absorptive pathways located along the nerve roots; the remainder ascends to join the main stream as it passes to the cerebral convexities to reach the superior sagittal sinus. The passage of CSF from the arachnoid villi to the superior sagittal sinus is governed by a passive, pressure-dependent mechanism; for normal CSF absorption, the venous pressure must be lower than the CSF pressure. Thus, raised venous pressure (e.g., in cases of superior sagittal sinus thrombosis and superior vena cava occlusion) can impair CSF absorption. The result is a backup of CSF in the subarachnoid spaces and the ventricles, which creates extraventricular obstructive hydrocephalus or communicating hydrocephalus, also known as FUNCTIONAL HYDROCEPHALUS (Fig. 3). This is further exemplified by achondroplasia wherein stenotic jugular foramina impair flow through the jugular veins, producing communicating hydrocephalus (Fig. 4).

In obstructive conditions, besides transependymal extravasation of CSF into adjoining extracellular spaces, other sites take part in CSF absorption. These sites include leptomeninges, choroid plexus and absorptive pathways along cranial and spinal nerves.

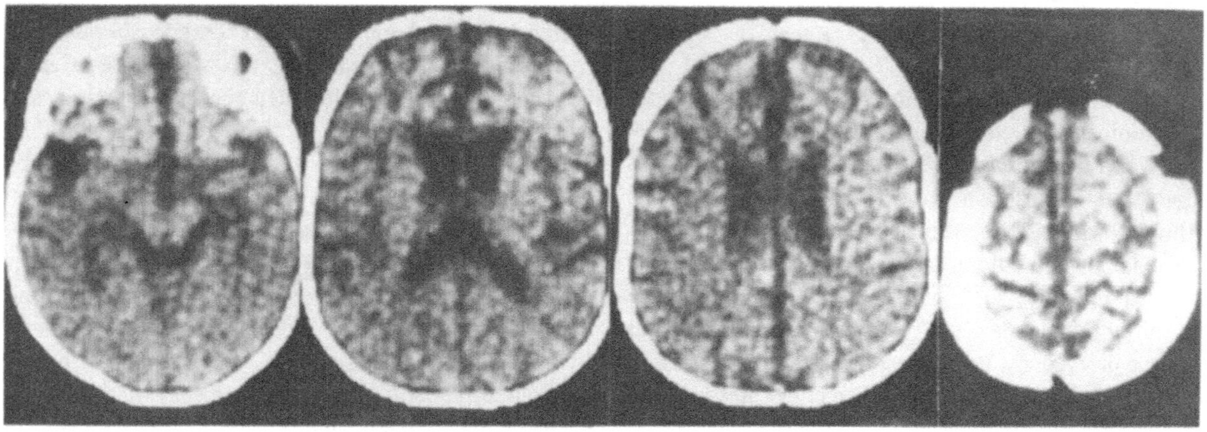

Figure 1. Benign external hydrocephalus in a 6-month-old child with an enlarged head. Note generalized enlargement of the non-ventricular subarachnoid spaces and cisterns. There is mild ventricular dilation as well.

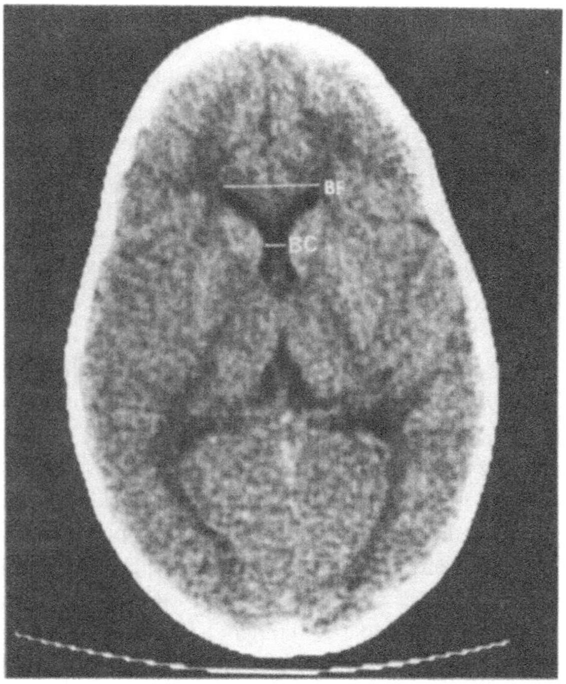

Figure 2. Normal CT scan slice at lateral ventricular level. One-year-old child. Bifrontal (BF) ratio is measured by measuring the span of the frontal horns divided by brain width at the same level. Bicaudate (BC) ratio is determined by measuring the span between the lateral ventricles where the caudate nuclei indent them divided by brain width at the same level. Bifrontal and bicaudate ratios greater than 40 percent and 20 percent, respectively, may be considered abnormal.

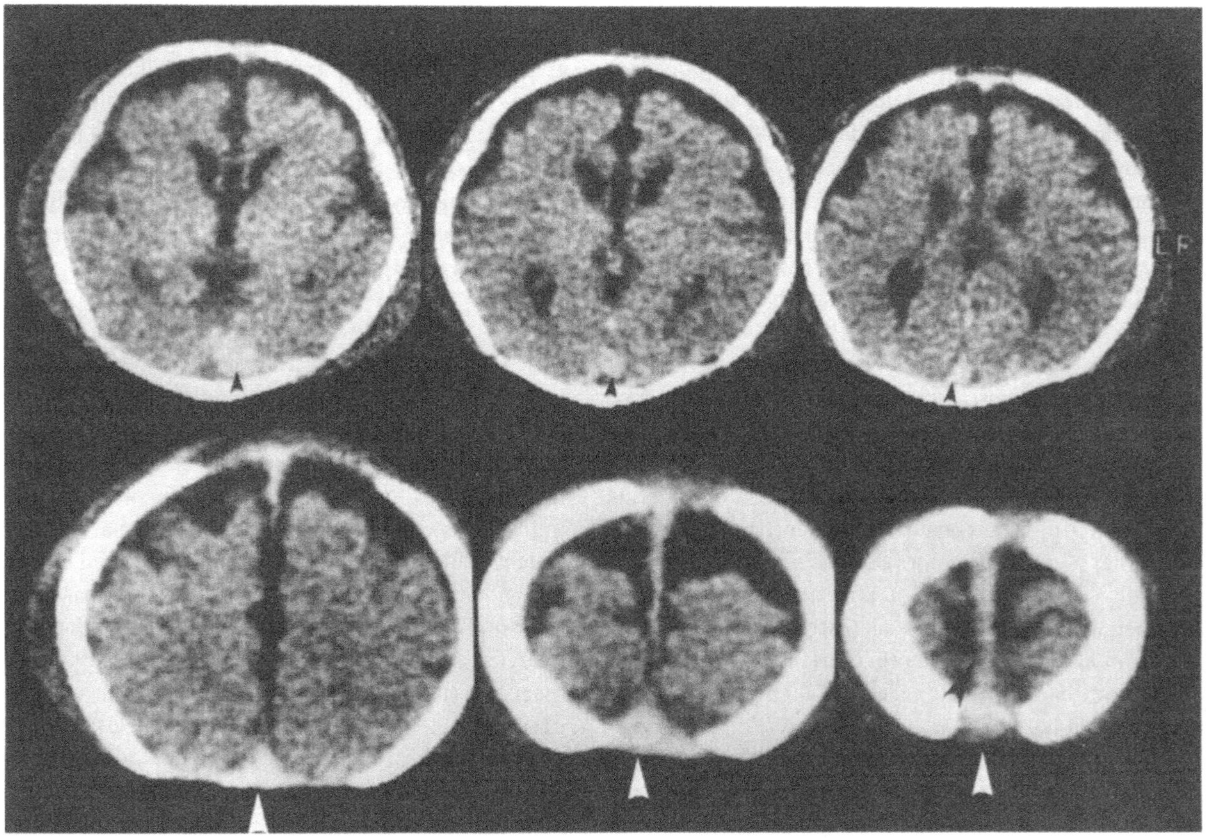

Figure 3. External hydrocephalus in a newborn. Note considerable enlargement of the subarachnoid spaces over the brain surface. There is slight ventriculomegaly as well. This newborn had superior vena occlusion and intracranial sinus thrombosis manifested by increased density in their expected locations (**arrowheads**).

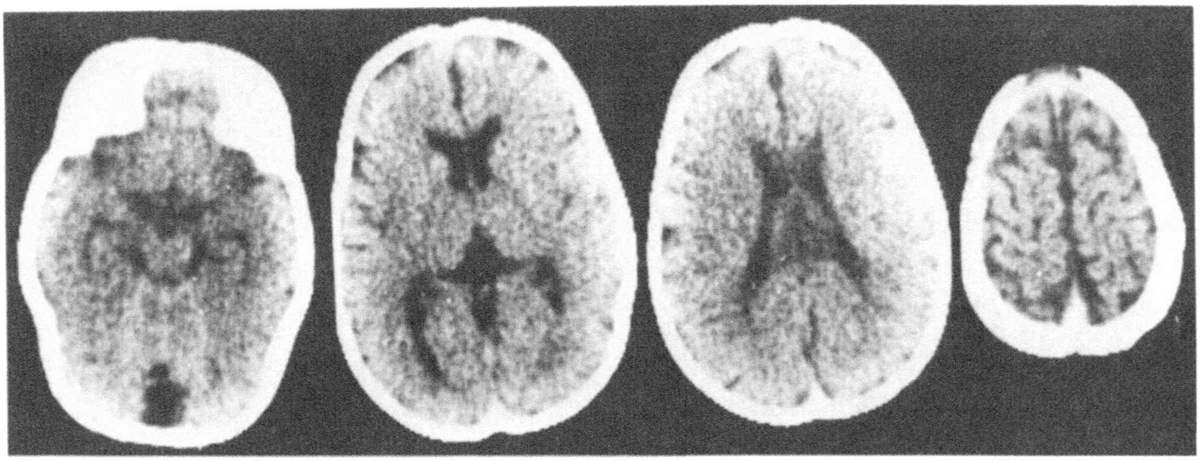

Figure 4. A 2-month-old child with achondroplasia and head circumference measurement of more than 95th percentile. Note prominent subarachnoid spaces. The lateral ventricles are only minimally enlarged. It is possible that megalencephaly (large brain) may partly account for large head seen in these patients.

FACTORS INFLUENCING MORPHOLOGY OF HYDROCEPHALUS

Normal ventricular asymmetry (14) (the left lateral ventricle usually is larger) partially accounts for the asymmetric hydrocephalus. However, any process that impedes or lowers the endoventricular CSF pulse pressure will result in less enlargement of that ventricle. For example, the shunted lateral ventricle is invariably smaller than its counterpart, since part of the CSF pulse pressure is absorbed by the shunt tubing and, therefore, not available for ventricular distention (15) (Fig. 5).

Frontal horns normally are smaller than the atria and occipital horns. This partly accounts for almost constantly observed disproportionate enlargement of the atria and the occipital horns in hydrocephalus. Applying LaPlace's law (force = pressure x area) and considering that the hydrostatic pressure in the ventricular system is the same, it readily becomes obvious that a greater force is available for distension of atria and occipital horns. Further, it has been suggested that basal ganglia along the frontal horns offer more resistance to ventricular expansion than the white matter adjoining the atria and the occipital horns.

In considering the hydrocephalic ventricular morphology, it is essential to understand the interplay of various forces, including brain elastance and resistance offered by dura mater and calvarium. While calvarium is molded by and responds to change in volume of its contents (brain and CSF), it does possess an inherent resistance to stretching or expansion. That part of the ventricular system near which the calvarial resistance is least, is more likely to distend the most. This, again, accounts for greater enlargement of atria and occipital horns, since the skull gapes more widely at the vertex than at the base or frontally in hydrocephalus (16,17). In addition, the ventricle adjoining an area of durectomy and/or craniectomy dilates the most. This same principle explains why one may see massive ventriculomegaly in children in whom the skull is thin and sutures separable as opposed to in adults in whom the bone is thicker and the sutures closed.

NEURAL TISSUE CHANGES IN HYDROCEPHALUS (18-23)

The parenchymal changes in hydrocephalus are borne principally by white matter. In acute to subacute hydrocephalus, the insult sustained by white matter is reflected in the production of white matter edema, which usually is most pronounced near the frontal horns. Ventricular distension also causes separation, or even rupture, of the ventricular ependymal lining leading to extravasation of CSF into the adjoining extracellular spaces. Transependymal CSF absorption, through intact ependyma that occurs in hydrocephalus, has been demonstrated, as well. All of these pathologic changes are seen as periventricular lucency on CT scan and are most noticable anteriorly (Fig. 6). Most are reversible after shunting, although the return to normal of these changes lags behind clinical improvement. If ventricular shunting is delayed or the white matter damage has been severe prior to shunt therapy, the periventricular lucency

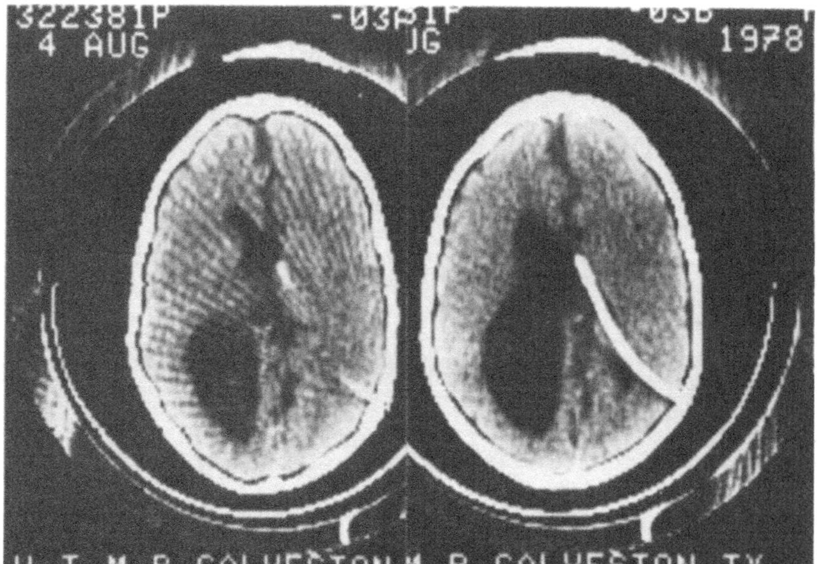

Figure 5. Smallness of the lateral ventricle containing the shunt. This child had Arnold-Chiari Type malformation.

can become areas of gliosis and cavitation. White matter lucency, therefore, constitutes an indication for shunt therapy. As stated, this periventricular lucency occurs in acute to subacute clinical states; examples include meningitis and the presence of posterior fossa neoplasm in children.

In contrast to acute or subacute hydrocephalus, periventricular lucency is minimal or absent in chronic hydrocephalus. When present, it usually is generalized and not confined to the neighborhood of the frontal horns. Aqueductal stenosis is a typical example (Fig. 7).

Occasionally, the CSF can escape through the ependymal lining and infiltrate the brain substance along the track of a malfunctioning shunt (Fig. 8). This CSF edema subsides following successful shunt revision (24).

Unmitigated hydrocephalus occasionally causes so much attenuation of the ependymal lining (Fig. 9) and overlying cortical mantle (Fig. 10) that a ventricular diverticulum may form at area/s of developmental weakness (25) (Figs. 11,12). These areas include the inferomedial atrial wall and the anterior and posterior walls of the third ventricle. If the overlying pia mater gives in, the diverticulum may communicate freely with the subarachnoid space.

Massive ventriculomegaly cannot displace the falx and the tentorium once they have acquired their normal fixation on the calvarium at 12 weeks of gestation (26,27). Their eccentric placement or abnormal location indicates that hydrocephalus has occurred before that period (Fig. 13). For example, higher placement of the torcular in Dandy-Walker syndrome indicates that it occurred before 12 weeks of gestation.

VENTRICULAR, CALVARIAL AND BRAIN MORPHOLOGY FOLLOWING SHUNTING (28-33)

In the pediatric age group, especially up to 2 to 3 years of age when the brain is rapidly attaining its maturity, the calvarium follows closely the changes in volume of its contents. As the ventricular size becomes smaller following shunting, the pliable calvarium collapses to fill in the space created. However, this reduction in volume of the calvarial cavity is not sufficient. The subarachnoid spaces and the brain substance themselves have to partake as well. This participation is manifested by passive enlargement of the subarachnoid spaces and of the cortical mantle. Part of the subarachnoid space growth is due to compressive atrophy of the brain (Fig. 7). The thickening of the cortical mantle is due partly to reexpansion of the previously compressed extracellular space and partly to rearrangement and thickening of the axonal fibers, which had been markedly stretched and compressed. This cortical thickening is preempted if the white matter has suffered irreversible damage. The CSF accumulation on the brain surface may be focal. Subsequent brain growth will obliterate these prominent subarachnoid spaces.

If the ventricular decompression is relatively rapid, the bridging cortical veins can rupture to produce subdural hematoma. Fortunately, this does not happen frequently. The extracerebral hematoma, usually small and self limiting, occurs relatively more frequently in adults in whom the rigid skull does not collapse.

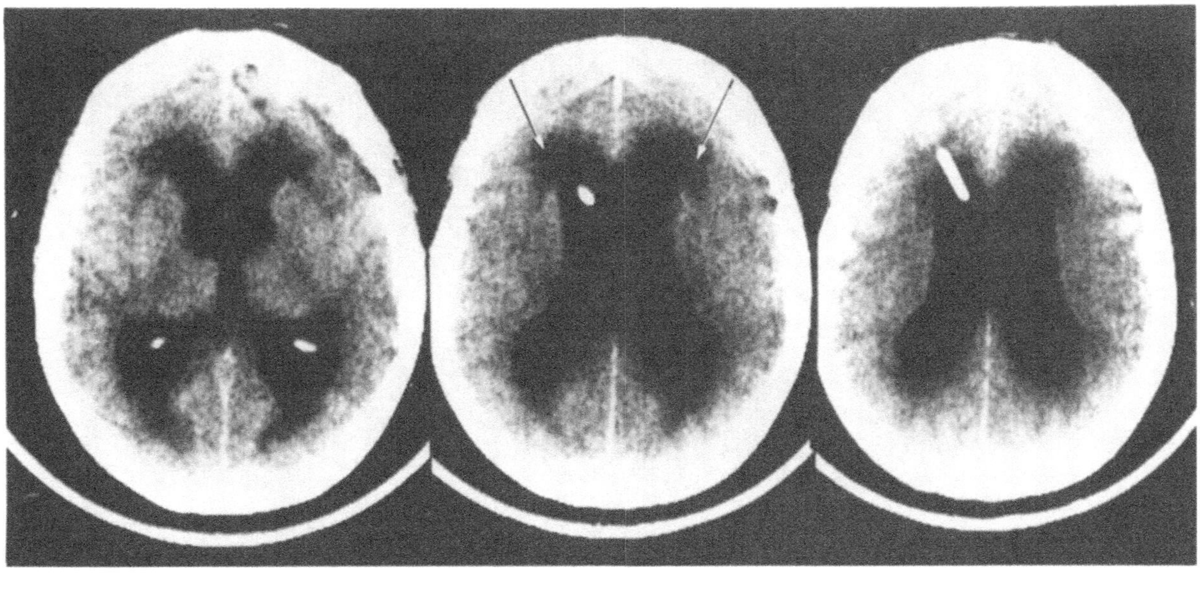

Figure 6. Periventricular lucency (**arrows**) of acute hydrocephalus in a 57-year-old woman with tentorial meningioma.

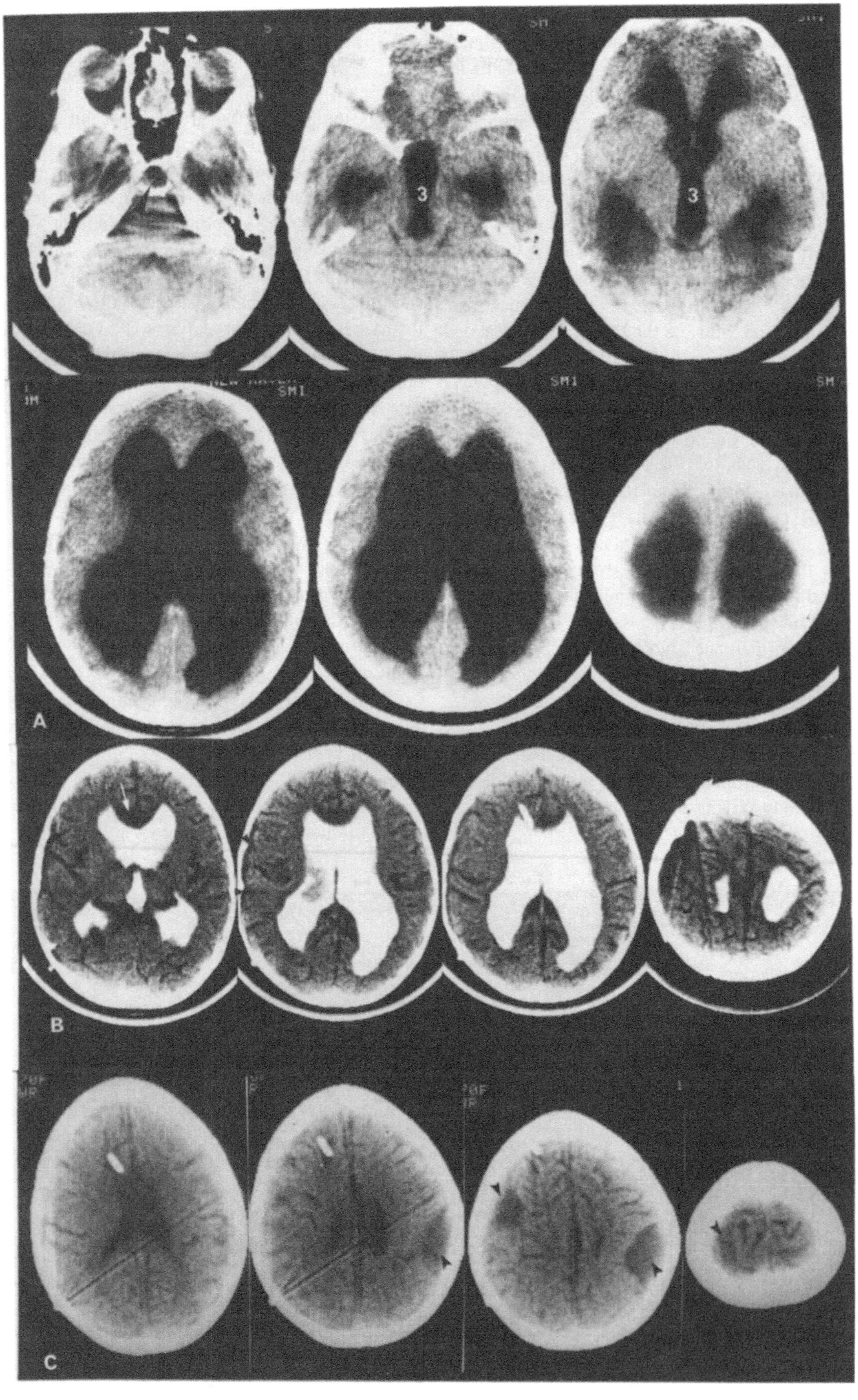
3
3
A
B
C

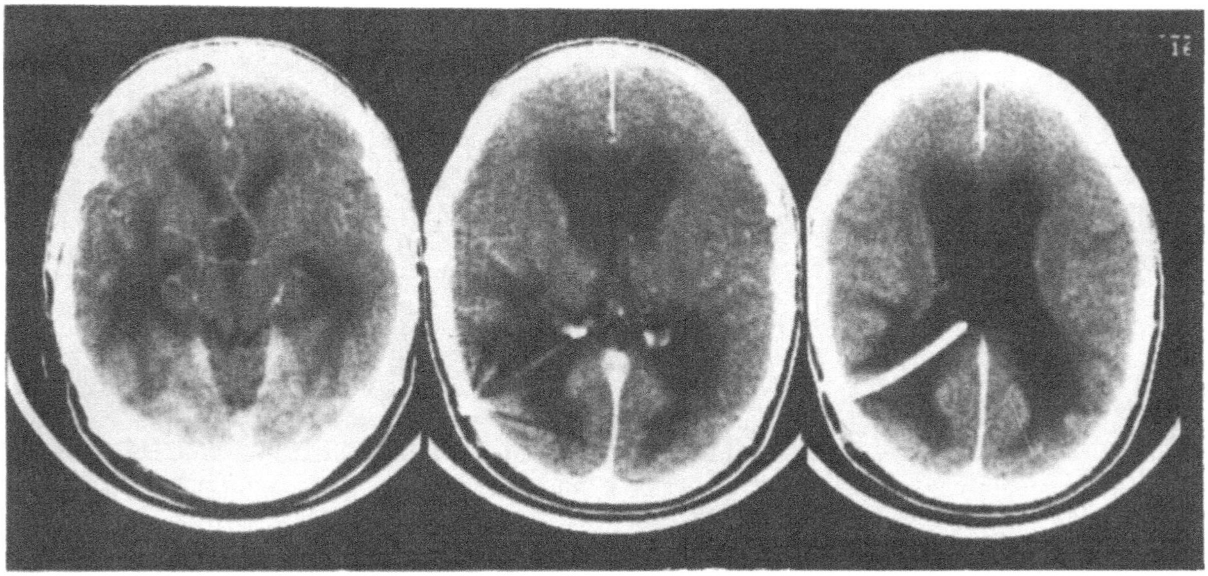

Figure 8. CSF edema in a 50-year-old man with possible aqueductal stenosis. CSF edema (hypodensity) is seen along the path of the ventricular shunt. Also note mild generalized periventricular lucency.

←

Figure 7. Chronic hydrocephalus due to aqueductal stenosis in a 10-year-old child.
A. CT scan obtained on October 14, 1982. There is massive ventriculomegaly with minimal to no periventricular lucency. Markedly distended third ventricle (3) resides in an enlarged sella turcia (**arrowhead**).
B. CT scan obtained on October 27, 1982, after ventricular shunting. Concomitant with reduction in size of lateral ventricles, there is enlargement of the subarachnoid spaces. Peripheral lucency (**arrowheads**) should not be confused with chronic subdural hematoma. Hypodensity of corpus callosum (**arrow**) denotes compression dysmorphology.
C. CT scan obtained in January 1983 shows pools of CSF (**arrowheads**) due to retraction of the brain parenchyma. These should not be misinterpreted as loculated chronic subdural hematomas.

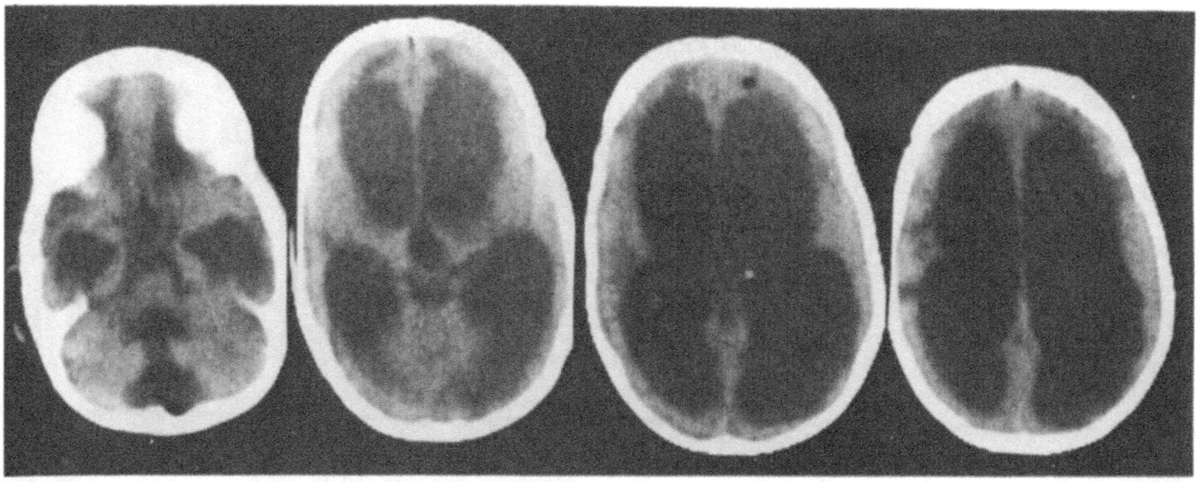

Figure 9. Extraventricular obstructive (communicating) hydrocephalus in a child. The ventricular system, as well as the cisterna magna, is enlarged. Small areas of lucency along the lateral ventricular walls very likely represent focal ependymal rupture with extravasation of CSF.

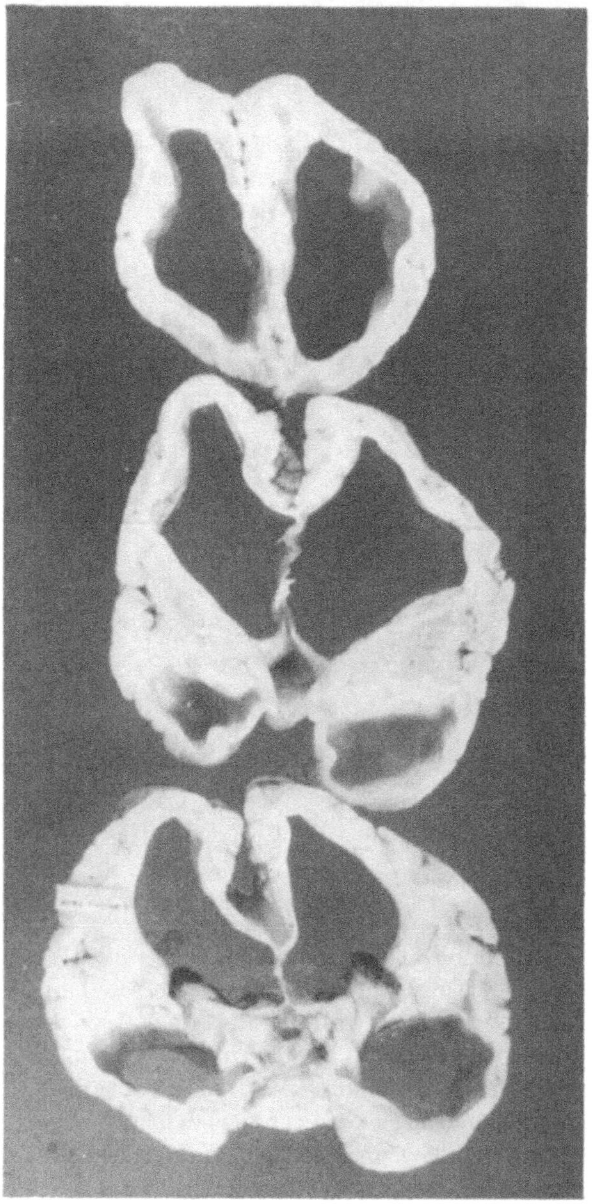

Figure 10. Pathologic specimen of hydrocephalus. Note thinned cortical mantle.

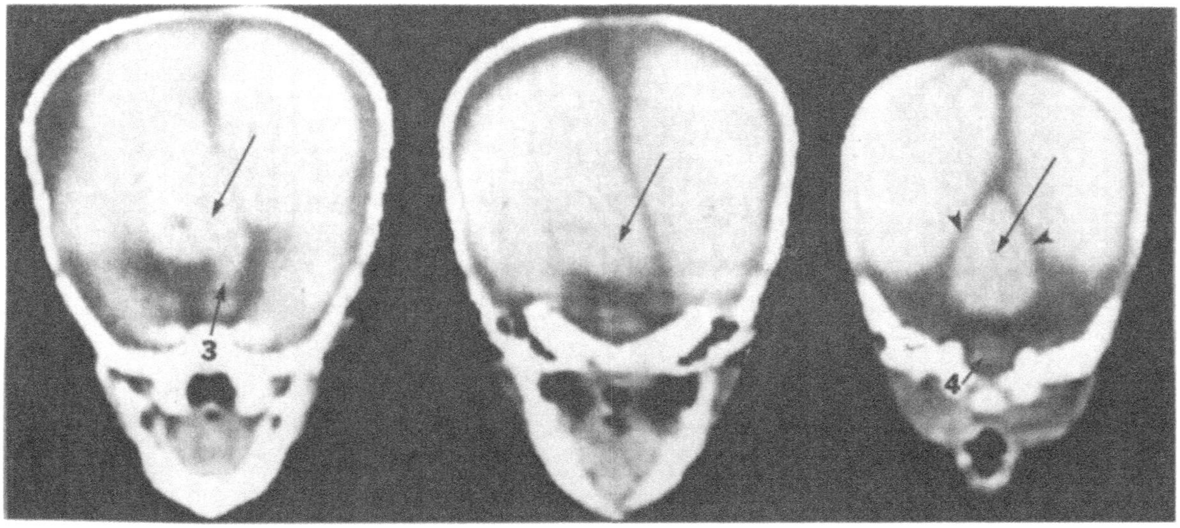

Figure 11. Atrial diverticulum (**arrowhead**) in hydrocephalus.

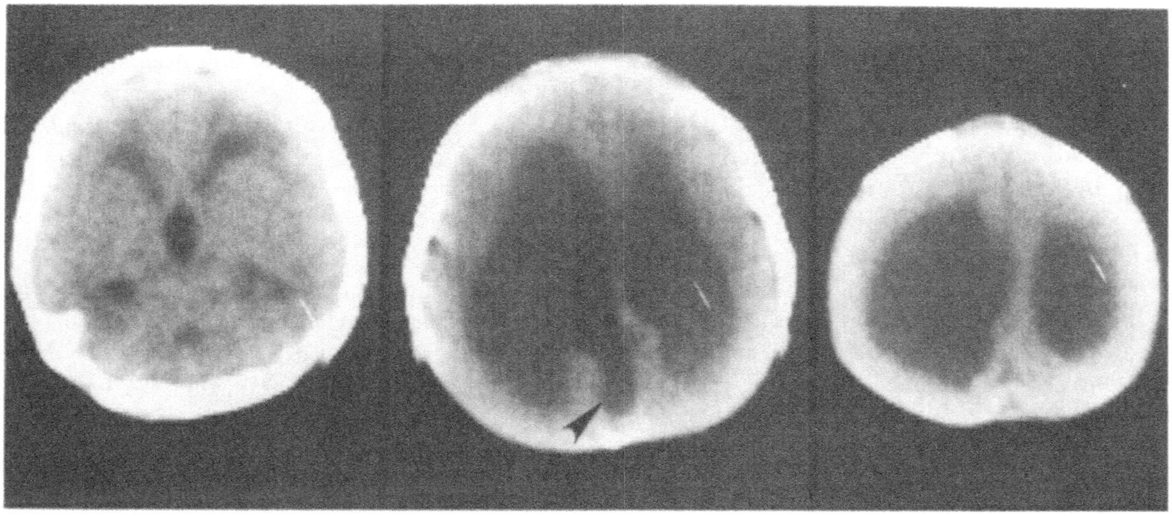

Figure 12. Atrial diverticulum in an infant with congenital hydrocephalus. Coronal CT scans after introducing metrizamide into the lateral ventricle. The diverticulum (**arrows**) extends from the supratentorial to the infratentorial compartment. The third ventricle (3) is shifted contralaterally, and fourth ventricle (4) displaced downward. **Arrowheads** = tentorial leaves. [From (25) with permission.]

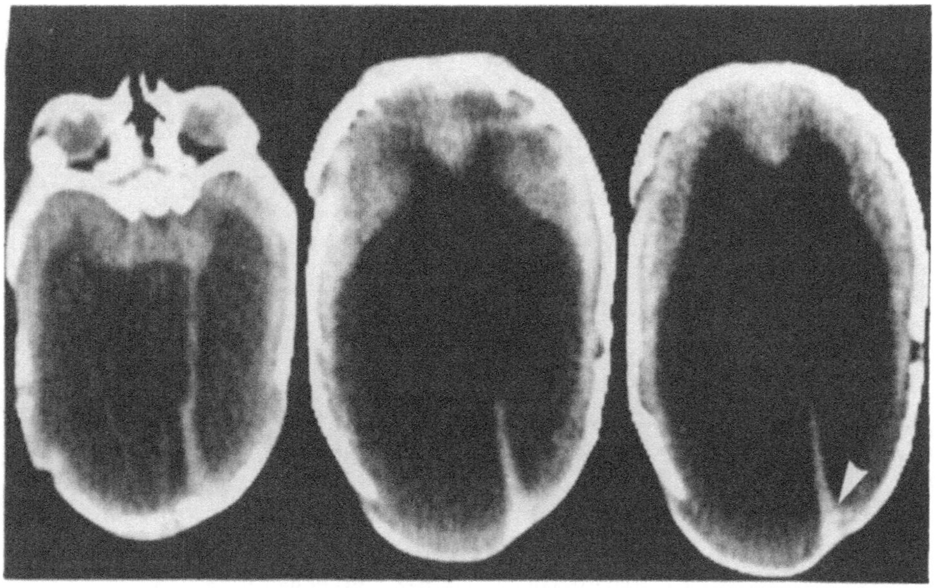

Figure 13. Massive ventriculomegaly with eccentric placement of falx indicating that hydrocephalus occurred before 12 weeks of gestation. There is disproportionate enlargement of atria and occipital horns.

If the calvarium caves in too much following size reduction of the ventricles, overriding of the bones at the sutures and even premature fusion can occur. The latter happens most frequently at the sagittal suture, accounting for scaphocephaly seen frequently in such chidlren. If the brain subsequently does not grow or grows poorly, the calvarium becomes thicker than normal due to lack of stimulus for reexpansion from the underlying brain.

If infection has complicated the shunting procedure, areas of porencephaly and cystic leuko- or encephalomalacia may be seen. Hemorrhage along the shunt tubing or in the ventricles also may occur. Parenchymal hemorrhage can develop into areas of porencephaly on resorption of the clot. Ventriculitis/ependymitis may cause irregularity of the ventricular contours. Obstruction at the aqueduct and occlusion of the outlet foramina of the fourth ventricle may isolate or entrap the fourth ventricle (see Chapter 6), which can attain a considerable size and require separate shunting to alleviate signs of posterior fossa compression.

A peculiar, poorly understood ventricular state is called SLIT-LIKE VENTRICLES. Such ventricles remain very small, even while the ventricular shunt is malfunctioning and the child is symptomatic of intracranial hypertension. This disorder probably is associated with the inability of the ventricular walls to expand; subependymal fibrosis has been suggested as one explanation. Increased brain compliance and enhanced resistance to ventricular distension from dura and calvarium may be additional contributing factors.

Etiology

1. Congenital malformations:
   a. Stenosis or maldevelopment of aqueduct
   b. Dandy-Walker malformation
   c. Posterior fossa extra-axial cyst
   d. Arnold Chiari malformation
   e. Destructive lesions:
      1) Hydrencephaly
      2) Porencephaly
2. Inflammatory lesions:
   a. Meningoencephalitis

Prenatal:	Bacterial:	Syphilis
	Viral:	CID, Rubella
	Parasitic:	Toxoplasmosis
Postnatal:	Bacterial:	Neonatal meningitis
		H. Inf. meningitis
		Tuber. meningitis
	Viral:	Mumps
	Fungal:	Torulosis
	Parasitic:	Cysticercosis

3. Expanding intracranial mass lesions:
   a. Neoplastic: (In childhood, 75% intra-axial)
      1/3 supratentorial:
         Choroid plexus papilloma
         Craniopharyngioma
         Teratoma
         Optic nerve glioma
      2/3 infratentorial:
         Cerebellar astrocytoma
         Medulloblastoma
         Ependymoma
         Brain stem glioma
   b. Vascular:
      Subdural hematoma
      Vein of Galen "aneurysm."
   c. Inflammatory:
      Abscess
      Granuloma
4. Intracranial bleeding:
   a. Birth wt. 2500 grams or more:
      Subarachnoid hemorrhage, usually traumatic
   b. Birth wt. 1600 grams or less:
      Germinal matrix hemorrhage
   c. Infancy:
      A-V malformation
      Aneurysm, usually cortical
   d. Older children:
      Aneurysm
5. Trauma and its complications

FUNCTIONAL (NEUROLOGIC) IMPAIRMENT IN HYDROCEPHALUS (34-37)

Neurologic impairment results from associated malformations and hydrocephalus per se. Hydrocephalus causes stretching of the overlying cerebral mantle resulting in axonal attenuation and defective myelination. Such adverse effects are most pronounced at areas of maximal ventricular distension, i.e., vertex and occipital region. This results in visual impairment, which is further aggravated by abnormality of gaze due to tectal plate compression. Fine motor control is impaired due to disturbed kinesthetic-proprioceptive basis of hand control, as well as bimanual motor function due to stretching of the corpus callosum fibers. All of these factors combine to cause low nonverbal intelligence.

Cortical mantle thickness (defined as the shortest distance between the frontal horn and the inner table of the skull) of at least 28 mm results in normal intelligence quotient (IQ). Cortical mantle thickness of 10 mm or less may be expected to cause severe IQ deficit. The presence of myelodysplaisa causes a poorer prognosis. Shunting before 6 months of age carries a far better prognosis. Also, the faster the ventricular size diminishes after shunting, the better the neurologic recovery and prognosis. Multiple shunt revisions and associated complications, mainly infection, adversely affect the neurologic function.

REFERENCES

1. Ment LR, Duncan CC, Geehr R: Benign enlargement of the subarachnoid spaces in the infant. *J Neurosurg, 54:*504-508, 1981.
2. Volpe JJ, Pasternak JF, Allan WC: Ventricular dilation preceding rapid head growth following neonatal intracranial hemorrhage. *Am J Dis Child, 131:*1212-1215, 1977.
3. Pedersen H, Gyldensted M, Gyldensted C: Measurement of the normal ventricular system and supratentorial subarachnoid space in children with computed tomography. *Neuroradiology, 17:*231-237, 1979.
4. Hahn FJY, Rim K: Frontal ventricular dimensions on normal computed tomography. *AJR, 126:* 593-596, 1976.
5. Cutler RWP, Page L, Galicich J, *et al.*: Formation and absorption of cerebrospinal fluid in man. *Brain, 91:*707-720, 1968.
6. Milhorat TH: The third circulation revisited. *J Neurosurg, 42:*628-645, 1975.
7. Rubin RC, Henderson ES, Ommaya AK, *et al.*: The production of cerebrospinal fluid in man and its modification by acetazolamide. *J Neurosurg, 25:* 430-436, 1966.
8. Fishman RA: *Cerebrospinal Fluid in Diseases of the Nervous System.* W.B. Saunders, Philadelphia, 1980.
9. Stewart DR, Johnson, DG, Myers GG: Hydrocephalus as a complication of jugular catheterization during total parenteral nutrition. *J Pediat Surg, 10:*771-777, 1975.
10. Di Rocco C, Di Trapani G, Pettorossi VE, *et al.*: On the pathology of experimental hydrocephalus induced by artificial increase in endoventricular CSF pulse pressure. *Childs Brain, 5:*81-95, 1979.
11. Drapkin AJ, Sahar A: Experimental hydrocephalus: Cerebrospinal fluid dynamics and ventricular distensibility during early stages. *Childs Brain, 4:* 278-288, 1978.
12. Rosman NP, Shands KN: Hydrocephalus caused by increased intracranial venous pressure: A clinicopathological study. *Ann Neurol, 3:*445-450, 1978.

13. Bering EA, Salbi B: Production of hydrocephalus by increased cephalic-venous pressure. *J Neurol & Psychiat, 81:*693, 1959.
14. LeMay M: Morphological cerebral asymmetrics of modern man, fossil man, and nonhuman primate *Annals New York Acad Sciences, 280:*349-366. 1976.
15. Linder M, Diehl JT, Sklar FH: Significance of post shunt ventricular asymmetries. *J Neurosurg, 55:* 183-186, 1981.
16. Hochwald GM, Epstein F, Malhan C, *et al.*: The role of the skull and dura in experimental feline hydrocephalus. *Dev Med Child Neurol,* [Suppl] *27:*65-69, 1972.
17. Naidich TP, Epstein F, Lin JP, *et al.*: Evaluation of pediatric hydrocephalus by computed tomography. *Radiology, 119:*337-345, 1976.
18. Pasquini U, Bronzini M, Gozzoli E, *et al.*: Periventricular hypodensity in hydrocephalus: a clinico-radiological and mathematical analysis using computed tomography. *J Comput Assist Tomogr, 1:*443-448, 1977.
19. Hiratsuka H, Fujiwara K, Okada K, *et al.*: Modification of periventricular hypodensity in hydrocephalus with ventricular reflux in metrizamide CT cisternography. *J Comput Assist Tomogr, 3:* 204-208, 1979.
20. Di Chiro G, Arimitsu T, Brooks RA, *et al.*: Computed tomography profiles of periventricular hypodensity in hydrocephalus and leukoencephalopathy. *Radiology, 130:*661-666, 1979.
21. Moseley IF, Radu EW: Factors influencing the development of periventricular lucencies in patients with raised intracranial pressure. *Neuroradiology, 17:*65-69, 1979.
22. Hopkins LN, Kakay L, Kinkel WR, *et al.*: Demonstration of transventricular CSF absorption by computerized tomography. *Acta Neurochir, 39:* 151-157, 1977.
23. Naidich TP, Schott LH, Baron RL: Computed tomography in evaluation of hydrocephalus. *Rad Cl N Amer, 20:*143-167, 1982.
24. Chiba, Y, Takagi H, Nakajima F, *et al.*: Cerebrospinal fluid edema: a rare complication of shunt operation for hydrocephalus. Report of three cases. *J Neurosurg, 57:*697-700, 1982.
25. Naidich, TP, McLone DG, Hahn YS, Hanaway J: Atrial diverticula in severe hydrocephalus. *AJNR, 3:*257-266, 1982.
26. Nixon GW, Ravin CE: Malposition of the attached portion of the falx cerebri and the superior sagittal sinus: an indicator of severe cerebral maldevelopment. *AJR, 122:* 44-51, 1974.
27. Wolpert SM: Dural sinus configuration: measure of congenital disease. *Radiology, 92:*1511-1516, 1969.
28. Shellinger D, McCullough DC, Pederson RT: Computed tomography in the hycrocephalic patient after shunting. *Radiology, 137:*693-704, 1980.
29. Rubin RC, Hochwald G, Liwnicz B: The effect of severe hydrocephalus on size and number of brain cells. *Dev Med Child Neurol, 14*[Suppl 27] :117-120, 1972.
30. Rubin RC, Hochwald G, Tiell M, *et al.*: Reconstitution of the cerebral cortical mantle in shunt-corrected hydrocephalus. *Dev Med Child Neurol,* [Suppl 35] :151-156, 1975.
31. Rubin RC, Hochwald GM, Tiell M, *et al.*: Hydrocephalus: I. Histological and ultrastructural changes in the pre-shunted cortical mantle. *Surg Neurol, 5:*109-114, 1976.
32. Rubin RC, Hochwald GM, Tiell M, *et al.*: Hydrocephalus: II. Cell number and size, and myelin content of the pre-shunted cortical mantle. *Surg Neurol, 5:*115-118, 1976.
33. Rubin RC, Hochwald GM, Tiell M, *et al.*: Hydrocephalus: III. Reconstitution of the cerebral cortical mantle following ventricular shunting. *Surg Neurol, 5:*179-183, 1976.
34. Raimondi AJ, Soare P: Intellectual development in shunted hydrocephalic children. *Am J Dis Child, 127:*664-671, 1974.
35. Lorber J: The results of early treatment of extreme hydrocephalus. *Dev Med Child Neurol, 16:*21-29, 1968.
36. Young HF, Nulsen FE, Weiss MH, Thomas P: The relationship of intelligence to cerebral mantle in treated infantile hydrocephalus. *Pediatrics, 52:* 38-54, 1973.
37. Dennis M, Fitz CR, Netley CT, *et al.*: The intelligence of hydrocephalic children. *Arch Neurol, 38:*607-615, 1981.

8

Neurocutaneous Syndromes (Phakomatoses)

This group of inherited disorders is characterized primarily by skin and central nervous system (CNS) lesions. They are also known as phakomatoses, in reference to the associated skin lesions, a relationship that is explained by the common origin of ectoderm and neuroectoderm. Visceral lesions (mesodermal dysplasia) also may be present. These disorders are autosomally dominant and show a great propensity to develop neoplasia.

The following is a list of important types of phakomatoses:

1. Neurofibromatosis (von Recklinghausen disease)
2. Sturge-Dimitri-Weber syndrome (encephalofacial angiomatosis)
3. Tuberous Sclerosis (Bourneville disease)
4. Von-Hippel-Lindau disease
5. Ataxia-telangiectasia (Louis-Bar syndrome)
6. Miscellaneous

NEUROFIBROMATOSIS (von Recklinghausen disease: VRD)

General Considerations

This hereditary and progressive disorder of unknown etiology results from dysplasia of neuroectodermal and mesodermal tissue. The disease was named after von Recklinghausen (1882), but he credited Tilesius (1793) with the first description of the cutaneous fibromata. Its frequency is about 1 in 3,000. It is transmitted by an autosomal dominant gene with about 50 percent mutation. Since the histologic pattern of lesions in this disease varies considerably, controversy exists with regard to the cell or cells of origin.

The classic clinical presentation consists of cutaneous cafe au lait spots, multiple soft cutaneous tumors and neurofibromata of the peripheral nerves. According to Crowe *et al.* (1956) the presence of six or more cafe au lait spots, each exceeding 1.5 cm at its broadest diameter, probably indicates neurofibromatosis. Almost any organ can harbor a neoplasm because of the great tendency for tumor development in this disorder.

Central Nervous System Lesions

The major lesions of neurofibromatosis pertaining to CNS are as follows:

- Optic glioma
- Bilateral acoustic schwannomas
- Intraventricular (particularly in the temporal horn) meningioma or multiple meningiomas
- Meningiomatosis
- Tumors (gliomas) at other parts of the brain, especially in the hypothalamus
- Pulsatile proptosis due to herniation of the temporal lobe into the globe through dysplastic sphenoid wing
- Lamboid defect (more commonly on the left side) is virtually pathognomonic of this disease. Other skull defects (e.g., parietal foramina) also may be present
- Hypertrophy of skull (Maki *et al.*, 1981)
- Bilateral enlargement of the internal auditory canals whether due to schwannoma (very commonly) or dural ectasia (rarely)
- Arterial stenosis or occlusion (Hilal *et al.*, 1971)
- Basal ganglia calcification
- Aqueduct stenosis (very rare) (Till, 1971)
- Ventriculomegaly

CT Scan Findings

The CT scan findings reflect the expected CNS lesions. Of the neoplasms, optic gliomas and bilateral acoustic schwannomas are the most common (Fig. 1). **Optic glioma** manifests as a fusiform enlargement of the optic nerve(s). Posterior extension of the neoplasm(s) into the optic chiasm and along the optic tracts also can be evaluated (Fig. 2). Whereas contrast enhancement of the intraorbital part of the tumor may be difficult to appreciate, that of the chiasmal and optic tract component of the lesion usually is profound. With thin-cuts and high resolution CT scanning, enlargement of the optic canals can be readily appreciated. In every case of optic glioma, evidence of neurofibromatosis must be sought diligently (association: approximately 20-50%).

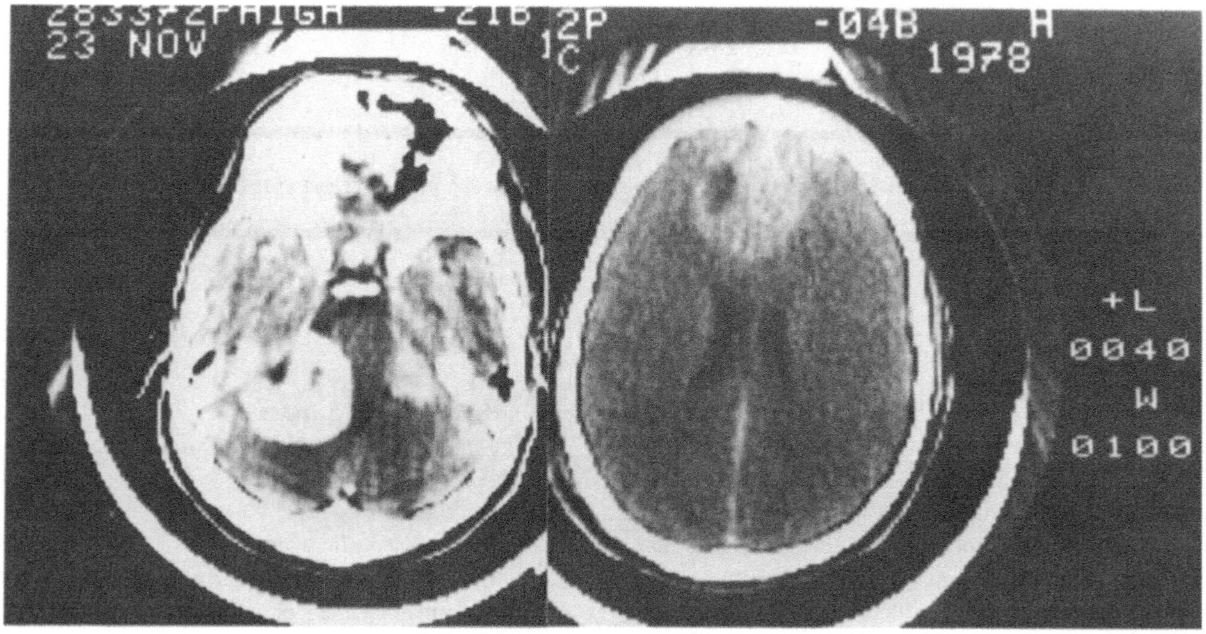

Figure 1. A 22-year-old mentally retarded male with neurofibromatosis. He has bilateral acoustic schwannomas, far larger on the right side. He also has a partly cystic frontal falx meningioma. Contrast CT scans.

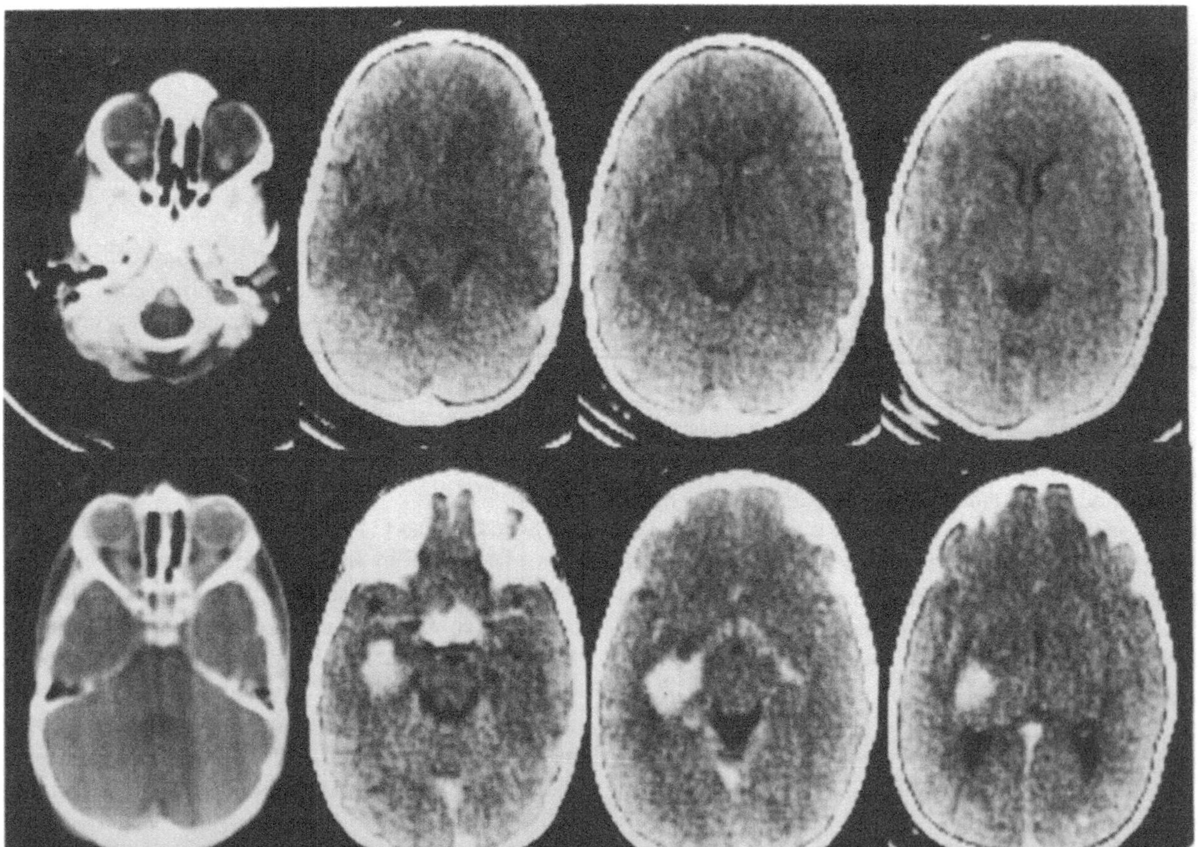

Figure 2. Bilateral optic gliomas with intracranial extension along the optic pathways. A) non-contrast and B) contrast CT scan. Note that the intracranial portion of the neoplasm is not recognizable in the non-contrast CT scan.

This 2-year-old boy presented with seizures and impaired vision. At least one cafe au lait spot was seen on the skin. (From Morristown Memorial Hospital, NJ.)

In children under 7 years of age, **enlargement of the internal auditory canal** very likely is explained by dural ectasia rather than acoustic schwannoma; the latter has not been reported under this age to my knowledge. In older patients, the internal auditory canal enlargement overwhelmingly results from the presence of acoustic schwannoma. While only about ten percent of patients with VRD have acoustic schwannomas, the presence of bilateral acoustic schwannomas usually is pathognomonic of VRD. Not only can the enlargement of internal auditory canals (IAC) be visualized on the CT scan, these contrast enhancing schwannomas are easily identifiable on the contrast CT scan.

The **temporal horn calcification** occurring alone (Modic *et al.*, 1980) or in association with meningioma, also is characteristic of VRD. Meningiomas usually are isodense to slightly hyperdense lesions with or without associated calcification. All of them show profuse and homogeneous contrast enhancement, unless there is an associated cystic component, which occurs in about one to three percent of cases.

Meningomatosis also is a rather typical lesion of VRD. It is composed of abundant proliferation of blood vessels and collagenous tissue. Such proliferation can assume the appearance of "meningioma en plaque" in the involved part of the cerebral tissue. Calcification and irregular streaky densities may appear on the contrast CT scan (Kasantikul and Brown, 1981); angiogram may show small clusters of abnormal vessels.

Sphenoid wing dysplasia (a manifestation of sphenoid bone dysplasia and consequent herniation of the temporal lobe into the orbit) resulting in pulsatile exophthalmos, is another characteristic feature of VRD (Fig. 3). The involved orbit and superior orbital fissure become enlarged. On coronal CT sections, dysplasia of the body of the sphenoid bone results in excessive tilt of the sella turcica floor.

Major arterial stenosis and/or occlusion at the skull base, a relatively rare manifestation of VRD, will result in typical CT findings of cerebral infarction. Angiographically occult arterial lesions causing multiple small infarcts might account for a relatively high incidence of non-obstructive ventriculomegaly seen in this disorder (Patronas *et al.*, 1982). Unilateral ventriculomegaly may be related to unilateral megalencephaly. Bilateral megalencephaly can cause macrocrania (Holt and Kuhns, 1976).

The calvarial defects are best studied by viewing the images at bone settings.

STURGE-DIMITRI-WEBER SYNDROME

History

The classic description of this entity was provided in 1879 by Sturge. His epileptic and hemiparetic patient had facial nevus and buphthalmos (congenital galucoma), as well. The first published description of gyriform calcification was written by Dimitri in 1923, although Wissing had shown a typical radiograph in 1921 at a Copenhagen meeting. In 1929, Weber published a radiograph showing cortical calcification. Krabbe (1932, 1934) correctly pointed out that the radiographically visible calcifications were intracortical and not calcification of the anomalous pial vessels (angiomatosis).

Clinical Characteristics

The following are the major clinical characteristics of this syndrome:

Cutaneous vascular (capillary) nevus which affects the face, particularly its upper part, is almost invariably present.

Seizure disorder in almost every case beginning in early life.

Homonymous hemianopia and mental retardation of various degrees is present in most of the cases.

Hemiplegia

Buphthalmos

It now is generally agreed that intracranial calcifications must be concurrently present with facial nevus, which must at least involve the first division of the trigeminal nerve (upper face), before this syndrome can be diagnosed.

Pathologic Considerations

The essential pathologic features of this disorder include facial cutaneous nevus and the leptomeningeal angiomatosis, which consists of a network of pial venules aggregated on the brain surface. This collection of venules may be so dense and large in certain areas that it completely conceals the underlying brain. The syndrome is invariably unilateral and predominantly affects the occipital lobe, although the adjoining temporal and parietal lobes and sometimes the entire cerebral hemisphere also may be involved. The cerebellum is rarely affected. The involved cerebral lobe(s) is atrophied to various degrees.

The thin-walled abnormal vessels usually are not larger than 140 microns. They may form single or multiple (four to five deep) layers at the crown of the gyri, with greatest concentration at the superficial and widest portion of the sulci. Rarely do these vessels penetrate the gray matter.

Calcifications

The nature and size of calcifications seen in this disorder must be understood. The calcifications involve the cortex (Fig. 4) and the arteries on the brain surface. (Calcifications are more pronounced in the deeper layers of the cortex.) The classic gyriform calcifications seen on the plain skull film are calcifications of the cortex itself, not of the vessels. While arterial calcification does exist, it appears almost exclusively on the brain surface and is unrelated to the gyri calcification. Only rarely, and to a mild extent, do the capillaries of the deeper cortex (layer 4, 5) show droplet calcifications.

The calcifications of the cortex (gyri) are believed a consequence of local oxygen deficiency due to poor functioning, stasis and/or thrombosis of the vessels partaking in angiomatosis and of adjoining cortical veins and superior sagittal sinus (Bentson *et al.*, 1971).

The gross appearance of the leptomeningeal angiomatosis suggests that it is persistence of Streeter's primordial plexus. This concept seems to be supported by the observation of slow and nondirectional blood flow at surgery.

The relationship of facial nevus and occipital lobe angiomatosis can be explained by reviewing some relevant facts of early embryogenesis. In the early period of development, the ectoderm, which is destined to form the skin of the upper part of the face, overlies that part of the neural tube that is ordained to form the occipital lobe and the adjacent cerebrum. Similarly, in the embryo, the vascular supply to the telencephalon, eye and overlying integuments is approximated. Subsequent posterior migration of the parieto-occipital lobe carries the cerebral part of the malformation backwards (Ronne, 1937).

CT Scan Findings

Calcification is the hallmark of CT scan findings. It is seen commonly in the occipital lobe, but can involve adjacent temporal and/or parietal lobes, or the entire cerebral hemisphere, as well (Figs. 5,6). Invariably, the calcification is unilateral. The classic gyriform pattern of calcification on skull films is not seen on the axial CT scan images. Instead, the calcification usually assumes a rather homogeneous character. Because of anoxic atrophy, there is enlargement of the ipsilateral lateral ventricle most pronounced close to the area of calcification; the adjacent sulci also are widened, and adjoining calvarium is thickened. All of these changes are secondary to shrinking volume of the cerebral tissue. On the contrast CT scan, some enhancement (which may be larger than the area of calcification) and prominent deep veins (e.g., basal vein of Resenthal) may be noted due to poor functioning, stasis and/or thrombosis of the vascular channels forming the angiomatosis and of adjoining cortical veins and/or superior sagittal sinus (Fig. 7). Part of the enhancement may be related to the leptomeningeal angiomatosis itself.

TUBEROUS SCLEROSIS
(Bourneville Disease)

Von Recklinghausen, in 1863, provided one of the earliest accounts of this disorder in an infant with multiple cardiac rhabdomyomas and cerebral sclerosis. However, it was Bourneville and his colleagues (between 1880 and 1900) who further elaborated on the disease and described the association of "tuberous sclerosis of cerebral convolutions" with idiocy. Vogt, in 1908, outlined the characteristic clinical triad of this syndrome, and in 1913 Berg reported on its hereditary nature. The blastomatous character of the disorder was elucidated by Bielschowsky in 1924, and in 1942 Moolten underlined its hamartomatous nature in view of the multiplicity of organs involved.

Clinical Presentation

The clinical triad consists of a cutaneous lesion ("adenoma sebaceum"), mental deficiency and seizures. These features become manifest between the ages of 2 and 6. "Adenoma sebaceum" probably is a misnomer, since hyperplasia of sebaceous glands is neither a prominent nor a constant feature of the cutaneous lesion, and present only occasionally or not at all. Its more common characteristics include the presence of connective and vascular tissue – the latter may be so abundant that the cutaneous lesion histologically resembles an angiofibroma. These angiofibromas occur in about 90% of cases and may be a more precise term than adenoma sebaceum. The cutaneous lesions may be present at birth, but they become more prominent and numerous with increasing age. Other types of cutaneous lesions seen in tuberous sclerosis are shagreen patches, cafe au lait spots, and angiomas.

The characteristic ophthalmologic lesion of tuberous sclerosis consists of the retinal "phakoma," which commonly occurs at the posterior pole of the globe. Histologically, these phakomas are composed of glial fibres with central hyaline material or calcifications. These retinal tumors usually do not interfere with vision. Other ophthalmologic lesions include retinal hemangioblastoma and choroidal angioma.

Tuberous sclerosis shows an irregular dominant inheritance mode. Its exact incidence is difficult to ascertain, but has been estimated at approximately 1 in 300,000 to 500,000 of the total population and at 0.1 - 0.5 percent of patients admitted to psychiatric institutions.

Pathologic Anatomy of the Brain

Characteristic lesions consist of: a) cortical tubers (for which the disease was named); b) aggregates of heterotopic cells in the white matter; and c) periventricular nodules (Fig. 8).

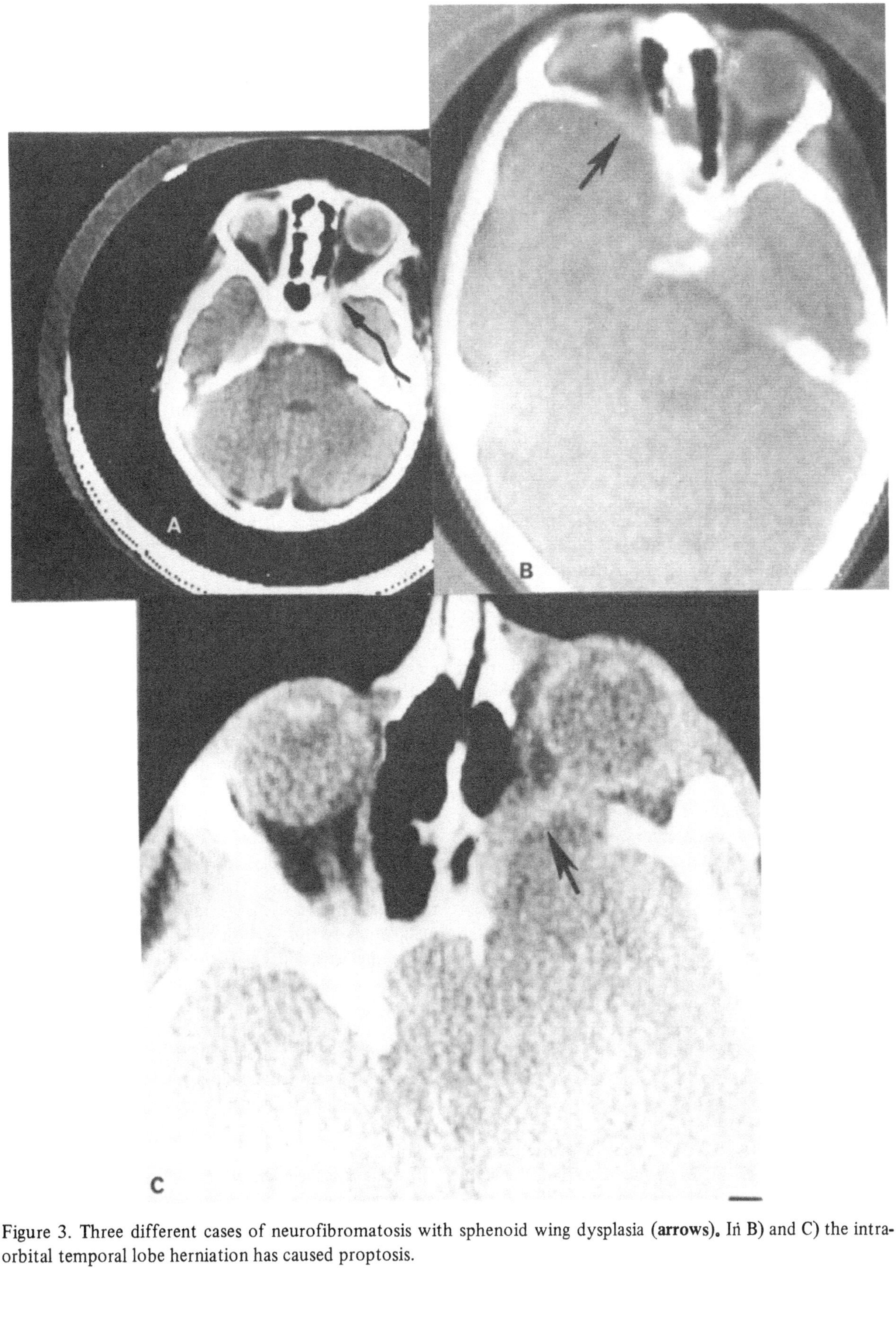

Figure 3. Three different cases of neurofibromatosis with sphenoid wing dysplasia (**arrows**). In B) and C) the intraorbital temporal lobe herniation has caused proptosis.

Figure 4. Histologic section of brain of a patient with Sturge-Weber syndrome. Note that the calcification (arrowheads at only a few calcifications) is in the cortex and not in the leptomeningeal angiomatosis. (Courtesy Dr. Schochet.)

The cortical tubers are composed primarily of fibrillary gliosis. They are rarely cystic and calcification is far less common than that in periventricular nodules.

The heterotopia of neurons is a manifestation of their impaired migration during embryogenesis. The heterotopic cells are mostly oriented in a radial pattern between the subependymal nodules and the cortical tubers. That is, these heterotopic neurons are arrested at points along the path of their normal migration.

Subependymal (periventricular) nodules usually are present and most often are discovered at the striatothalamic sulcus. Variable in size, they may become larger than a tangerine and can obstruct the interventricular foramen and cause hydrocephalus. These subependymal nodules have a strong tendency toward calcification which can progress with advancing age.

Infratentorial, mainly cerebellar, lesions are far less common than those that are supratentorial. Of the visceral type, hamartomatous lesions (mainly angiomyolipoma) of the kidney (seen in approximately 80% of cases) are of particular note.

The subependymal giant-celled astrocytoma at the interventricular foramen level also is a characteristic lesion in this disorder.

CT Scan Findings

The characteristic CT finding is periventricular calcified tubers (Fig. 9). These tubers are not visible on the skull films in the first 2 to 4 years of life, but they can be visualized at an earlier age on the CT scan because of its markedly enhanced sensivity. The 50 percent reported incidence of calcification on skull films can be expected to be higher on the CT scan. These calcified lesions are multiple in at least 75 percent of the patients and bilateral in 50 percent. The parenchymal tubers also may calcify (Fig. 10). The degree of tuberous calcification bears no direct relationship to the severity of mental retardation and epilepsy. The non-calcified parenchymal tubers are not recognizable as they are small and do not cause sufficient change in attenuation. However, parenchymal and periventricular tubers may become recognizable only on the contrast CT scan (Fig. 11). Such a situation does indicate the feasibility of routine contrast CT scan on all patients with seizure disorder. Somewhat larger tubers may be expected to betray themselves as hyperdense lesions. A parenchymal hypodense lesion conceivably may result from infarction, since arterial occlusive lesions may be encountered in tuberous sclerosis (Hilal, 1971). Occasionally, a mild but normal irregularity of the ventricular borders may be difficult to distinguish from lesions of tuberous sclerosis; clinical history and follow up CT scans will help resolve such a dilemma. It should be noted that periventricular calcification is not pathognomonic of tuberous sclerosis; it can be seen in various inflammatory lesions as well.

With more refinement in CT scanning, it may be possible to identify the retinal and choroidal lesions of this disease.

The concurrence of periventricular calcification and a neoplasm at the interventricular foramen level (subependymal giant-celled astrocytoma) is almost pathognomonic of this disease (Figs. 12,13). Calcified tubers do not show contrast enhancement, but the calcified periventricular and/or ventricular gliomas do.

The occasional finding of micrencephaly and/or cortical atrophy (large ventricles and sulci) may be a manifestation of generalized poor development of the brain. Rarely observed hypodense areas in the white matter may be focal areas of demyelination (Nova *et al.*, 1981 and Giarrick *et al.*, 1979), which are known pathologically to occur.

Intracranial calcifications before the appearance of cutaneous lesions have been described (Burkhart *et al.*, 1981 and Barry *et al.*, 1977). Prominent choroid plexus, hemangioma of choroid plexus and calcified branches of middle cerebral artery in infants have been reported (Welch *et al.*, 1980).

VON HIPPEL-LINDAU DISEASE

Among other authors, Von Hippel brought attention to retinal angiomatosis in 1904 and in 1911. However, it was Lindau who, in a 1926 monograph, provided a coherent description of this entity which has retinal, cerebral and visceral components, and is transmitted as an autosomal dominant trait. By definition, the disorder is characterized by cerebellar hemangioblastoma with one or more of the following associated anomalies:

- Retinal hemangioblastoma
- Spinal cord hemangioblastoma
- Pancreatic cysts
- Renal abnormalities (cyst, tumor)

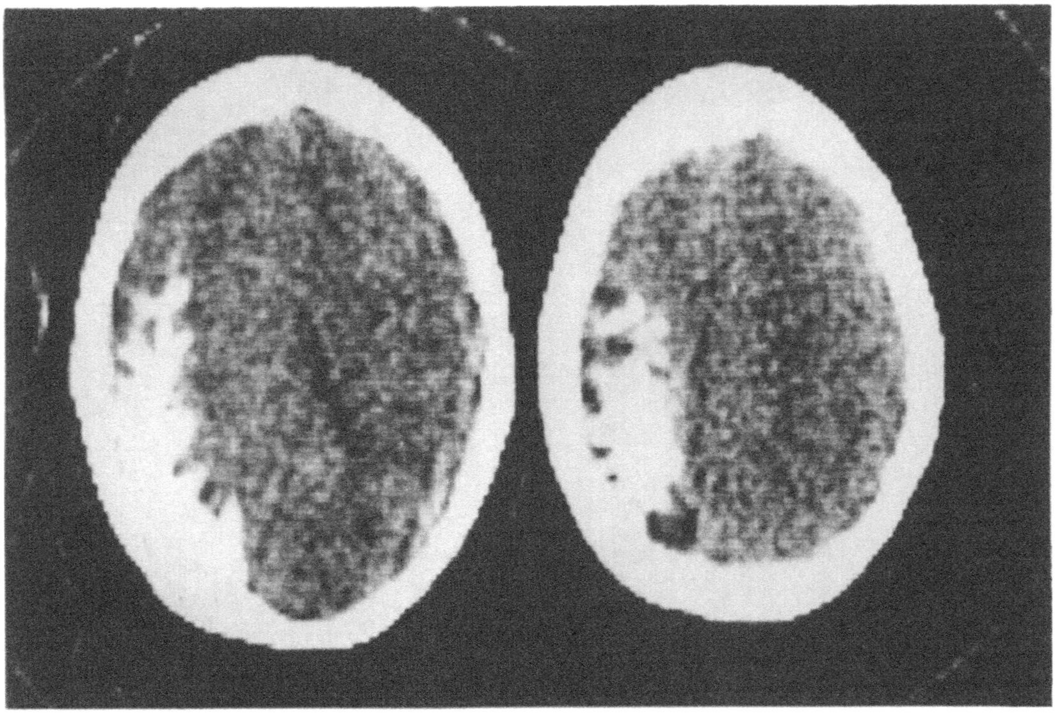

Figure 5. Sturge-Weber syndrome. Cerebral calcification in the parieto-occipital lobe. Note that the calcification extends from the brain surface deep into the cortex. The adjoining bone is slightly thickened and there is focal enlargement of the sulci, both findings indicating anoxic brain atrophy.

This 10-year-old child had facial nevus and seizures.

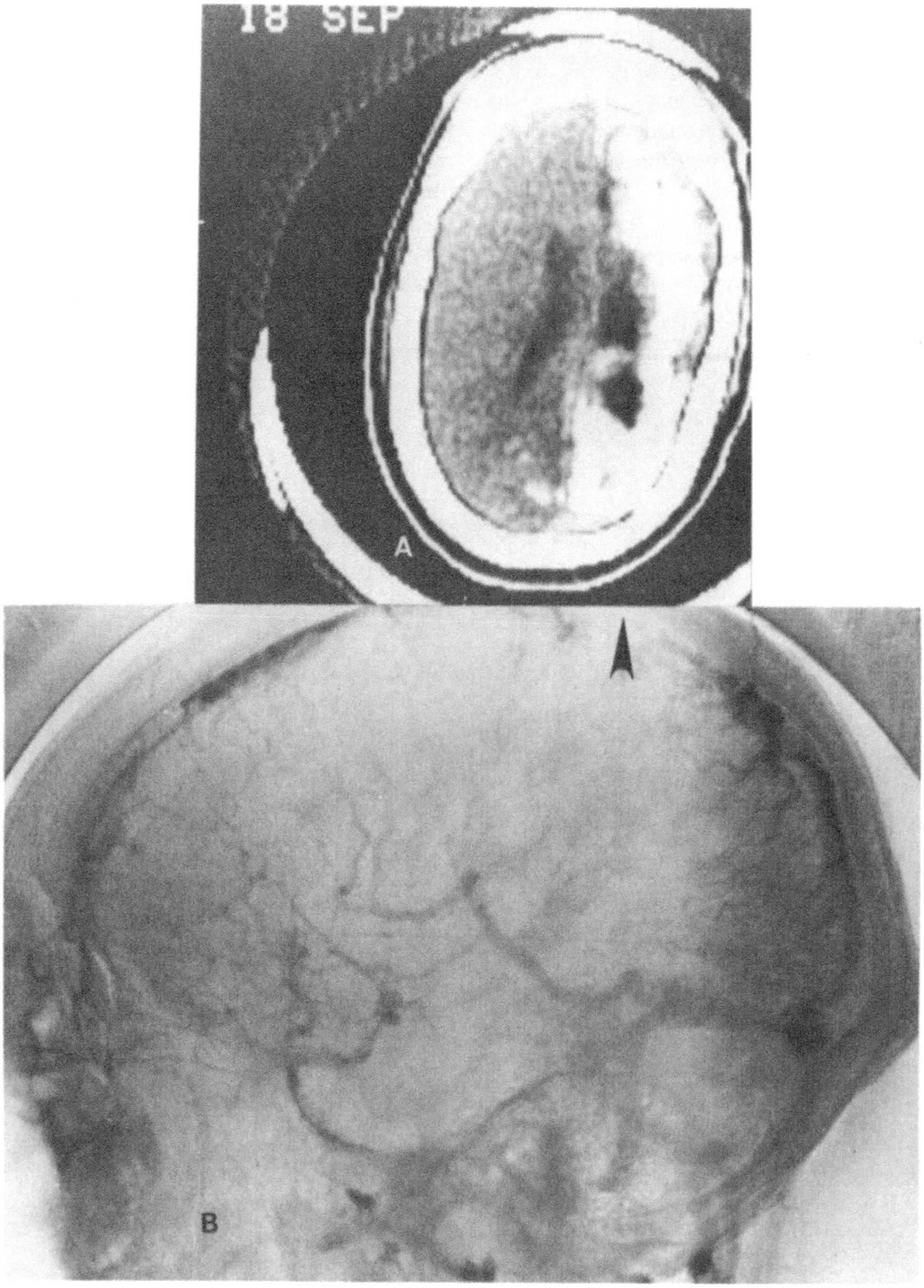

Figure 6. A 25-year-old male with Sturge-Weber syndrome.

A. CT scan. Note extensive calcification of the hypoplastic cerebral hemisphere. The ipsilateral lateral ventricle is slightly larger than its counterpart.

B. Venous phase of right carotid angiogram, lateral view. There is thrombosis of parietal portion of superior sagittal sinus (**arrowhead**) and of deep cerebral veins which are not opacified. Note prominent collateral veins.

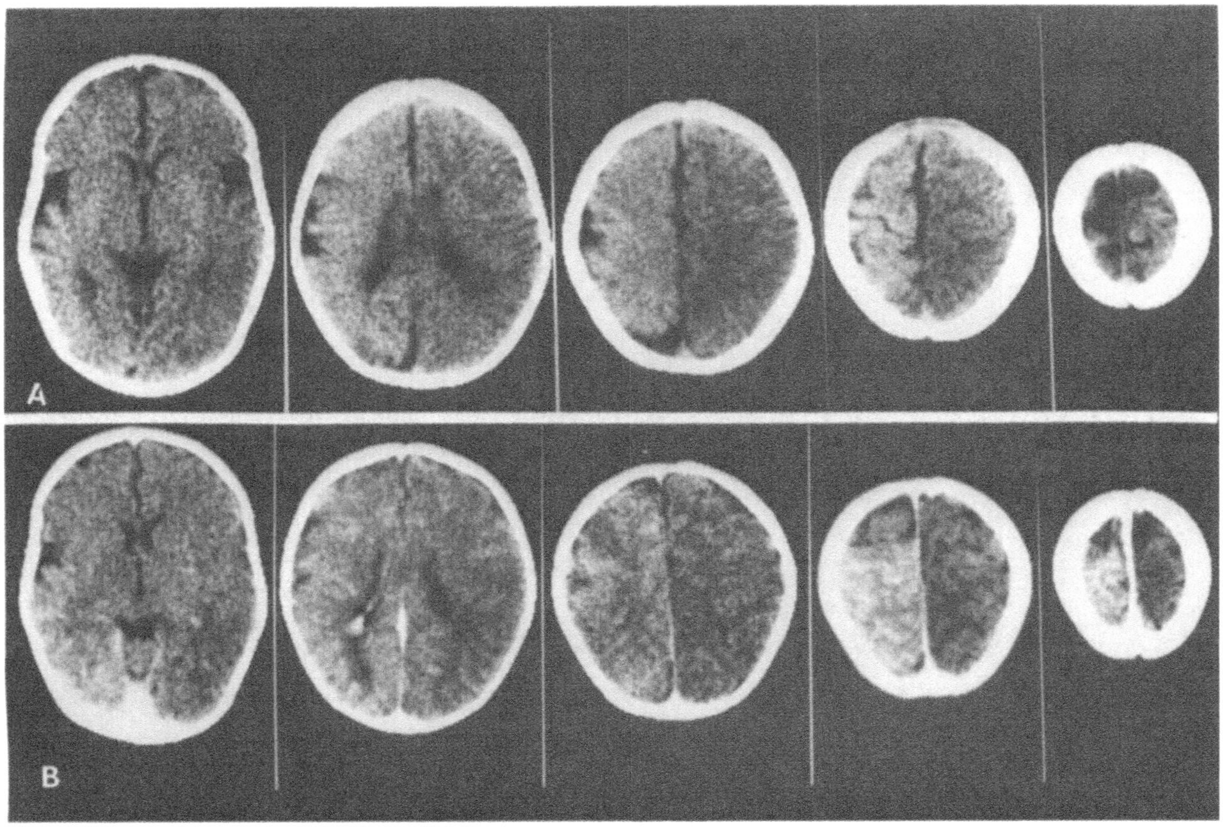

Figure 7. One-month-old with Sturge-Weber disease.
A. Non-contrast CT. There is increased density of the right cerebral hemisphere, mainly in the parieto-occipital lobe. This increased density is related partly to anoxic dystrophic calcification of gray-matter and possible partly to blood stasis in the leptomeningeal angiomatosis. The right cerebral hemisphere is slightly smaller than the left and the ipsilateral subarachnoid spaces are prominent compared with the other side.
B. Contrast CT. There is enhancement of the lesion that is most pronounced in the parieto-occipital lobe.

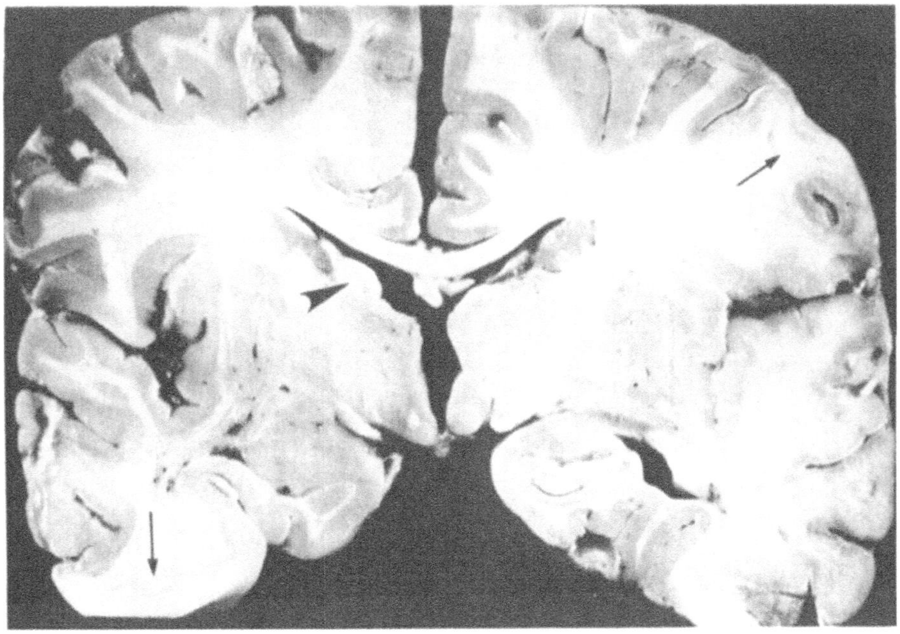

Figure 8. Pathologic specimen of a patient with tuberous sclerosis. Note periventricular tuber (**arrowhead**). Also observe loss of gray-white matter demarcation due to fibrillary gliosis (**arrows**). (Courtesy Dr. Schochet.)

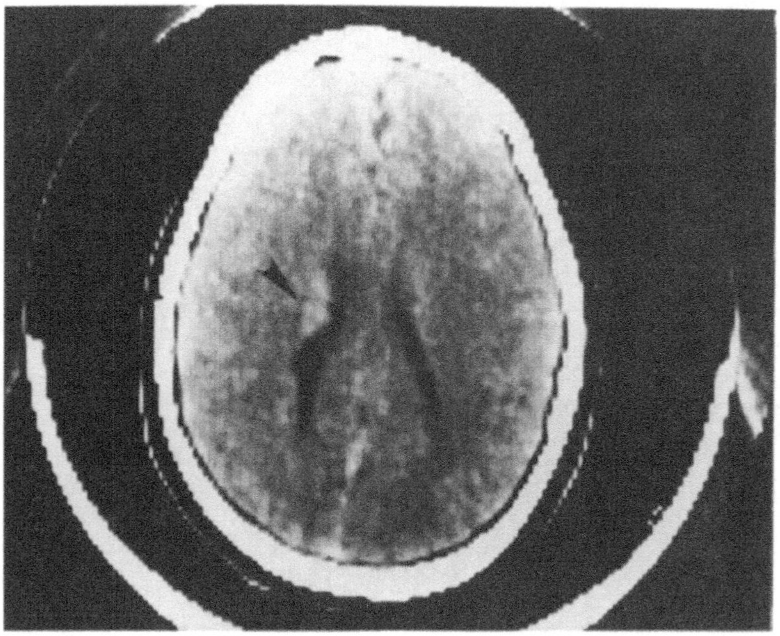

Figure 9. Tuberous sclerosis. A 10-year-old boy. Note a large lobulated periventricular lesion. Non-contrast CT scan.

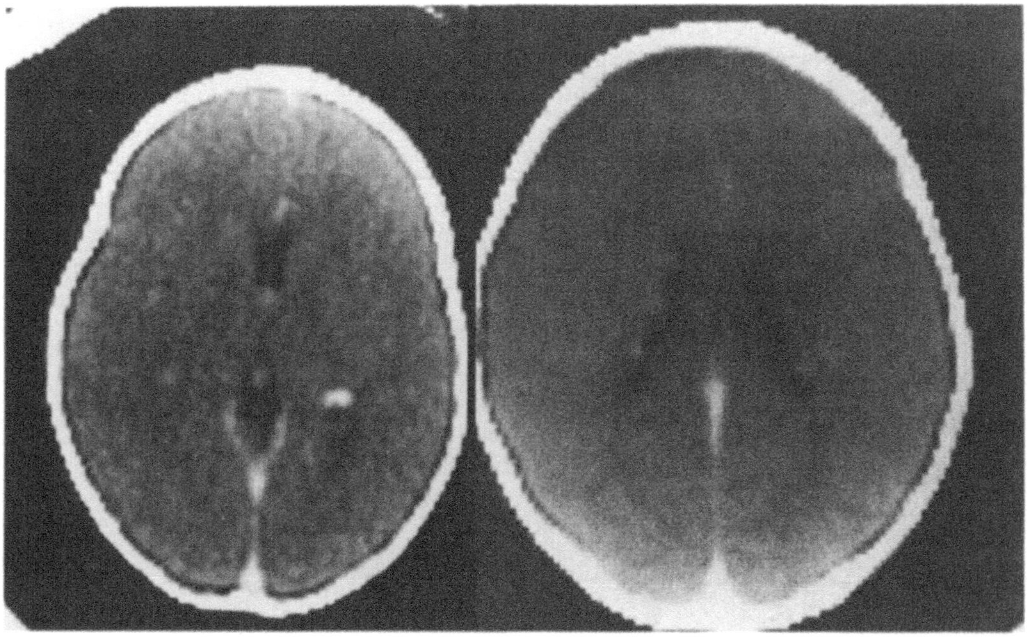

Figure 10. Tuberous sclerosis. 15-month-old child with seizures. There are both periventricular and parenchymal lesions, probably mildly calcified. Contrast CT scan; non-contrast CT scan was not done.

Since the cerebellar hemangioblastoma is commonly cystic with a variable sized mural nodule, the latter enhances profusely on the contrast CT (Fig. 14). Fourth ventricle and/or aqueductal compression cause hydrocephalus. At present, it is difficult to diagnose retinal hemangioblastoma with certainty on the CT scan.

ATAXIA-TELANGIECTASIA (Louis-Bar Syndrome)

The primary characteristics of this heredofamilial disorder include progressive cerebellar dysfunction (ataxia), progressive oculocutaneous telangiectasia and increased tendency to contract sinopulmonary infection because of an associated impaired immunocompetence (lymphoid hypoplasia). Neoplasia, particularly of the lymphoreticular system, tend to develop. In the absence of bronchopulmonary disease and lymphoreticular malignancy, the chance of survival increases considerably after the second decade of life. The main neuropathologic lesions are cerebellar cortical atrophy (Fig. 15), dentato-olivary degeneration and axonal swelling in the brain stem.

Transmitted as a simple autosomal recessive trait, ataxia-telangiectasia is a multisystem genetic disorder that predominantly affects children; males and females are equally affected. Nearly 500 cases have been described.

This syndrome should be considered particularly in young children when CT scan shows evidence of cerebellar degeneration – large fourth ventricle, large cerebellar cisterns and increased subarachnoid spaces around the cerebellum.

LINEAR NEVUS SEBACEOUS SYNDROME

Historical Background

In 1895, Jadassohn described lesions believed to be hamartomatous in nature, characterized by linear sebaceous nevus involving mainly the scalp and face. Schimmelpenning in 1957 (cited by Leonidas *et al.*) and Feuerstein and Mims in 1962 described a syndrome with sebaceous nevus of linear facial distribution associated with mental retardation and seizures – it is now considered a distinct neurocutaneous syndrome.

Definition and Characteristics

In addition to calvarial and CNS lesions, other skeletal system as well cardiac and renal malformations may occur. The most common radiographic findings include lesions of the skull and brain.

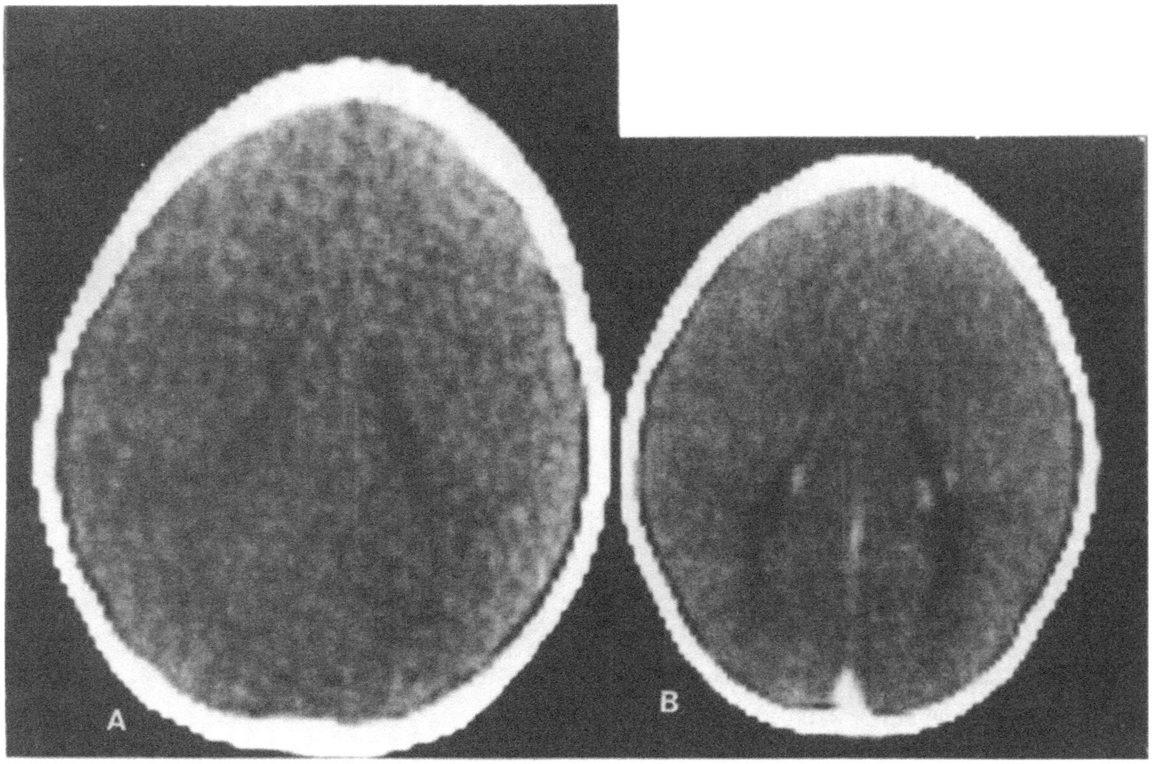

Figure 11. Tuberous sclerosis. 6-month-old infant. Note periventricular tubers becoming manifest only on the contrast CT scan. A) non-contrast and B) contrast CT scan.

Skull lesions include asymmetry which may or may not be associated with asymmetry of facial bones and orbits. Sellar and sphenoidal abnormalities have been reported. **CNS lesions** include cerebral atrophy or hemiatrohpy, hydrocephalus, porencephaly and intracranial hematomas. The spine anomalies include scoliosis.

NEUROCUTANEOUS MELANOSIS

This rare disorder is characterized by abnormal skin pigmentation and giant pigmented nevus. There is melanosis or melanoma only in the meninges and not in any other part of the body (Fig. 16).

It may be noted that on rare occasions overlap of cutaneous and cerebral lesions in these phakomatoses can occur. This is understandable in the light of recent embryologic work suggesting that these neurocutaneous syndromes represent a generalized dysplasia of neural crest cell origin in which one or more elements of skin and central nervous system may be differently affected (Sagar *et al.*, 1983). For example, it is possible to have typical CT scan or pathologic features of Sturge-Weber disease in the brain without concurrent typical facial stigmata or vice versa. A case of tuberous sclerosis with calcified white matter angiomatosis mimicking CT changes of Sturge-Weber disease has been reported (Maekawa *et al.*, 1979). Also, forme fruste in all types of phakomatoses can occur.

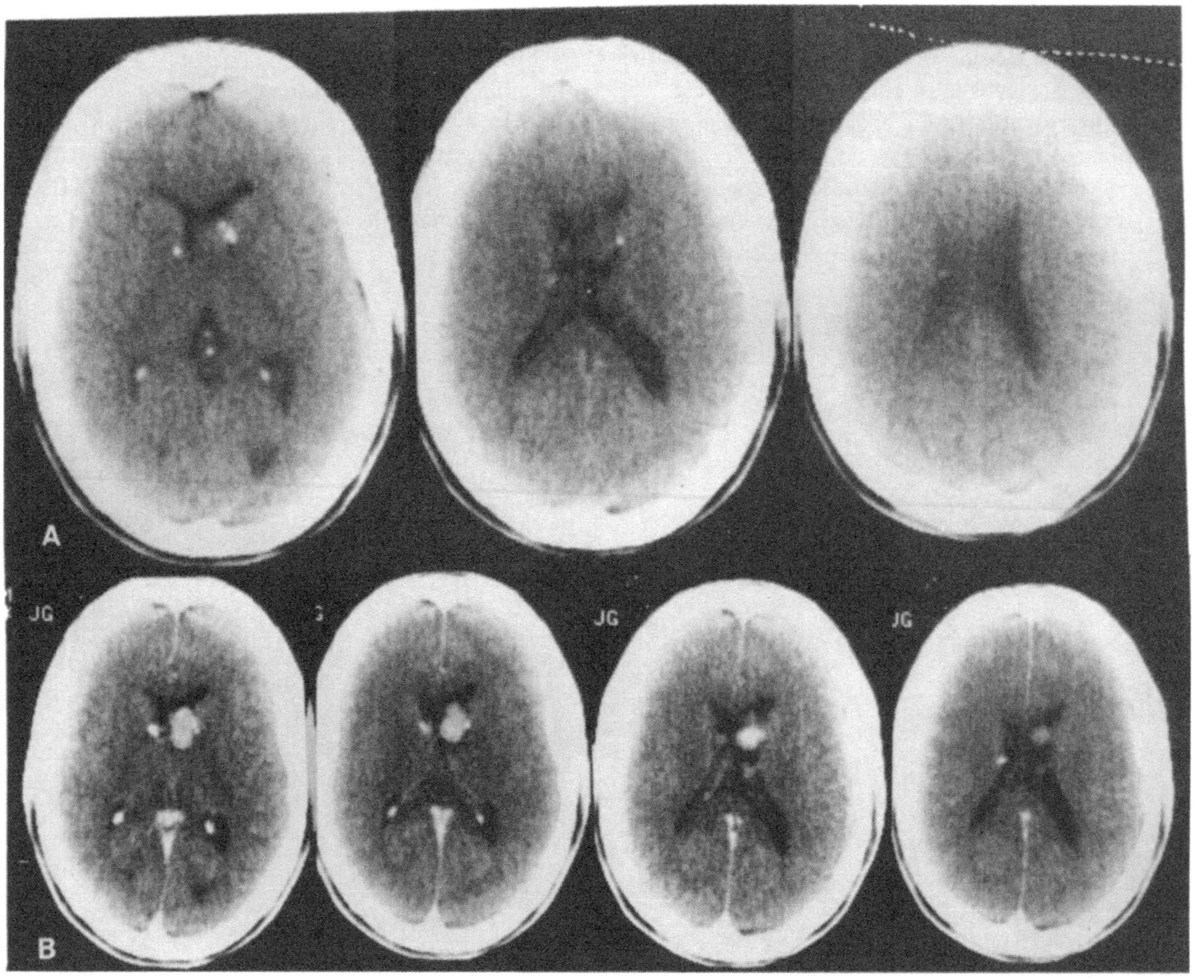

Figure 12. A 24-year-old man with tuberous sclerosis.

A. Non-contrast CT scan. Note small calcified periventricular tubers and calcified isodense (**arrowhead**) neoplasm near the interventricular foramen.

B.Contrast CT scan. Note enhancement of the neoplasm near the interventricular foramen. It was giant celled astrocytoma.

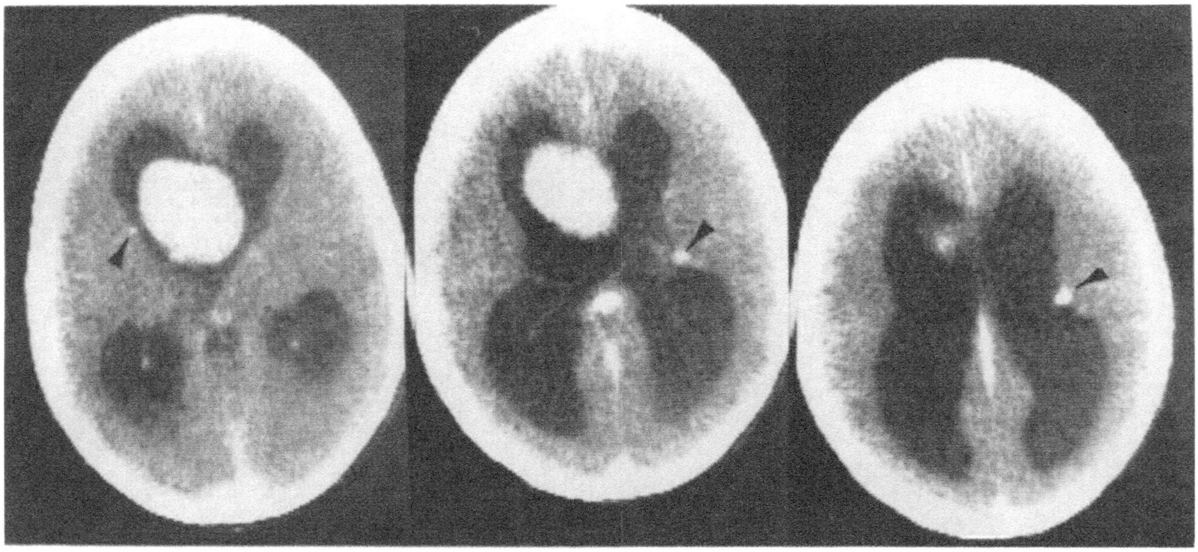

Figure 13. A 5-year-old boy with tuberous sclerosis. Contrast CT scan. Note a large subependymal giant-celled astrocytoma located near the interventricular foramina. It has caused obstruction at these foramina resulting in hydrocephalus. Note also small periventricular tubers (**arrowheads**).

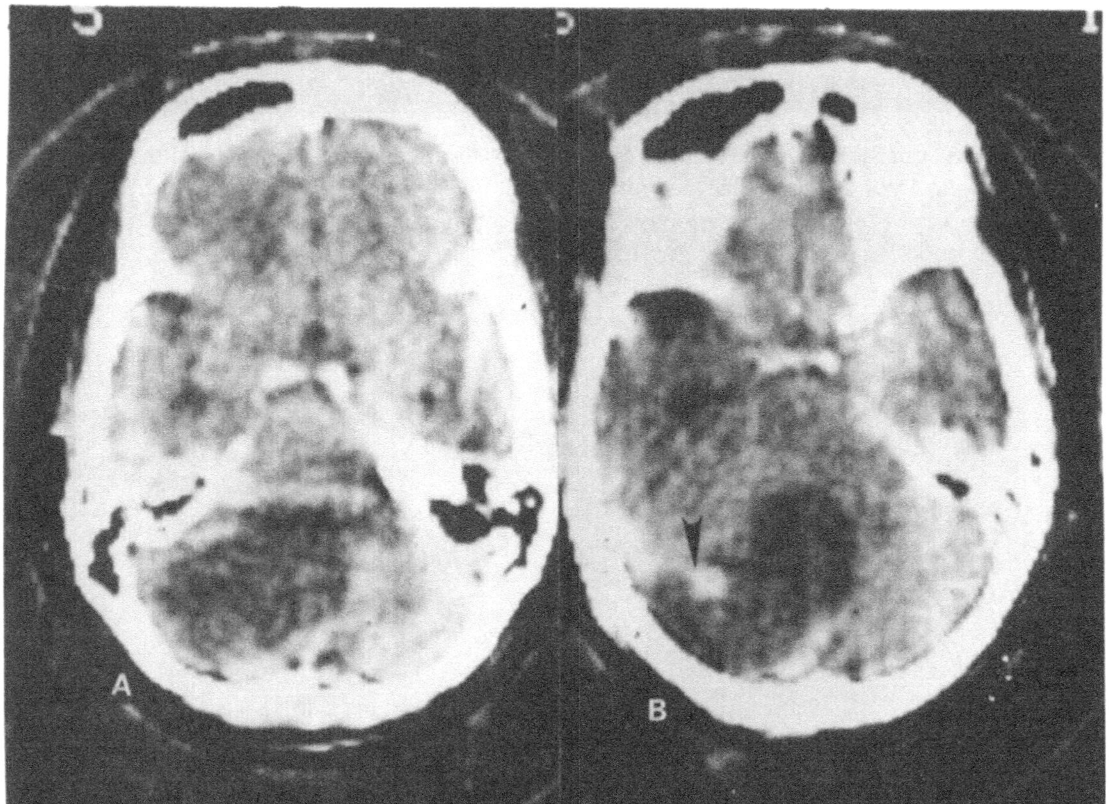

Figure 14. 55-year-old woman with predominantly cystic cerebellar hemangioglastoma. A) non-contrast and B) contrast CT scan. Note that this low density (cystic) lesion shows an enhancing nodule (**arrowhead**).

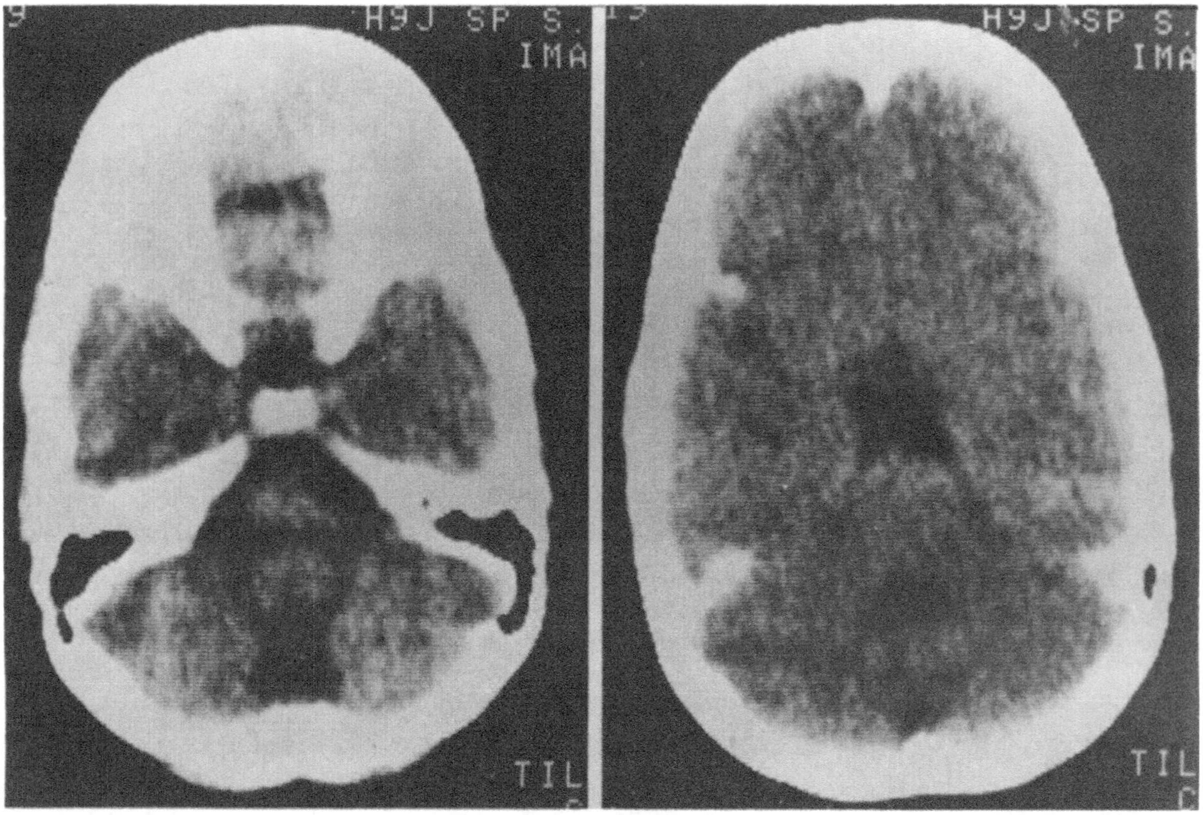

Figure 15. Ataxia-telangiectasia in a 4½-year-old boy with gait disturbance since age 10 months and conjunctival telangiectasia noted at 1 year of age. He had been afflicted with frequent infections. Non-contrast CT scan. See large fourth ventricle suggestive of cerebellar atrophy. Large cisterna magna may be incidental or part of cerebellar atrophy. (From Assencio-Ferreira *et al.*, with permission.)

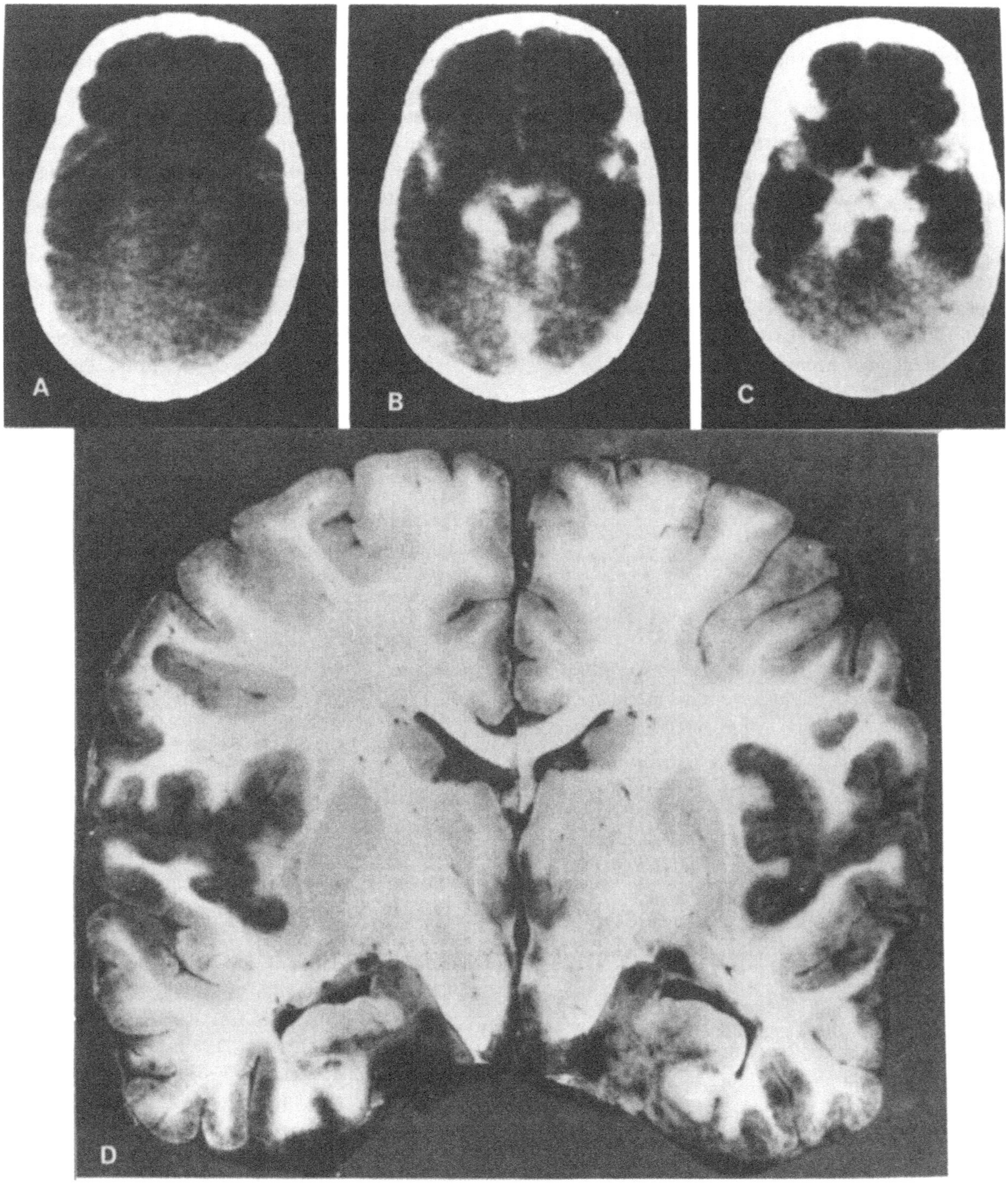

Figure 16. Neurocutaneous melanosis in a 16-month-old boy who presented with clinical history and CSF findings suggesting bacterial meningitis.

A. Non-contrast CT scan. Note non-visualization of the basal CSF spaces due to the presence of mainly isodense lesions in them.

B, C. Contrast CT scan. There is profuse enhancement in the subarachnoid spaces because of infiltration of meninges by melanosis. Same type of CT appearances can be seen in granulomatous and fungal meningitis and in meninges with melanosis and tumor. (From Kudel *et al.*, with permission.)

GENERAL REFERENCES

Neurocutaneous syndromes. *Seminars in Roentgenology, 2* (1): 1976.

Vinken PJ, Bruyn GW, eds: *Handbook of Clinical Neurology. The Phakomatosis.* Vol. 14, North-Holland Publishing Co., Amsterdam, 1972.

Yakovlev PI, Guthrie RH: Congenital ectodermoses (neurocutaneous syndromes) in epileptic patients. *Arch Neurol Psychiat, 26:*1145-1194, 1931.

Neurofibromatosis (von Recklinghausen disease)

Binet EF, Kieffer SA, Martin SH, Peterson HO: Orbital dysplasia in neurofibromatosis. *Radiology, 93:* 829-833, 1969.

Bruwer AJ, Kierland RR: Neurofibromatosis and congenital unilateral pulsating and nonpulsating exophthalmus. *Arch Ophthalmol, 53:*2-12, 1955.

Crowe FW, Schull WJ, Neel JV: *A Clinical, Pathological, and Genetic Study of Multiple Neurofibromatosis.* Publication No. 281, American Lecture Series. Monograph in the Bannerstone Division of American Lectures in Dermatology. Published by Charles C Thames, Publisher, Springfield, Ill., 1956.

Hilal SK, Solomon GE, Gold AP, Carter S: Primary cerebral arterial occlusive disease in children. Part II: Neurocutaneous syndromes. *Radiology, 99:* 87-94, 1971.

Holt JF: Neuhauser lecture: Neurofibromatosis in children. *Am J Roentgenol, 130:*615-639, 1978.

Holt JF, Kuhns LR: Macrocrania and macroencephaly in neurofibromatosis. *Skeletal Radiology, 1:*25-28, 1976.

Jacoby CG, Go RT, Beren RA: Cranial CT of neurofibromatosis. *Am J Roentgenol, 135:*553-557, 1980.

Kasantikul V, Brown WJ: Meningiomatosis in the absence of von Recklinghausen disease. *Surg Neurol, 15:*71-75, 1981.

Maki Y, Enomoto T, Nose T *et al.*: Computed Tomography in von Recklinghausen's disease. *Childs Brain, 8:*452-460, 1981.

Modic MT, Weinstein MA, Rothner AD *et al.*: Calcification of the choroid plexus visualized by computed tomography. *Radiology, 135:*369-372, 1980.

Patronas NJ, Zelkowitz M. Levin K: Ventricular dilatation in neurofibromatosis. *J Comp Ass Tomogr, 6:*598-600, 1982.

Pearce J: The central nervous system pathology in multiple neurofibromatosis. *Neurology, 17:*691-697, 1967.

Riccardi VM: Von Recklinghausen neurofibromatosis. *NEJM, 305:*1617-1626, 1981.

Rosman NP, Pearce J: The brain in multiple neurofibromatosis (von Recklinghausen's disease). A suggested neuropathological basis of the associated neural defect. *Brain, 90:*829-838, 1967.

Saha MM, Agarwal KN, Bhardwaj OP: Calvarial bone defects in neurofibromatosis. *Am J Roentgenol, 105:*319-321, 1969.

Sarwar M, Swischuk LE: Bilateral internal auditory canal enlargement due to dural ectasia in neurofibromatosis. *AJR, 129:*935-936, 1977.

Till K: *Pediatric Neurosurgery for Pediatricians and Neurosurgeons.* Blackwell Scientific Publications, London, 1975, p. 213.

Tomsick TA, Lukin RR, Chambers AA: Neurofibromatosis and intracranial arterial occlusive disease. *Neuroradiology, 11:*229-234, 1976.

Sturge-Weber Syndrome

Alexander GL: Sturge-Weber syndrome. In: *Handbook of Clinical Neurology, The Phakomatosis.* Vol. 14, Eds: Vinken PJ and Bruyn GW. North-Holland Publishing Co., Amsterdam, 1972, p. 223.

Alexander GL, Norman RM: *The Sturge-Weber Syndrome.* William and Wilkins, Baltimore, 1960.

Bentson JR, Wilson GH, Newton TH: Cerebral venous drainage of the Sturge-Weber syndrome. *Radiology, 101:*111-118, 1971.

Coulam CM, Brown LR, Reese DF: Sturge-Weber syndrome. *Seminars in Roentgenology, 11* (1):55, 1976.

DiChiro G, Lindgren E: Radiographic findings in 14 cases of Sturge-Weber syndrome. *Acta Radiol, 35:* 387-399, 1951.

Enzmann DR, Hayward RW, Norman D, Dunn RP: Cranial computed tomographic scan appearance of Sturge-Weber disease: Unusual presentation. *Radiology, 122:*721-724, 1977.

Lichtenstein BW: Sturge-Weber-Dimitri syndrome. Cephalic form of neurocutaneous hemangiomatosis. *Arch Neural Psychiat, 71:*291-301, 1954.

Maki Y, Semba A: Computed tomography of Sturge-Weber disease. *Childs Brain, 5:*51-61, 1979.

Ronne: A case of Sturge-Weber's disease. *Acta Derm-Venerol (Stockh), 18:*591, 1937.

Segall HD, Ahmadi J, McComb JG *et al.*: Computed tomographic observations pertinent to intracranial venous thrombotic and occlusive disease in childhood. State of the art, some new data, and hypotheses. *Radiology, 143:*441-449, 1982.

Welch K, Naheedy MH, Abroms IF, Strand RD: Computed tomography of Sturge-Weber syndrome in infants. *J Comp Asst Tomogr, 4:*33-36, 1980.

Tuberous Sclerosis

Barry JF, Harwood-Nash DC, Fitz CR, Byrd SE: Unrecognized atypical tuberous sclerosis diagnosed with CT. *Neuroradiology, 13:*177-180, 1977.

Burkhart, CG, El-Shaar A: Computerized axial tomography in the early diagnosis of tuberous sclerosis. *J Am Acad Dermatol, 4:*59-63, 1981.

Cooper JR: Brain tumors in hereditary multiple system hamartomatosis (Tuberous sclerosis). *J Neurosurg, 34:*194-202, 1971.

Garrick R, Gomez MR, Houser OW: Demyelination of the brain in tuberous sclerosis: Computed tomography evidence. *Mayo Clin Proc, 54:*685-689, 1979.

Gomez MR, Kuntz NL, Westmoreland BF: Tuberous sclerosis, early onset of seizures and mental subnormality: study of discordant monozygotic twins. *Neurology, 32:*604-611, 1982.

Hilal SK, Solomon GE, Gold AP, Carter S: Primary cerebral arterial occlusive disease in children. Part II: Neurocutaneous syndrome. *Radiology, 99:* 87-94, 1971.

Kapp JP, Paulson GW, Odom GL: Brain tumors with tuberous sclerosis. *J Neurosurg, 26:*191-202, 1967.

Kuhlendahl HD, Gross-Selbeck G, Doose H *et al.*: Cranial computer tomography in children with tuberous sclerosis. *Neuropaediatrie, 8:*325-332, 1977.

Lee BCP, Gawler J: Tuberous sclerosis. Comparison of computed tomography and conventional neuroradiology. *Radiology, 127:*403-407, 1978.

Nova M, Castillo J, Castro A *et al.*: Computerized cerebral tomography in tuberous sclerosis. Study of 3 patients. *Med-Clin (Barc), 76:*150-153, 1981.

Osborn AG, Daines JH, Wing SD: The evaluation of ependymal and subependymal lesions by cranial computed tomography. *Radiology, 127:*397-401, 1978.

Pou-Serradell A, Pascula J, Ugarte A *et al.*: A study of 14 cases of Bourneville's tuberous sclerosis including two pathological reports and seven cases investigated by computer tomography. *Rev-Neurol (Paris), 135:*693-703, 1979.

Probst FP, Erasmie U, Nergardh A, Brun A: CT appearances of brain lesions in tuberous sclerosis and their morphological basis. *Ann Radiol (Paris), 22:* 171-183, 1979.

Ataxia-Telangiectasia Syndrome

Assencio-Ferreira VJ, Bancovsky I, Diament AJ *et al.*: Computed tomography in Ataxia-telangiectasia, *J Comp Assist Tomogr, 5:*660-661, 1981.

Oxelius VN, Berkel AI, Hanson LA: IGG_2 deficiency in ataxia-telangiectasia. *NEJM, 306:*515-517, 1982.

Scharnetzky M, Kohlschutter A, Kritsch H: Computerized tomographic findings in a case of ataxia-telangiectasia (Louis-Bar syndrome). *Neuropediatrics, 11:*384-387, 1980.

Linear Nevus Sebaceous Syndrome

Chalhub EG, Volpe JJ, Gado MH: Linear nevus sebaceous syndrome associated with porencephaly and nonfunctioning major cerebral venous sinuses. *Neurology* [Minneap] *25:*857-860, 1975.

Feuerstein RC, Mims LC: Linear nevus sebaceous with convulsions and mental retardation. *Am J Dis Child, 104:*675-679, 1962.

Gooskens RH, Verga-Pires JA, van Nieuwenhuizen O, Kaiser MC: CT of sebaceous nevus syndrome (Jadassohn disease). *AJNR, 4:*203-205, 1983.

Leonidas JC, Wolpert SM, Feingold M, McCauley RGK: Radiographic features of the linear nevus sebaceous syndrome. *AJR, 132:*277-279, 1979.

Neurocutaneous Melanosis

Fox H: Neurocutaneous melanosis. In: *Handbook of Clinical Neurology,* Vol. 14, eds. Vinken PH, Bruyn GW, New York, American Elsevier, 1972, pp. 414-428.

Haper CG, Thomas DGT: Neurocutaneous melanosis. *J Neurol Neurosurg Psychiat, 37:*760-763, 1974.

Kudel TA, Bingham WT, Tubman DE: Computed tomographic findings of primary malignant leptomeningeal melanoma in neurocutaneous melanosis. *AJR, 133:*950-951, 1979.

Maekawa K, Suga Y, Shirai I *et al.*: A case of tuberous sclerosis with calcification of angiomatous change in the white matter. *Brain and Develop, 1:*127-132, 1979.

Sagar HJ, Ilgren EB, Adams CBT: Nevus of OTA associated with meningeal melanosis and intracranial melanoma. Case report. *J Neurosurg, 58:*280-283, 1983.

9

Miscellaneous

ENCEPHALOCELE, MENINGOENCEPHALOCELE AND MENINGOCELE

These congenital anomalies connote protrusion of brain and its coverings through a calvarial defect. **Meningocele** implies herniation through the bone defect of the meninges, **meningoencephalocele** brain and meninges; **encepahlocele** only the brain. Encephalocele is the commonest and occurs mainly (75 percent or so) in the occipital region. The cerebral tissue contained in the encephalocele is usually dysplastic. **Basal encephaloceles** occur through defect in the skull base – cribriform plate, sphenoid bone, orbital fissures – and can present as nasopharyngeal "tumor" or "polyp." Frontoethmoid encephaloceles are particularly common in Thailand (6,7). Hydrocephalus is far more common in encephaloceles than in the others. Associated anomalies include dysgenesis of corpus callosum, chiari malformation, aqueductal stenosis, gray matter heterotopia, spinal dysraphism, and cerebellar dysplasia. If the herniated neural tissue is large, the skull becomes microcephalic.

Pathogenesis

The pathogenesis of encephalocele/meningoencephalocele is not fully explained. The embryologic evidence suggests that this malformation occurs at about 4 to 6 weeks of gestation and is a manifestation of defective development of the neuroectoderm. The neuroectoderm destined to form the cerebrum herniates through the membranous calvarium. In other words, the primary defect is impaired development of the neural tissue and not of the developing membraneous calvarium. As the herniated sac grows, it either perforates the developing superior sagittal sinus or pushes it lateral resulting in its eccentric location.

CT Scan Findings

The essential CT scan finding consists of herniation of the soft tissue beyond the calvarial defect (Figs. 1,2) The calvarial defect must be studied by bone shifts (Fig. 3). On the non-contrast CT scan, determination of Hounsfield (H) units of the herniated tissue might give a clue to its nature – whether CSF, brain or both. The CSF H. units should be 12 or less and those of the cerebral tissue somewhat between 15-45 or more. The averaging of CSF and neural tissue units may erroneously mask the presence of CSF. On the contrast CT scan the neural tissue will enhance to a varying degree. Whereas it is so essential to analyze the arterial and particularly the dural venous sinus morphology before the surgical repair, such information is not forthcoming to an acceptable degree even on high resolution contrast CT scanning.

Their correct diagnosis on CT scan is usually made without much difficulty. However, occasionally, if the clinically palpated lesion is not soft and cystic, other possibilities need to be considered. The most common such consideration is a dermoid (Fig. 4) especially if its contents does not contain enough tissue of fat density, is not calcified and has H. units mimicking those of an encephalocele.

PORENCEHPALY

Porencephaly (a term originally used by Heschl in 1859) is a non-neoplastic CSF-containing cavity within the brain (Fig. 5) [usually the cerebral hemishpere and rarely the cerebellum and brainstem], which commonly communicates with the verticular system. It can be termed a cyst when it produces significant mass effect. It is not lined by true ependyma and is devoid of choroid plexus. The increased tendency of the immature and the unmyelinated brain in the fetus and the infant to show greater and more rapid dissolution secondary to a necrotizing lesion explains the greater incidence of porencephaly in the young.

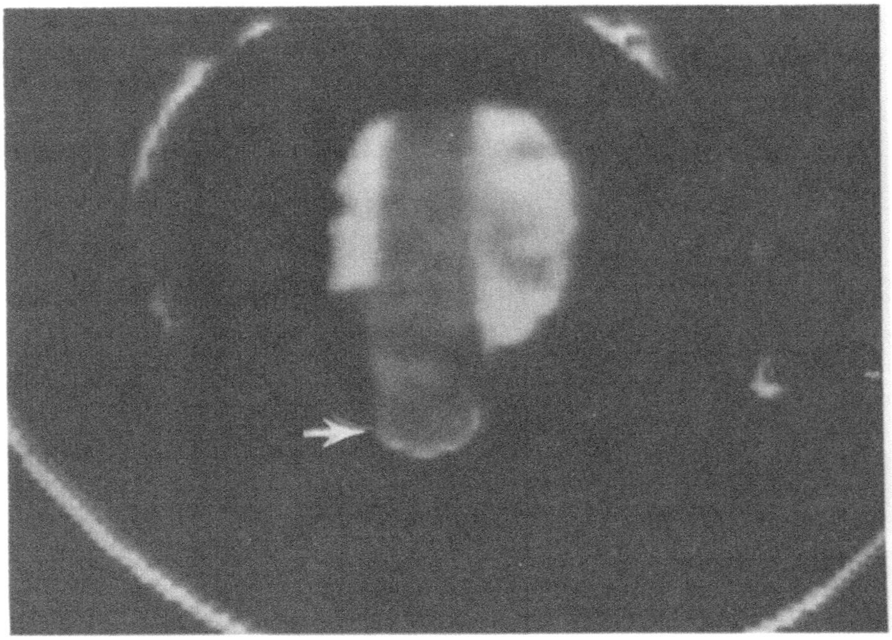

Figure 1. Meningoencephalocele (**arrow**) in a 2-day-old infant.

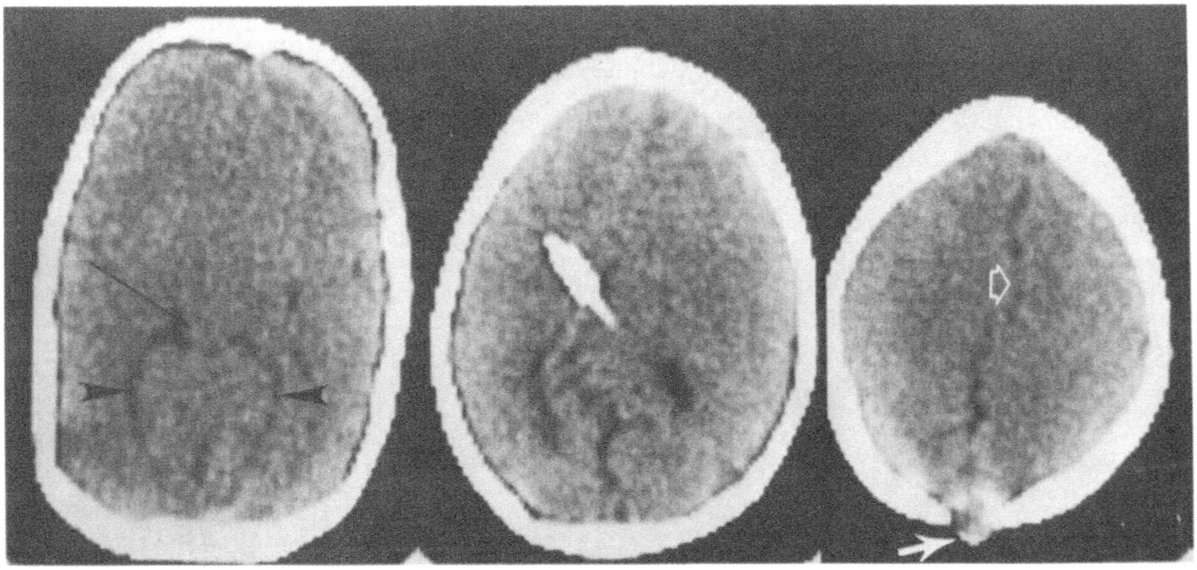

Figure 2. A small encephalocele (**white solid arrow**) and associated Arnold-Chiari malformation Type II manifested by mesencephalic beaking (**black solid arrow**), wide tentorial incisura (**arrowheads**), and interdigitating neural tissue (**open arrow**) at the interhemispheric fissure.

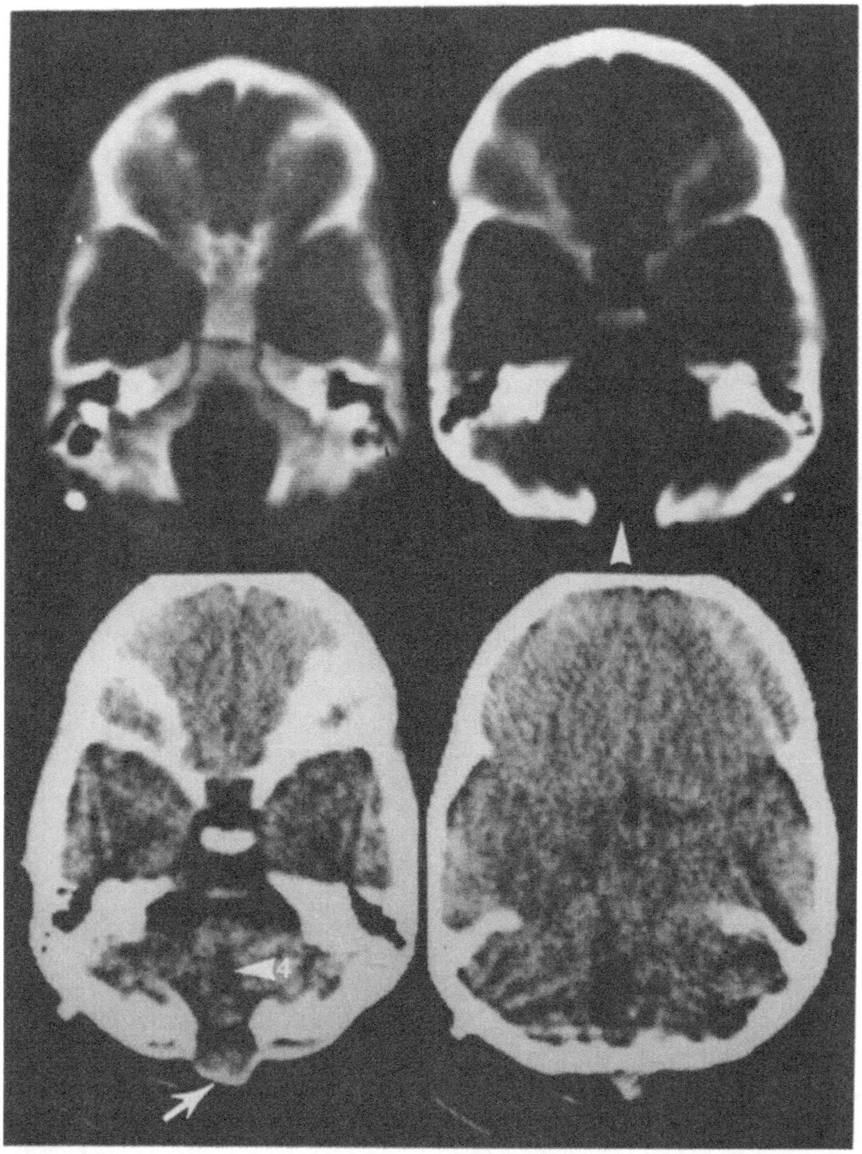

Figure 3. Recurrent or incompletely resected occipital encephalocele (**arrow**) in a 5-year-old male. Top row, bone shift images. The neural tissue herniates through the bony defect (**unlabelled arrowhead**). Note that the posterior fossa is small and the fourth ventricle (4) is pulled dorsally.

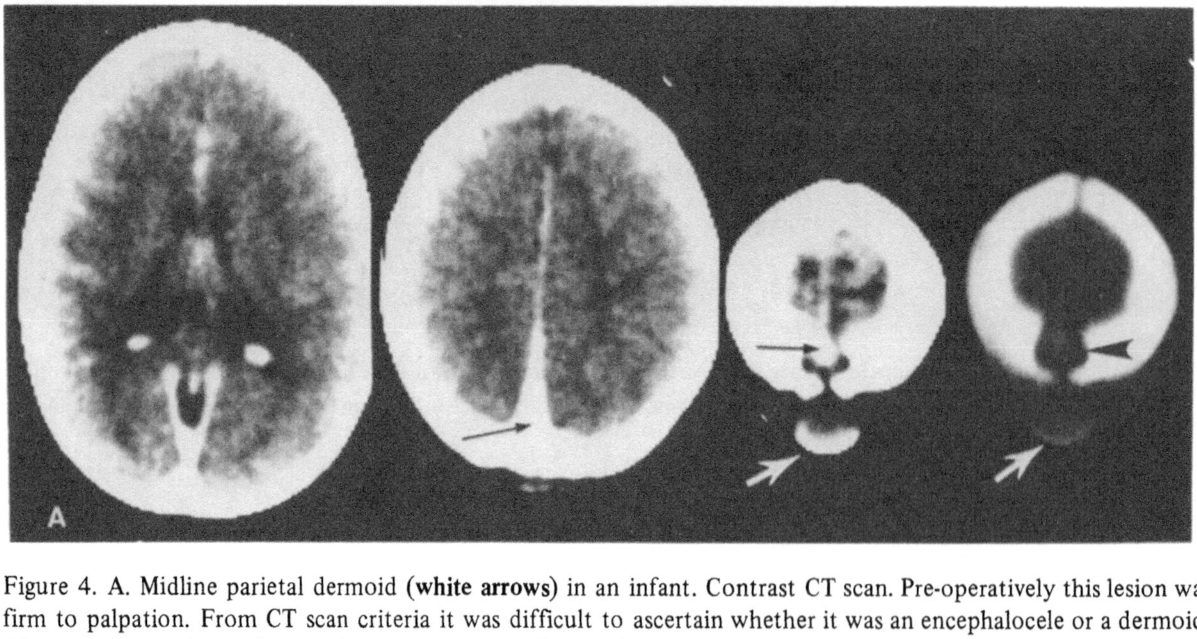

Figure 4. A. Midline parietal dermoid (**white arrows**) in an infant. Contrast CT scan. Pre-operatively this lesion was firm to palpation. From CT scan criteria it was difficult to ascertain whether it was an encephalocele or a dermoid. Also, its exact relationship to the superior sagittal sinus from contrast CT scan alone could not be determined.

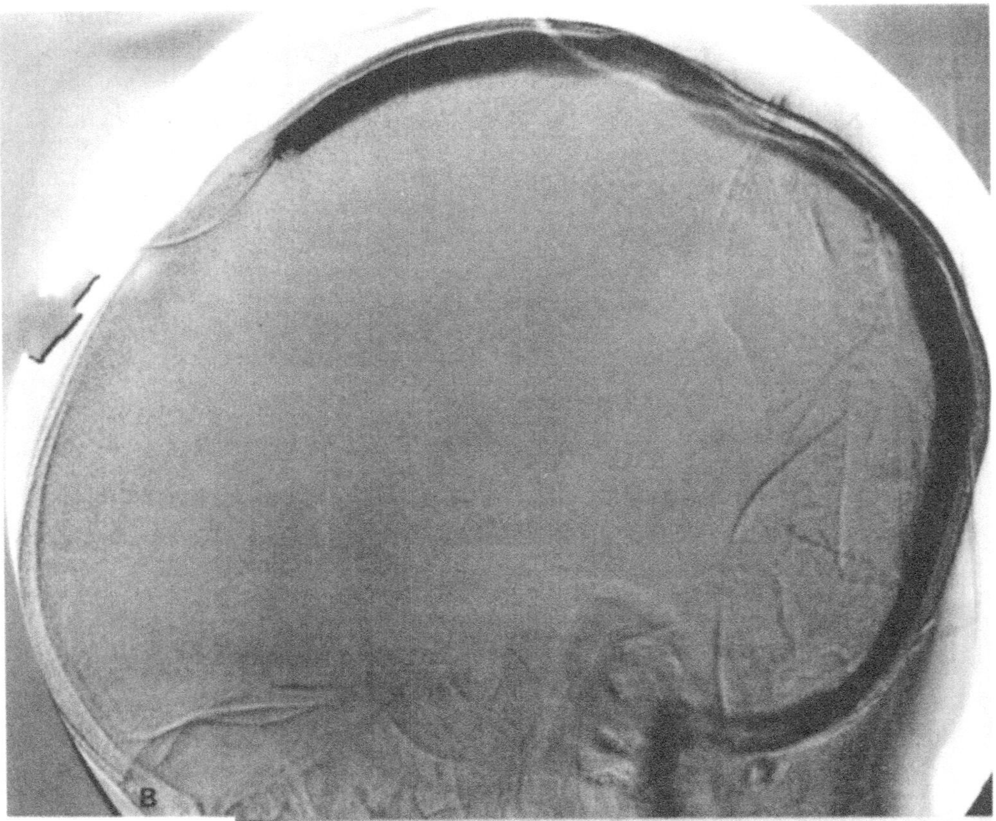

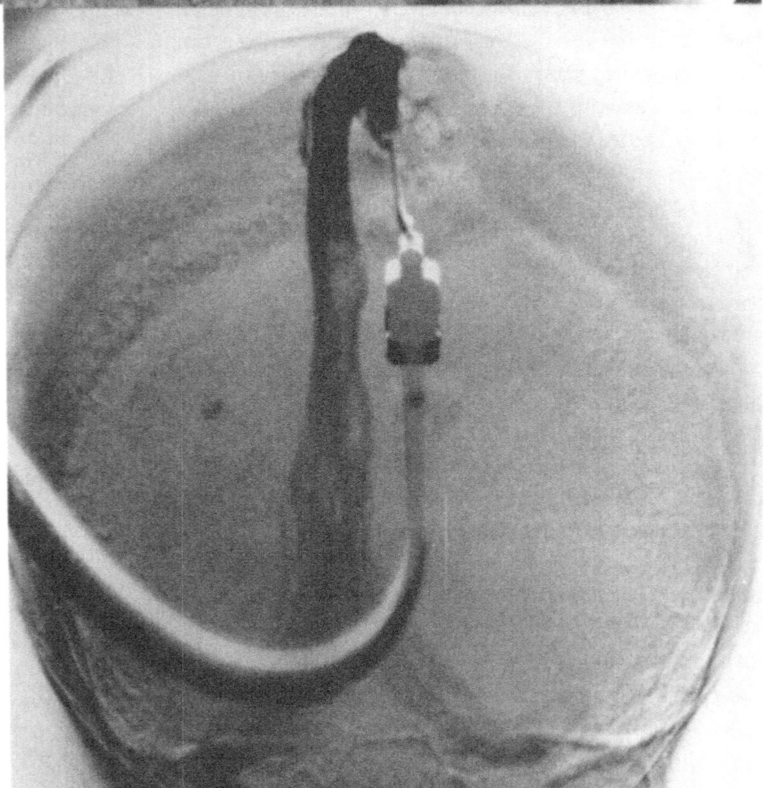

Figure 4. B and C. A sinugram was therefore done which did not reveal any cleft in the superior sagittal sinus. At surgery, a dermoid was encountered attached to the dura just to the left of the superior sagittal sinus which was slightly deviated to right. **Arrowhead** = bone defect associated with dermoid. **Black arrows** = superior sagittal sinus.

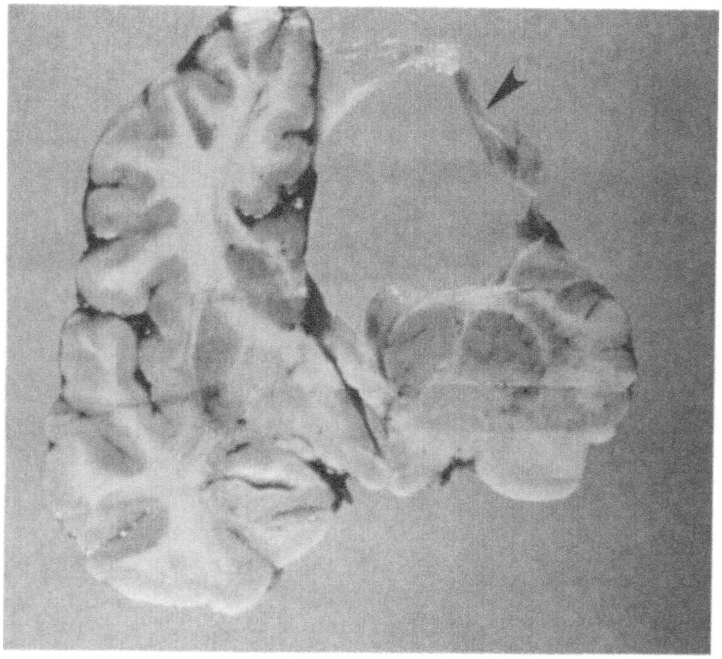

Figure 5. Porencephaly **(arrowhead)** shown on coronal section of a pathologic specimen. (Courtesy, W.F. McCormick, M.D.)

Yakovlev and Wadsworth (9) have divided them into two types. 1) **Schizencephaly**. It implies symmetrical clefts in the cerebral hemisphere wall resulting from a developmental error. The lips of the cleft may or may not fuse. They are commonly located along the primary cerebral fissures (Fig. 6). It may be difficult to recognize them as such on CT. Prominent sylvian fissures, in a malformed and hypoplastic brain, are difficult to characterize as being clefts or gaping fissures because of poor opercularization (covering) of the fissure. 2) **Encephaloclastic porencephaly**. They are formed by destruction of the previously normally formed neural tissue. They are the commoner ones and are usually seen in infants and children. They are secondary to occlusive vascular disease (ischemia), trauma, infarction, hemorrhage, or aroxia. They are usually located over the cortical surface of the cerebral hemisphere, commonly in the distribution of the middle cerebral artery.

The greater tendency of the white matter of the infant brain to show white matter necrosis can result in multiple small cavities (polyporencephaly) which may not communicate with the ventricular system (Fig. 7). The ependyma, mainly nourished by CSF, shows greater resistance to destruction than the surrounding neural tissue (Fig. 8).

Sometimes a porencephalic cyst that communicates with an hydrocephalic ventricle can progressively expand and enlarge the cranial cavity (10). Their shunting before age two can allow regaining of the near normal cortical thickness and result in amelioration of neurologic deficit.

On the CT scan, a porencephaly appears as a well-defined, CSF-containing cavity showing no contrast enhancement (11) Fig. 9).

MICROCEPHALY (MICRENCEPHALY)

It is defined as a head size which is smaller than the mean for age and sex by more than three standard deviations; an adult brain weighing less than 900 grams can be regarded as abnormal. The name implies only a disease process without specific etiology, whether destructive, malformative or degenerative. The main etiologic groups are indicated below with some examples of each group.

Developmental:
- Lissencephaly
- Holoprosencephaly
- Heterotopias

Genetic:
- Cockayne Syndrome
- (familial microcephaly with calcifications)
- Alper disease
- (progressive cerebral cortical atrophy)
- Phenylketonuria
- Sex-linked micorcephaly with aminoaciduria
- Kinky-hair disease

Chromosomal aberration:
- Down Syndrome
- (Trisomy 21)
- Trisomy 13
- Trisomy 17-18
- Cri-Du-Chat Syndrome
- Fanconi anemia

Intrauterine injuries and infections:
- Radiation
- Rubella
- Toxoplasmosis
- Diabetes mellitus
- Cytomegalic inclusion disease
- Fetal malnutrition
- Perinatal trauma or hypoxia

Perinatal and postnatal disorders:
- Multiple cystic encephalomalacia
- Encephalitis (for example, herpes simplex)

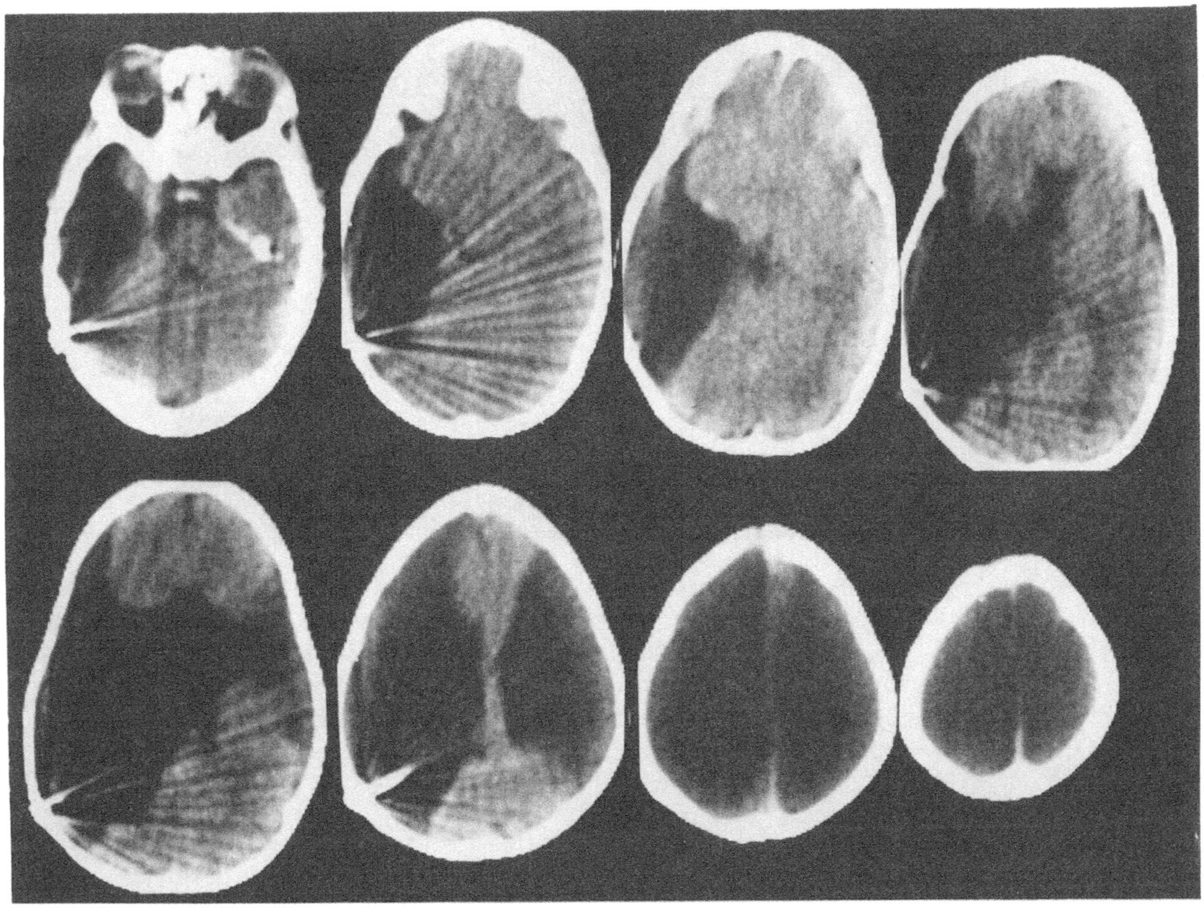

Figure 6A. Schizencephaly in an infant. Note large, symmetrical cerebral clefts that communicate with the lateral ventricles.

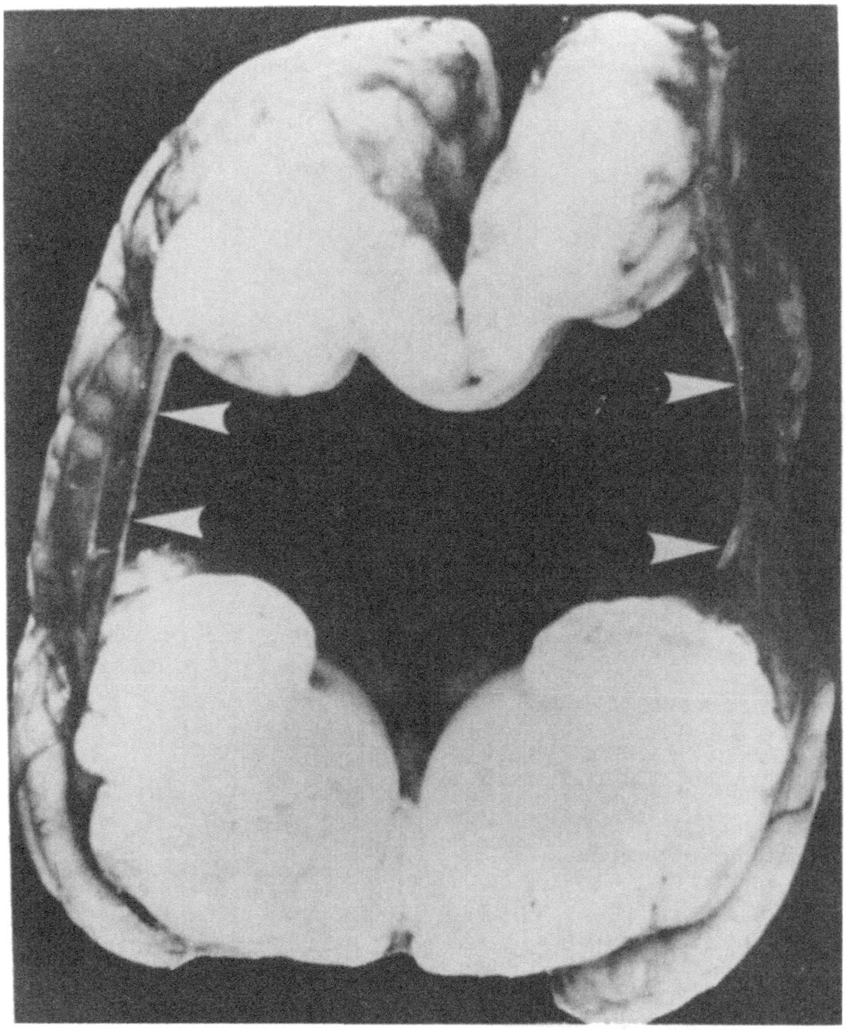

Figure 6B. Schizencephaly. Coronal section of the pathologic specimen (of another patient). Note the pia-ependyma lined (**arrowheads**) symmetric clefts merging with the abnormally developed ventricular system. (From Zimmerman *et al., Neuroradiology 25*:257, 1983, with permission.)

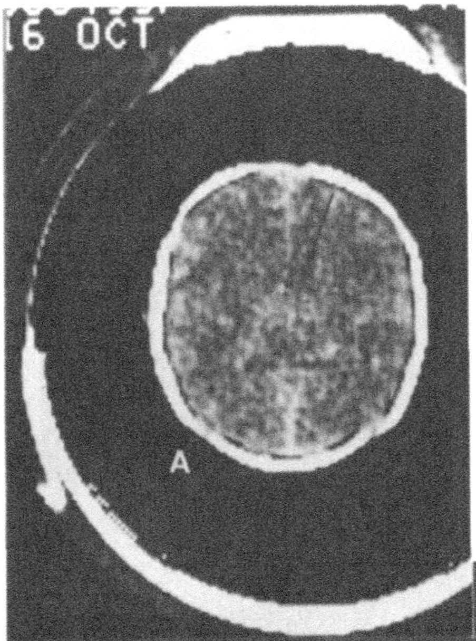

Figure 7. Anoxic spongy polyporencephaly in a newborn.

A. Non-contrast CT. There is generalized hypodensity of the brain such that it is barely distinguishable from the ventricular system (**arrow**).

B. Pathologic specimen. There are multiple porencephalies showing septation as well.

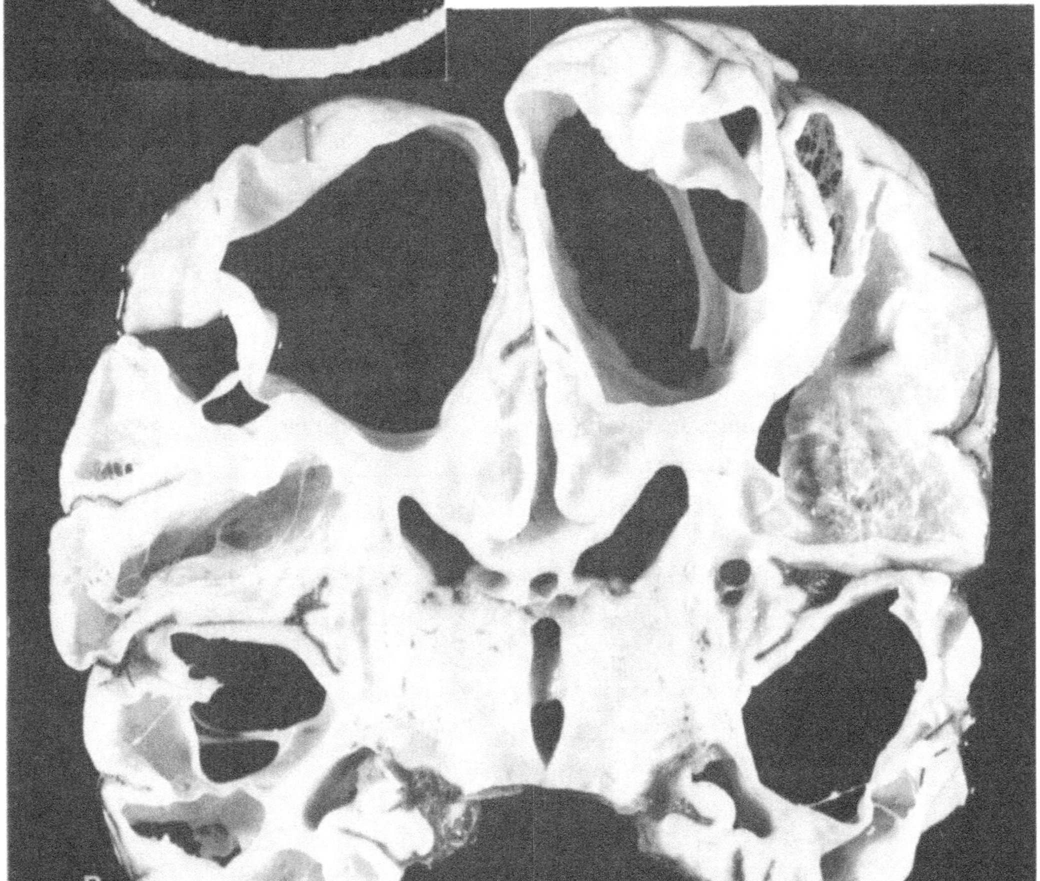

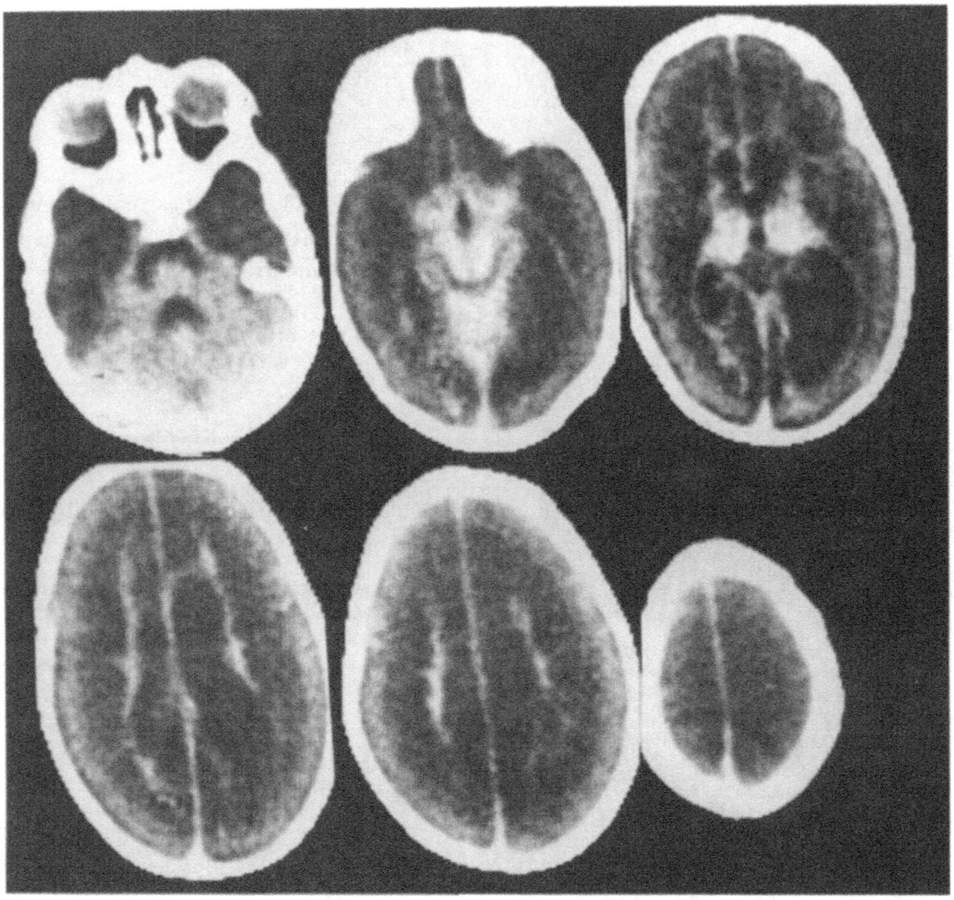

Figure 8. A full term neonate born with an Apgar of 4. She had severe hypoxic-ischemic brain injury. Non-contrast CT. There is marked hypodensity of the brain due to necrosis (polioencephalopathy). The ependyma, the basal ganglia and the posterior fossa structures are well-preserved and stand out in relief.

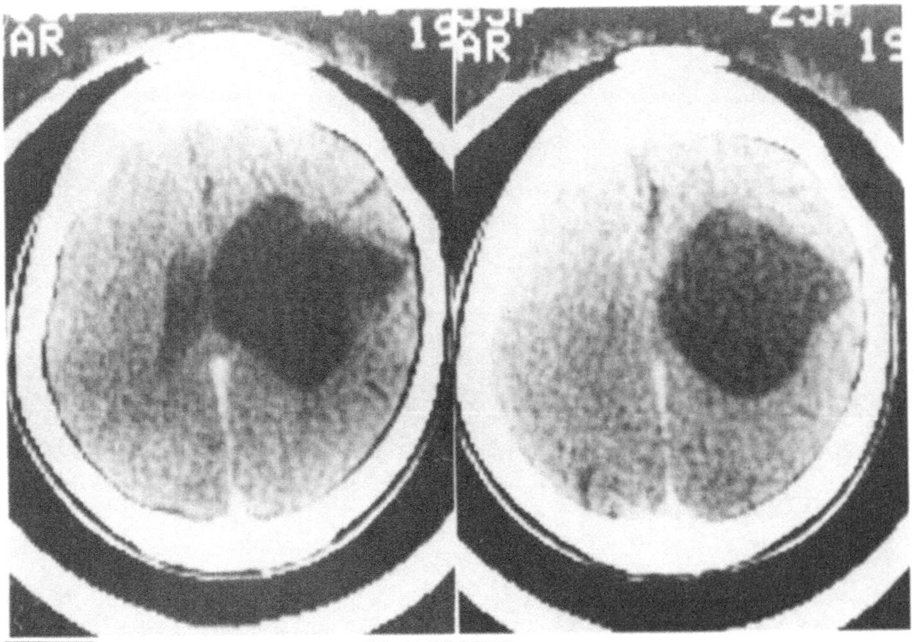

Figure 9. Post-traumatic porencephaly in a 38-year-old man. Contrast CT. There is no contrast enhancement of its wall. It communicates with the lateral ventricle.

CT Scan Findings

It is difficult to reliably assess head size from CT scans. One should rely on clinical head circumference measurements. CT scan, however, can provide a clue to the underlying cause of microcephaly. Periventricular and/or parenchymal calcifications can be seen in TORCH (toxoplasmosis, rubella, cytomegalic inclusion disease [Fig. 10], and herpes simplex encephalitis). Calcification in the basal ganglia and less often in the dentate nuclei is observed in Cockayne syndrome. Ventriculomegaly and sulcal enlargement (gyral atrophy) may be observed in conditions like Alper disease. CNS malformations like holoprosencephaly, will manifest their own characteristic features.

ANENCEPHALY (12)

The frequency of anancephaly in the United States and most of Eurpoe varies approximately from 0.5 to 2.0 per thousand births. Diagnosis of anencephaly is bovious at birth and always fatal. U.S. death rate from anancephaly is about 5 deaths per 100,000.

Most of these cases are born during the last trimester. There is a female preponderance of three or four to one.

Epidemiologic studies have not provided any convincing clue to an etiologic agent. Whereas no consistent abnormal chromosomal pattern has been identified, anencephaly has been observed coexistent with chromosomal anomalies on occasion.

Embryologic considerations suggest that this malformation occurs after the formation of the optic vesicle which occurs at about the eighteenth day of gestation. This observation stems from the fact that eyes have developed relatively normally in most instances. Anencephaly seems to occur at about the time of closure of the neural tube, that is, at about the fourth week of gestation.

This malformation may be considered as a manifestation of defective closure of the cephalad portion of the neural tube. There is absence of most or all of the brain. There is total deficiency (acrania) or underdevelopment of the squamous bones forming the cranial vault. The base of the skull is relatively preserved. The remnant "brain" consists of reddish, highly vascularized neural and mesenchymal tissue called the substantia cerebrovasculosa (Fig. 11). Sometimes the brain comprises of a pedunculated mass attached to the skull base.

Abnormality of the spine varies in degree from craniorachischisis (an open defect along the entire spine) to simple segmentation anomaly. Spinal cord is usually severely malformed and may be represented by a splayed-out layer of neural tissue: the central canal may be absent.

MEDIAN CLEFT FACE SYNDROME (13-15)

The median cleft face syndrome results from disturbance of the union of several structures in the median facial plane (Figs. 12,13). There is orbital hypertelorism. In most cases, the brain is normal or is only mildly abnormal (usually there is dysgenesis of corpus callosum). Whereas holoprosencephaly complex commonly occurs with midline facial defects and hypotelorism, it can rarely be seen in association with midline facial defects and hypertelorism. With CT, the facial defects and associated CNS malformations are likely to be detected more frequently and with greater clarity.

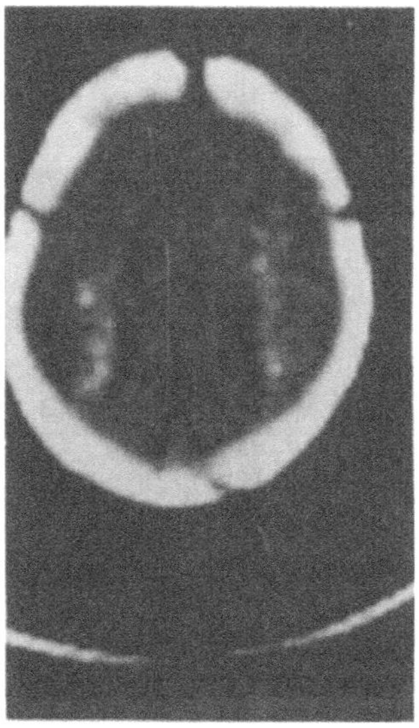

Figure 10. Widespread parenchymal and periventricular calcification related to cytomegalic inclusion disease in a 22-hour-old microcephalic infant.

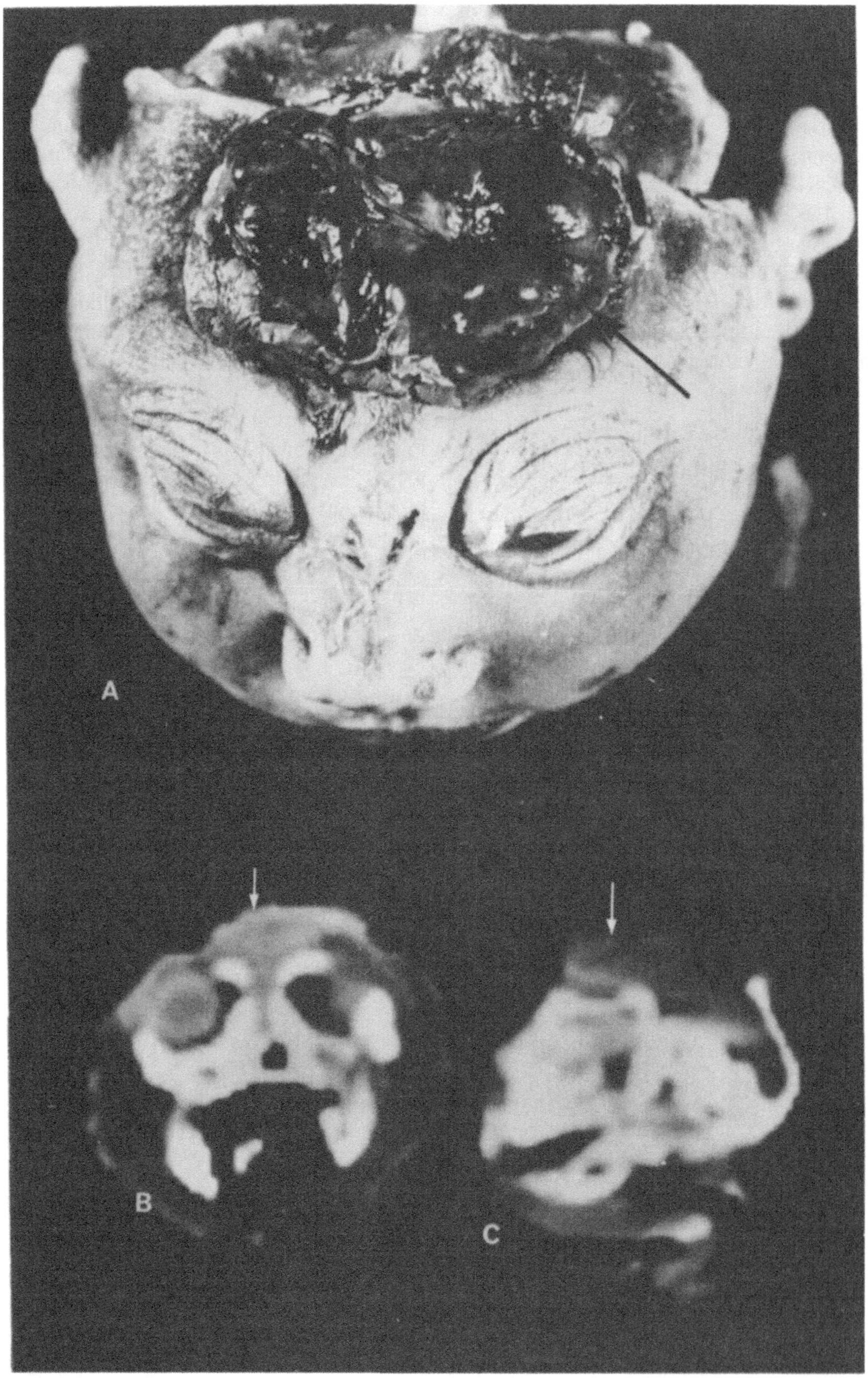

Figure 11. Anencephaly. A) Pathologic specimen. B) coronal, and C) sagittal CT scans of the pathologic specimen. **Arrows** = substantia cerebrovasculosa.

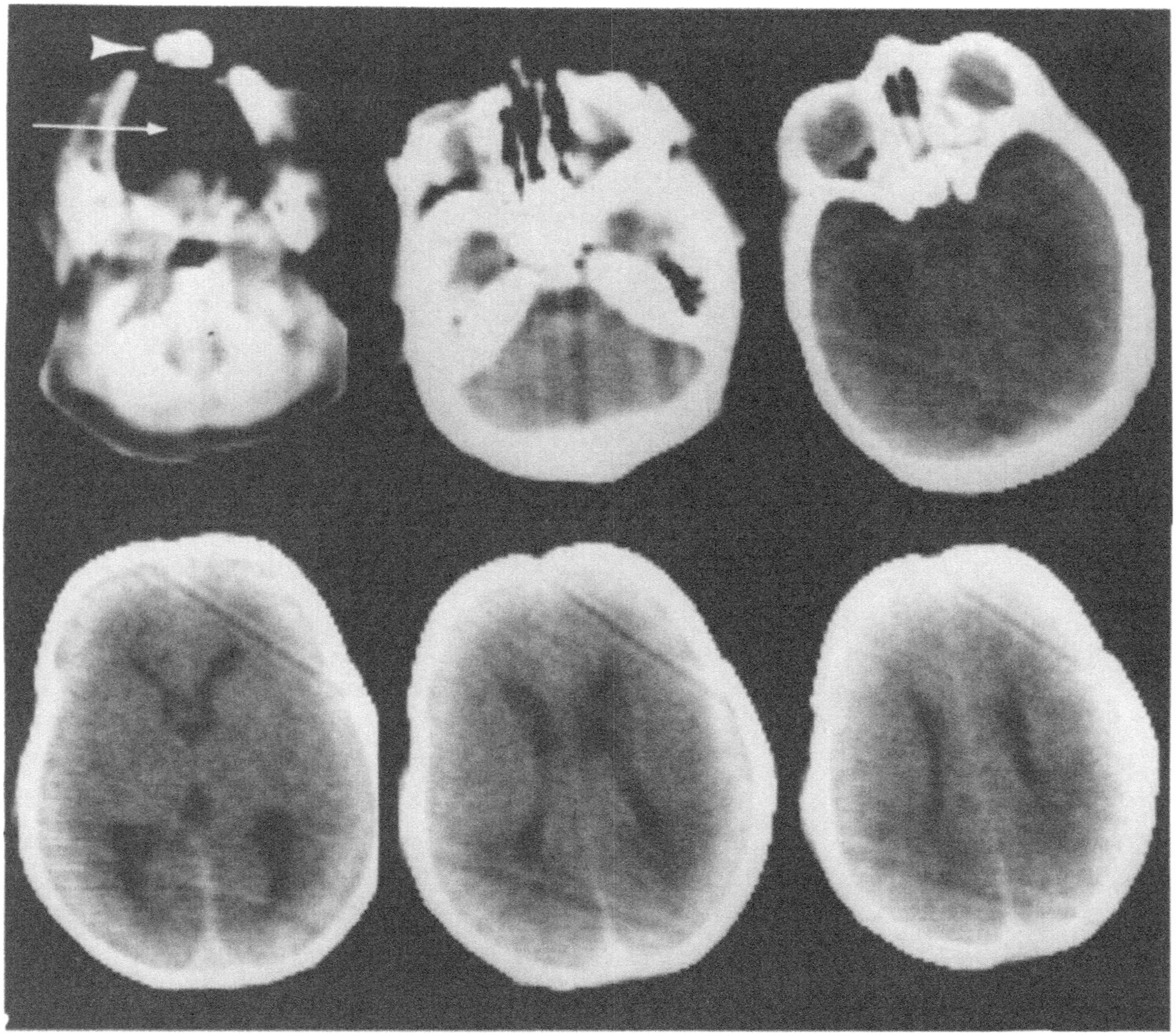

Figure 12. An infant with midline facial defects. Note cleft palate (**arrow**). There is minimal ventricular prominence. **Arrowhead** = premaxilla.

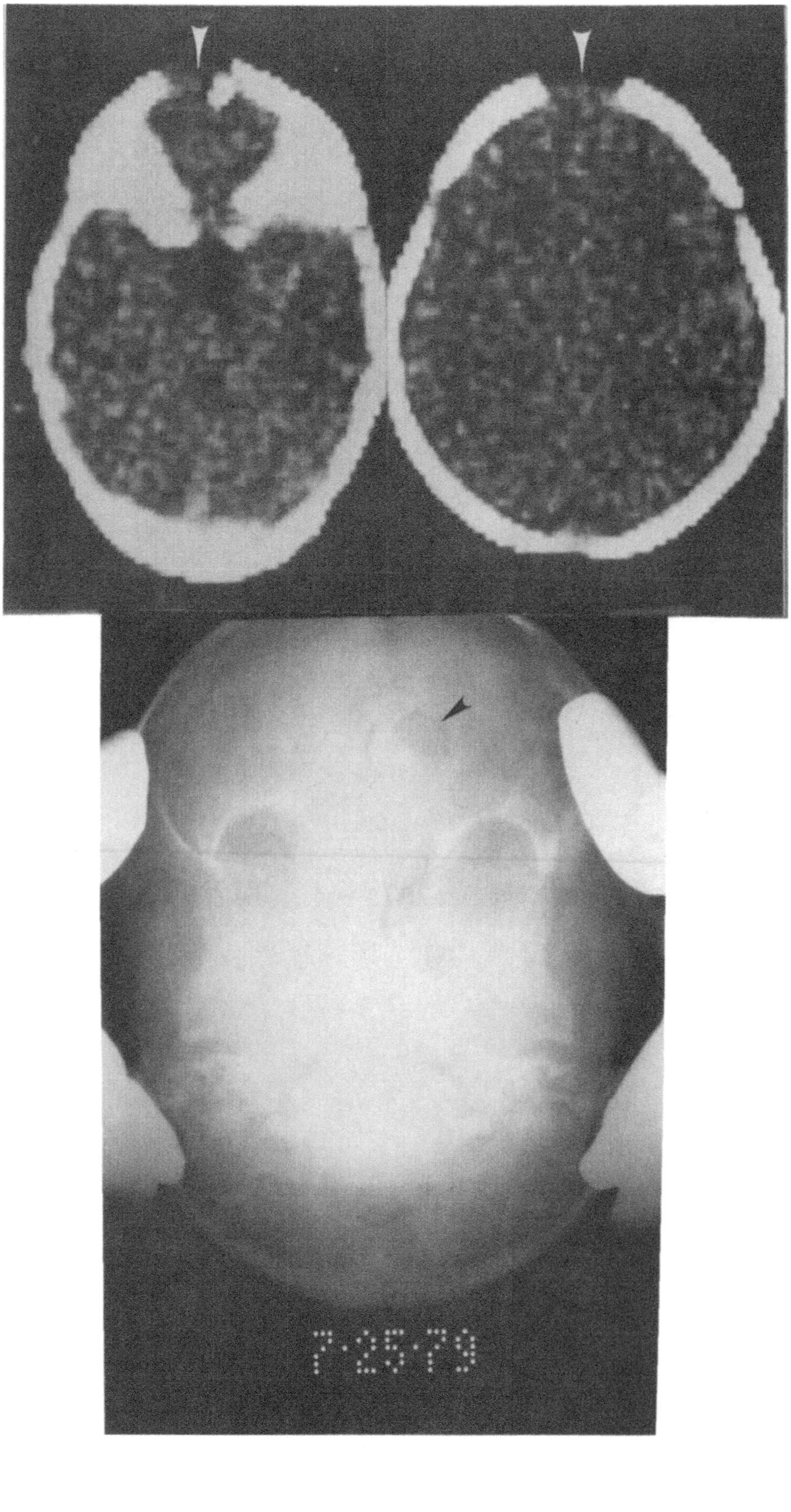

Figure 13. A 2-year-old child with median cleft face syndrome. Note median frontal bone defect **(arrowheads)**. There is hypertelorism on the skull film.

HYPERTELORISM

This implies abnormal increase in the interorbital distance. I am not aware of published reports on normal and abnormal interorbital distance on the CT scan. But, one can use the data provided by Currarino and Silverman in 1960 (15). Using the cursor, or taking into consideration the minification factor of the CT images, the interorbital distance between the medial orbital walls should be measured preferably on the bone shift images. The measurements should be compared with the ones provided in the chart by Currarino and Silverman. Under 5 years of age, interorbital distance greater than 25 mm may safely be considered to suggest hypertelorism.

In the early developmental stages, the eyes are wide apart, recapitulating phylogeny. As the fetus matures, the eyes come closer together. Hypertelorism may be primary or secondary. Secondary hypertelorism may be associated with the following conditions:

- Median cleft face syndrome
- Frontonasal and basal encephalocele or meningoencephalocele
- Cleidocranial dysostosis
- Cruzon disease
- Apert Syndrome
- Osteogenesis imperfecta
- Mucopolysaccharidoses type I and II.

HYPOTELORISM

Hypotelorism is characterized by decreased interorbital distance. The interorbital distance as measured on the CT scan should be compared with measurements provided in the chart by Currarino and Silverman. A distance less than 12 mm under 5 years of age may safely be considered to denote hypotelorism. In hypotelorism, there is hypoplasia of the ethmoids. It is commonly seen in: 1) holoprosencephaly complex; 2) trigoncephaly (triangular skull) occurring alone or in association with holoprosencephaly complex, due to premature closure of the metopic suture, and 3) Down syndrome (related mainly to ethmoidal hypoplasia).

LISSENCEPHALY (AGYRIA: PACHYGYRIA (16-20)

This rare condition denotes either complete absence of gyral formation leading to smooth-surfaced brain (agyria; Lissen = smooth) or to their incomplete development such that the gyri are coarse and broad separated by shallow sulci (pachygyria). These two types only reflect the varying severity of the disease. This defective development of the gyri is a manifestation of generalized hypoplasia of the brain (micrencephaly) and poor to no opercularization (covering) of the insulae by the cerebral hemispheres resulting in wide sylvian fissures. Large ventricles attest to the poor growth of the cerebral hemispheres (it may be recalled that at 20 weeks gestation 50 percent of the intracranial contents is ventricles; as the brain grows larger in size and the outlet foramina of the fourth ventricle become functional, the ventricles get progressively smaller). Since gyral formation becomes well defined at 26 to 28 weeks gestation and opercularization is noticable soon thereafter, it can be concluded that this malformation occurs before that period. Concurrent heterotopias reflect impaired neuroblastic migration.

Associated anomalies include colpocephaly (see colpocephaly); dysgenesis of corpus callosum is the commonest.

This condition has autosomal recessive inheritance. Clinically these children are microcephalic, have seizures and show severe psychomotor retardation.

CT Scan Findings

CT scan provides only strongly presumptive but by no means pathognomonic findings. The findings are: 1) ventriculomegaly; 2) wide sylvian fissures; and 3) absent or poorly recognizable cortical sulci (Fig. 14). Overall, the brain is hypoplastic.

COLPOCEPHALY (COLPOS = HOLLOW) (21-23)

This is a condition in which there is persistence of the fetal configuration of the occipital horns; they remain disproportionately enlarged (Fig. 15). This is very likely a manifestation of impaired morphogenesis (hypoplasia), primarily of the white matter, of the structures which determine the size and configuration of the occipital horns. They are optostriate nuclei, forceps major and tapetum of the corpus callosum and internal parietooccipital and calcarine fissures. It occurs before six months of gestation.

Such disproportionate enlargement of the occipital horns does not always indicate dysmorphogenesis. Similar occipital horn enlargement can occur in any condition (e.g., perinatal anoxia) which causes selective or predominant leukomalacia of the parieoccipital lobes. Also, occipital horns at young age show a tendency to enlarge more than the frontal horns in hydrocephalus (Fig. 16) [see Hydrocephalus chapter].

Clinically, these children are retarded and show a wide variety of motor, cranial nerve (particularly the optic system) and extrapyramidal system deficit.

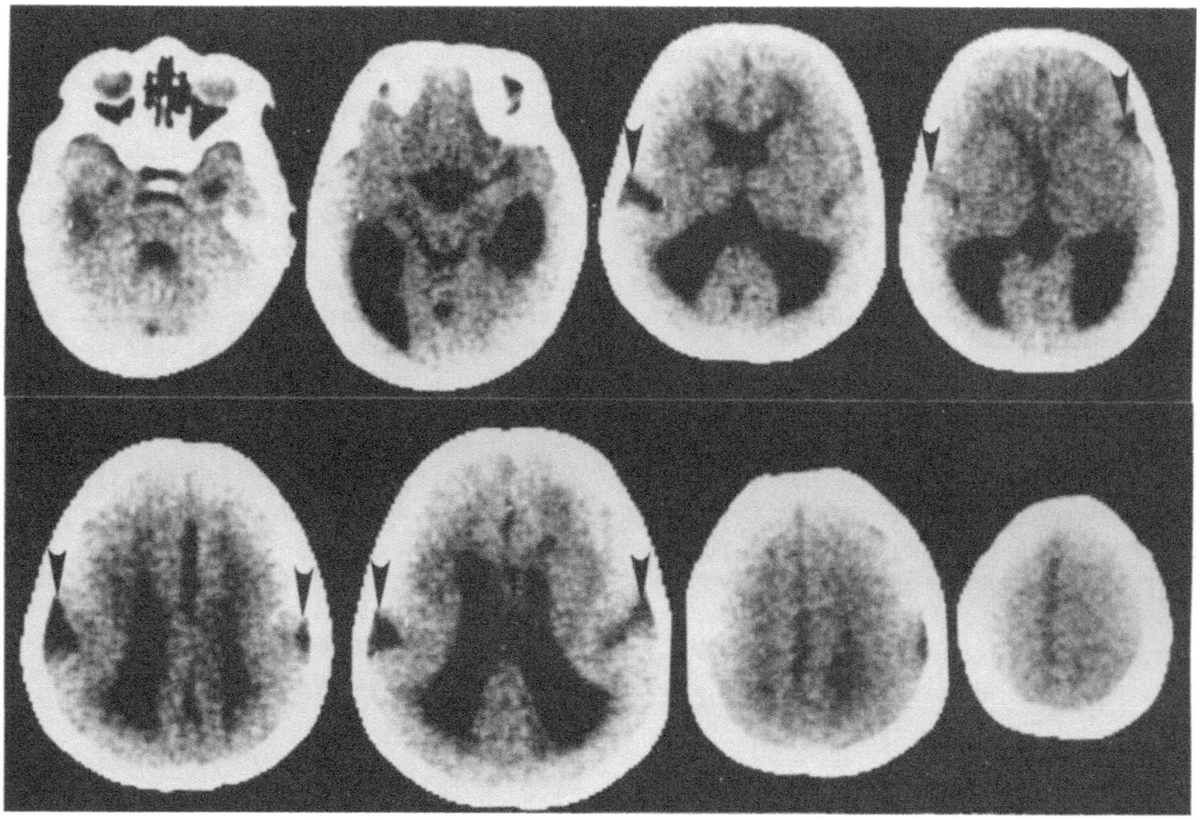

Figure 14. Probable lissencephaly in a 2-month-old infant with seizures and hypotonia. Note ventriculomegaly and wide sylvian fissures (**arrowheads**). There are hardly any recognizable cortical sulci. The gaping sylvian fissures are due to poor opercularization (overlapping) by the cerebral hemisphere lobes. The interhemispheric fissure also in prominent.

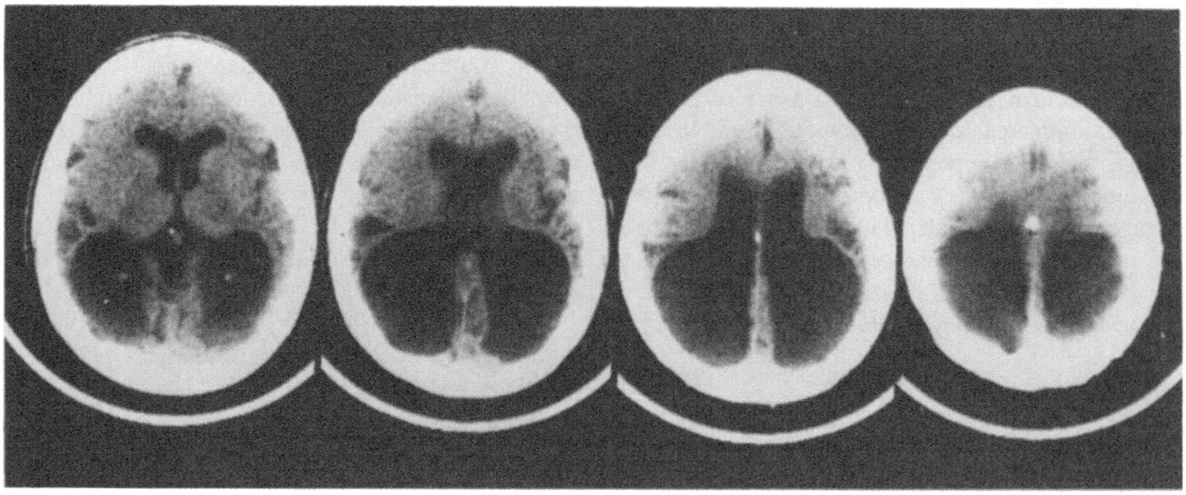

Figure 15. Colpocephaly. Note disproportionate enlargement of the occipital horns. This 24-year-old female was examined for mental retardation and long history of seizure disorder. Clinically, some chromosomal abnormality was suspected.

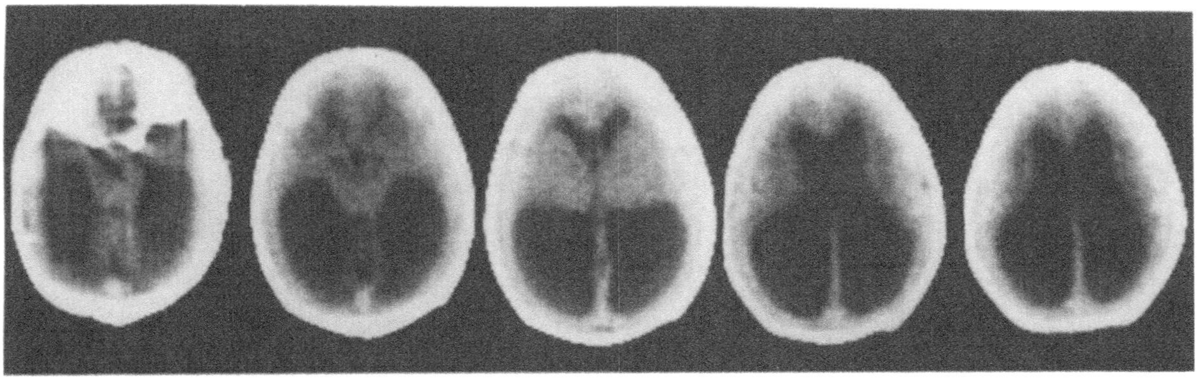

Figure 16. A 20-day-old infant with congenital hydrocephalus. Note disproportionate enlargement of the occipital horns.

FETAL ALCOHOL SYNDROME (24-26)

This syndrome afflicts about 30 to 45 percent of infants born to mothers who indulge in chronic, heavy daily drinking. Its incidence is about 1 to 1,000 live births in the western countries. Besides the teratogenic effect of ethanol, malnutrition and environmental factors probably play a role in the pathogenesis of this syndrome.

This is a multisystem disease which includes anomalies of the face and of the brain. The important facial malformations include short palpebral fissures, flat nasal bridge, flattened maxilla and mandibular hypoplasia. The brain dysmorphology usually consists of micrencephaly, neuronal heterotopia and generalized disorganization or dysgenesis of the neural tissue (Fig. 17). Anencephaly, porencephaly, and meningomyelocele also may occur.

ARACHNOID CYSTS (27, 26)

These arachnoid-lined cysts are of two types: primary and secondary. The **primary (congenital) arachnoid cysts** result from maldevelopment of the meninges such that an abnormal collection of CSF occurs in the fetal perimedullary mesenchyme. The **secondary (acquired) arachnoid cysts**, the commoner of the two, follow loculation of the subarachnoid space due to arachnoid adhesions from inlfammation or hemorrhage.

These cysts commonly occur in the middle and posterior fossae, over the cerebral convexity, parasellar region and near the collicular plate (paracollicular cysts). They cause the neurologic deficit due to an increase in their size from filtration, osmosis, or secretion of CSF into the cyst cavity.

On CT, they appear as well-defined CSF containing lesions without enhancement of their walls (Figs. 18,19). Metrizamide CT scanning may reveal whether or not they communicate with the adjacent subarachnoid space. The appropriate differential diagnosis includes an epidermoid or cystic astrocytoma.

MEGALENCEPHALY (29,30)

The term megalencephaly was introduced by Fletcher in 1900 and implies an enlarged brain weighing 1600 gm, or more, with normal sized or minimally enlarged lateral ventricles. DeMyer, in 1972, indicated that the definition should include any oversized and overweight brain irrespective of the quality of its neurological function and divided it into: a) anatomic and b) metabolic types. In **anatomic** megalencephaly, there is primary increase in the size or number of cells and there is no increased intracranial pressure. It can be associated, amongst other conditions, with achondroplasia, neurofibromatosis, tuberous sclerosis and Chiari malformation. In **metabolic type**, there is increase in cell size due to an accumulation of abnormal metabolic products; increased intracranial pressure is present. A few of the conditions in which it can be seen are the leukodystrophies, Tay-Sach's disease, gangliosidosis and mucopolysaccharidosis. Clinically, some kind of mental retardation is a usual feature and seizure disorder may be present.

CT scan usually is done in these patients to exclude hydrocephalus or extracerebral fluid collection as a possible cause of a large head. The diagnosis of megalencephaly is thus made by excluding these conditions. One can also make such a diagnosis if visually the head appears larger for age or the abnormal head size has been ascertained by some radiologic measurement. Some subarachnoid space and ventricular enlargement may be present in metabolic megalencephaly (Fig. 20).

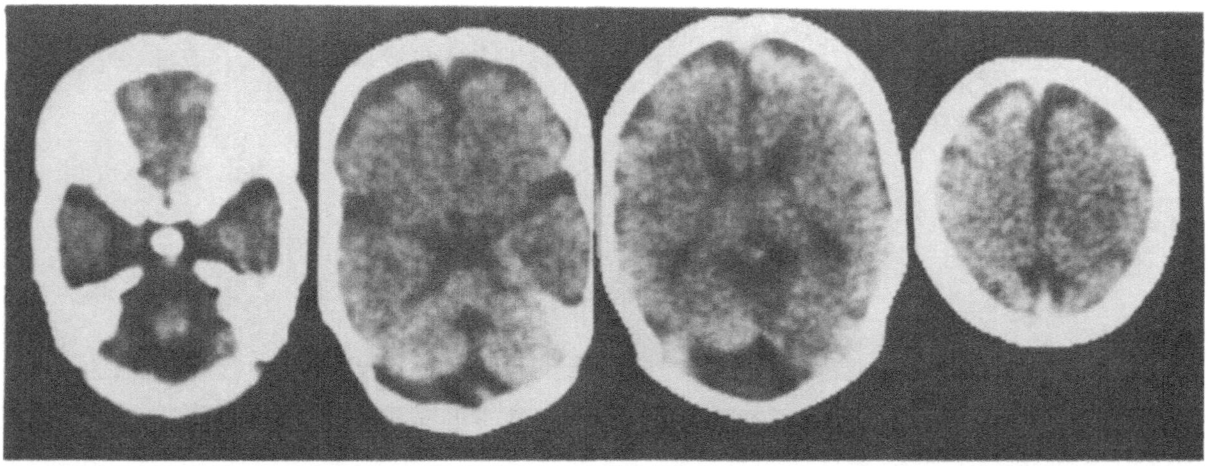

Figure 17. Fetal Alcohol Syndrome. Note generalized prominence of the subarachnoid spaces and of the ventricular system, both supra- and infratentorially, indicating brain hypoplasia.

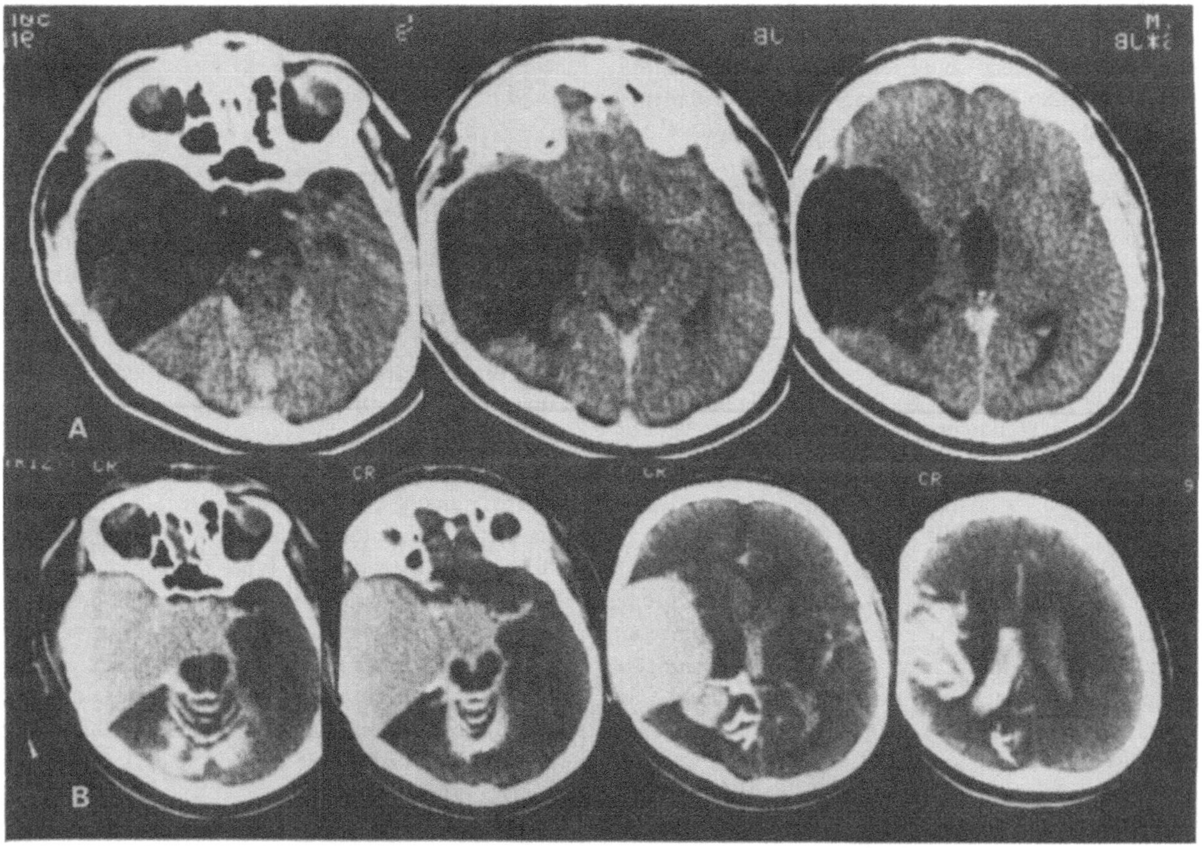

Figure 18. Middle fossa arachnoid cyst in a 21-year-old male with seizure disorder since age 3.

A. Contrast CT. The cyst enlarges the middle fossa. There is no contrast enhancement of its wall.

B. Metrizamide CT. The cyst communicates with the parasellar cistern. The ipsilateral cerebral peduncle is compressed and displaced posteriorly (**arrow**).

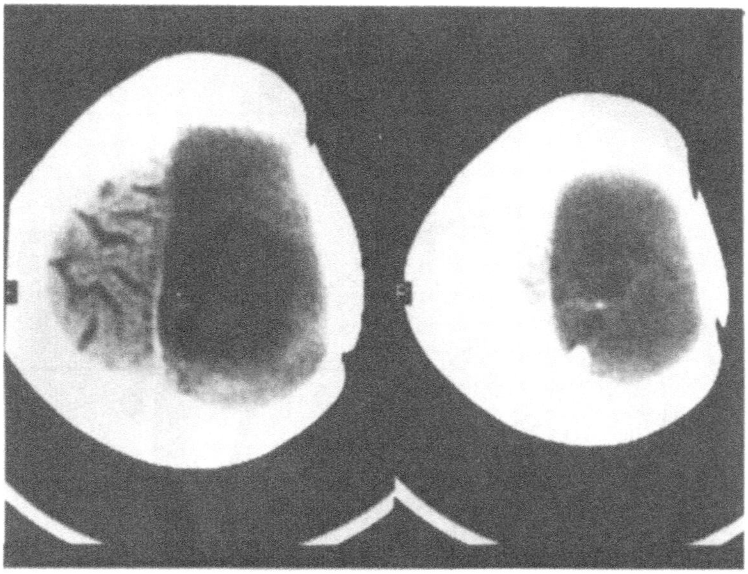

Figure 19. Hemispheric arachnoid cyst in a 13-year-old female. This had been diagnosed soon after birth.

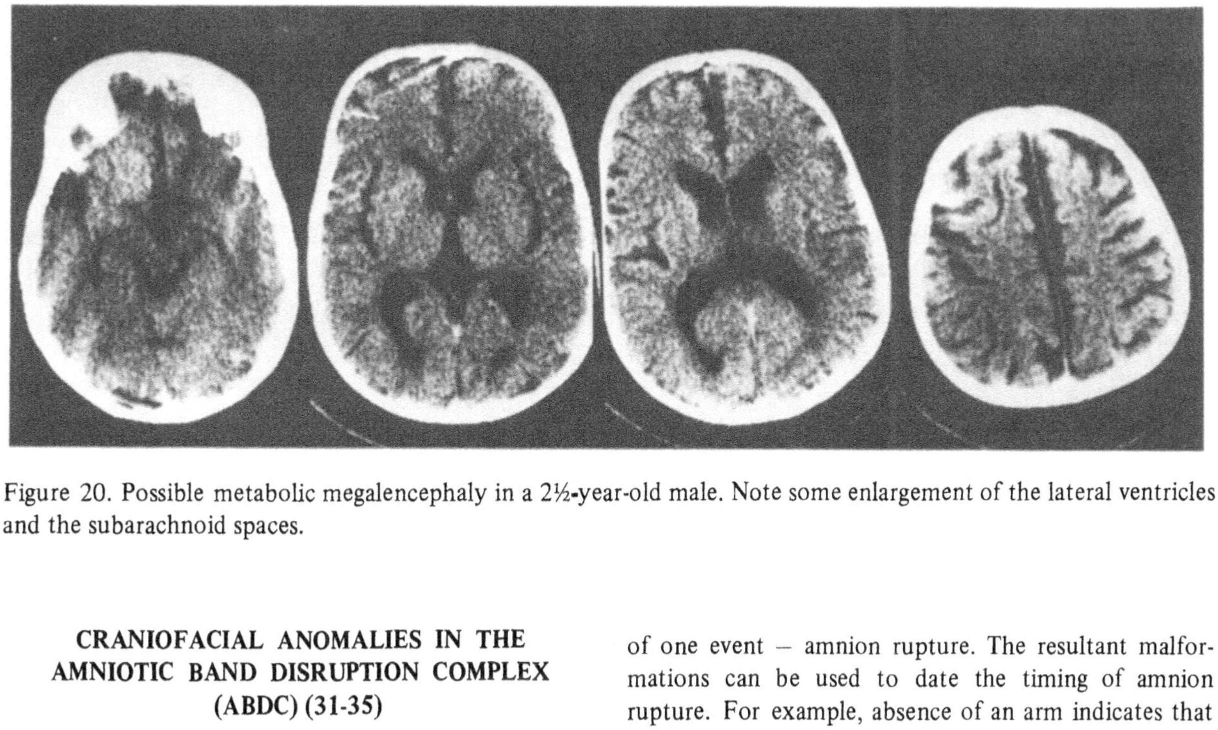

Figure 20. Possible metabolic megalencephaly in a 2½-year-old male. Note some enlargement of the lateral ventricles and the subarachnoid spaces.

CRANIOFACIAL ANOMALIES IN THE AMNIOTIC BAND DISRUPTION COMPLEX (ABDC) (31-35)

The basic premise of this entity, first recognized by Portal in 1685, is that the disruption of the amniotic sac due to an unexplained cause exposes the embryo or the fetus to the extrinsic compressive or constrictive effects of the amniotic bands (Fig. 21). Consequently, the nature and extent of the resulting malformations depend upon the stage of gestation at which the abnormal process occurs. The features of this complex anomaly range from the more common digital band constrictions to severe craniofacial defects, all sequelae of one event – amnion rupture. The resultant malformations can be used to date the timing of amnion rupture. For example, absence of an arm indicates that the amnion ruptured prior to 28 days of gestation, whereas ring constrictions and digit amputations result from later rupture of the amnion. The presence of these bands around the face and/or cranium result in craniofacial anomalies (Fig. 22). Interpositions of these bands between the apposing facial processes results in facial anomalies, such as hypertelorism, cleft lip and/or cleft palate. These facial clefts occur in bizarre, oblique planes that could not have simply resulted from intrinsic failure of the facial processes to appose.

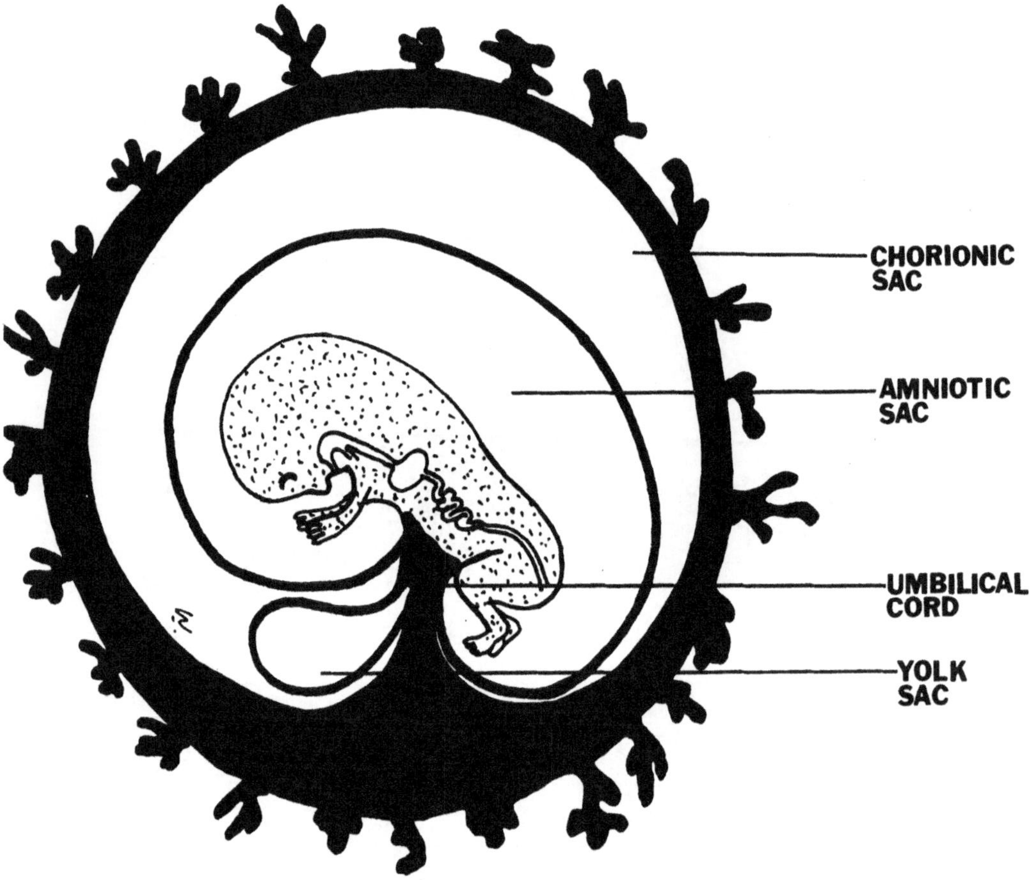

Figure 21. Drawing of a 10-week-old gestation fetus. (redrawn from Moore KL [1973], *The Developing Human,* W.B. Saunders Co., Philadelphia.)

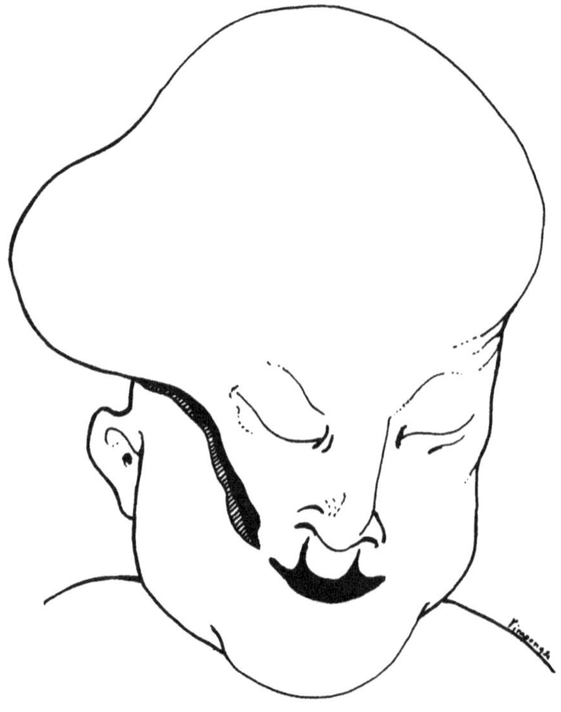

A

Figure 22. Amniotic Band Disruption Complex Syndrome in 2,900 gm, 37 week gestation neonate.

A. Diagrammatic representation of the facial appearance of the neonate. Note the right sided parietal soft tissue mass, the oblique deep facial furrow and the cleft lip.

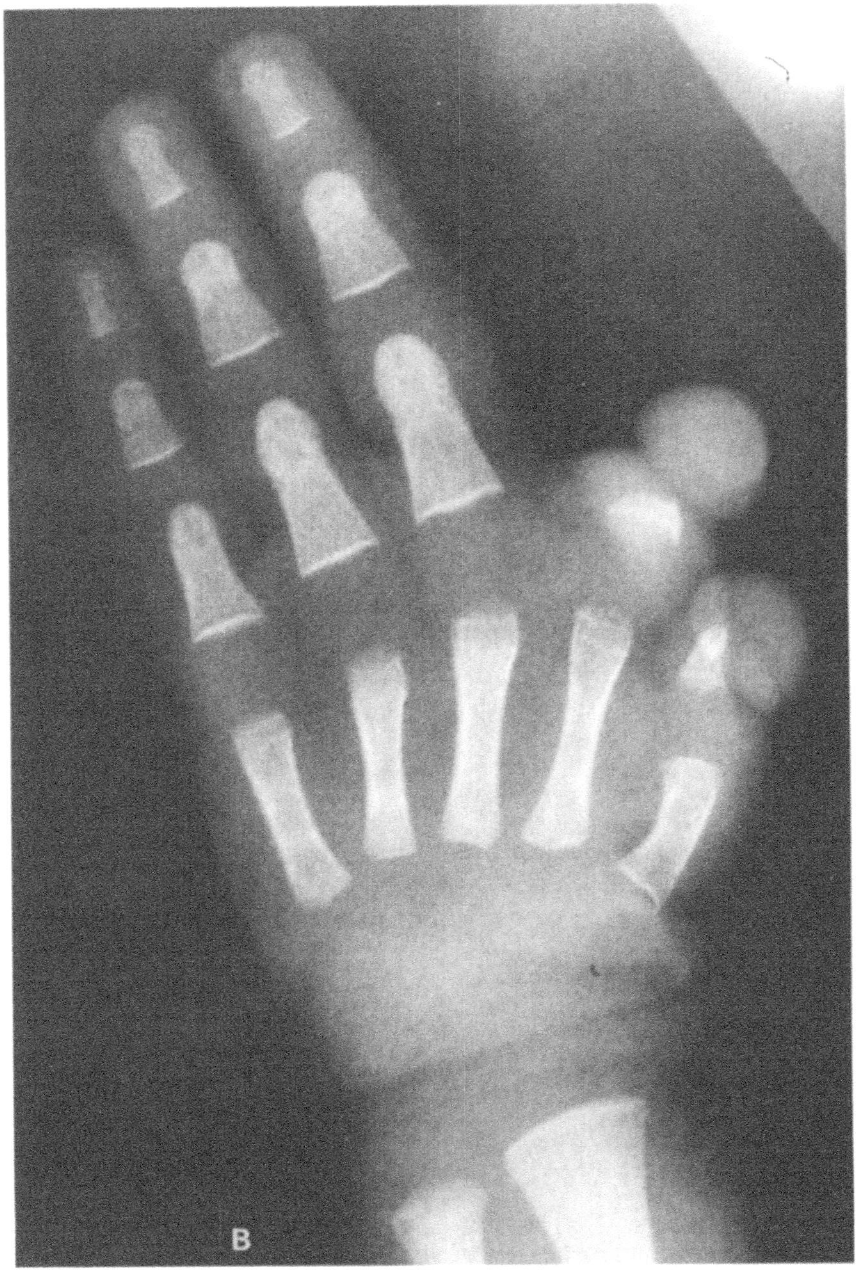

Figure 22. Amniotic Band Disruption Complex Syndrome in 2,900 gm, 37 week gestation neonate.

B. Radiograph of the right hand. Annular bands at the wrist, the thumb, and the index finger can be seen. No bone is present within the digits distal to the constriction deformity.

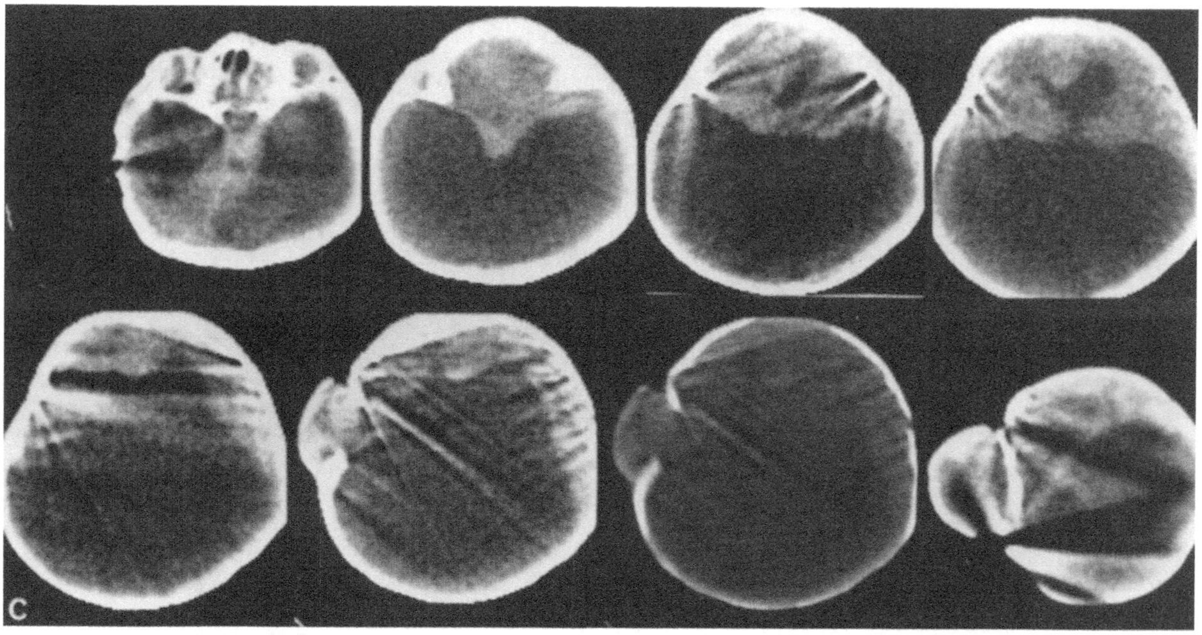

Figure 22. Amniotic Band Disruption Complex Syndrome in 2,900 gm, 37 week gestation neonate.

C. CT Scan. The sequential slices are shown from top left to bottom right. There is massive ventriculomegaly. Defect in the parietal bone and the associated encephalocele are shown.

Affected individuals have a common pathogenetic mechanism but are never quite alike since the timing of amniotic rupture and the extent to which fetal entanglement occurs is variable. There is no increased risk of recurrence in contrast to primary neural tube defects. The clinician and radiologist must recognize a pattern of malformations rather than a specific group of individual defects to identify the ABDC.

ANOMALIES OF THE SEPTUM PELLUCIDUM (36-39)

A. Cavum Septum Pellucidum (CSP)

Cavum septum pellucidum implies an enclosed cerebrospinal fluid (CSF) space between the two leaves of the septum pellucidum (Fig. 23). It usually measures 1 to 2 mm in thickness. Its posterior extension is called cavum vergae (CV); the latter is hardly ever present without the former.

CSP is physiologically present in all fetuses up to 8.5 months of age and 82% of full term neonates (36). This observation explains its very high incidence (at least 80-90%) in CT scans of premature infants. In a CT study of 1,050 infants and children, Nakano *et al.* (37) found that CSP and CV occurred in 10% under one year of age. The incidence gradually decreased with age: it was 5 to 6% at 2 to 5 years, 2.7% at 5 to 9 years, and 2.3% at 10 to 14 years. No statistically valid relationship between the presence of CSP-CV and neurologic dysfunction has been recognized.

B. Absence of Septum Pellucidum

Septum pellucidum may be congenitally absent or be secondarily thinned, and therefore unrecognizable, from increased pressure within hydrocephalic ventricles. It is absent as part of septo-optic dysplasia (de Morsier syndrome) (see Septo-optic Dysplasia for illustration). It also may be absent as part of other developmental defects (38).

C. Cyst of the Septum Pellucidum

When the CSF space between the frontal horns is contained within laterally bulging leaves of the septum pellucidum, it may be termed cyst of the septum pellucidum (Fig. 24). When large enough, it can separate the cloroid plexi of the lateral ventricles and depress the internal cerebral veins that lie on the third ventricle roof (39). It may become symptomatic.

CAVUM VELUM INTERPOSITUM
(Interventricular cavum)

Cavum velum interpositum is an anterior extension of the quadrigeminal cistern, seen most commonly

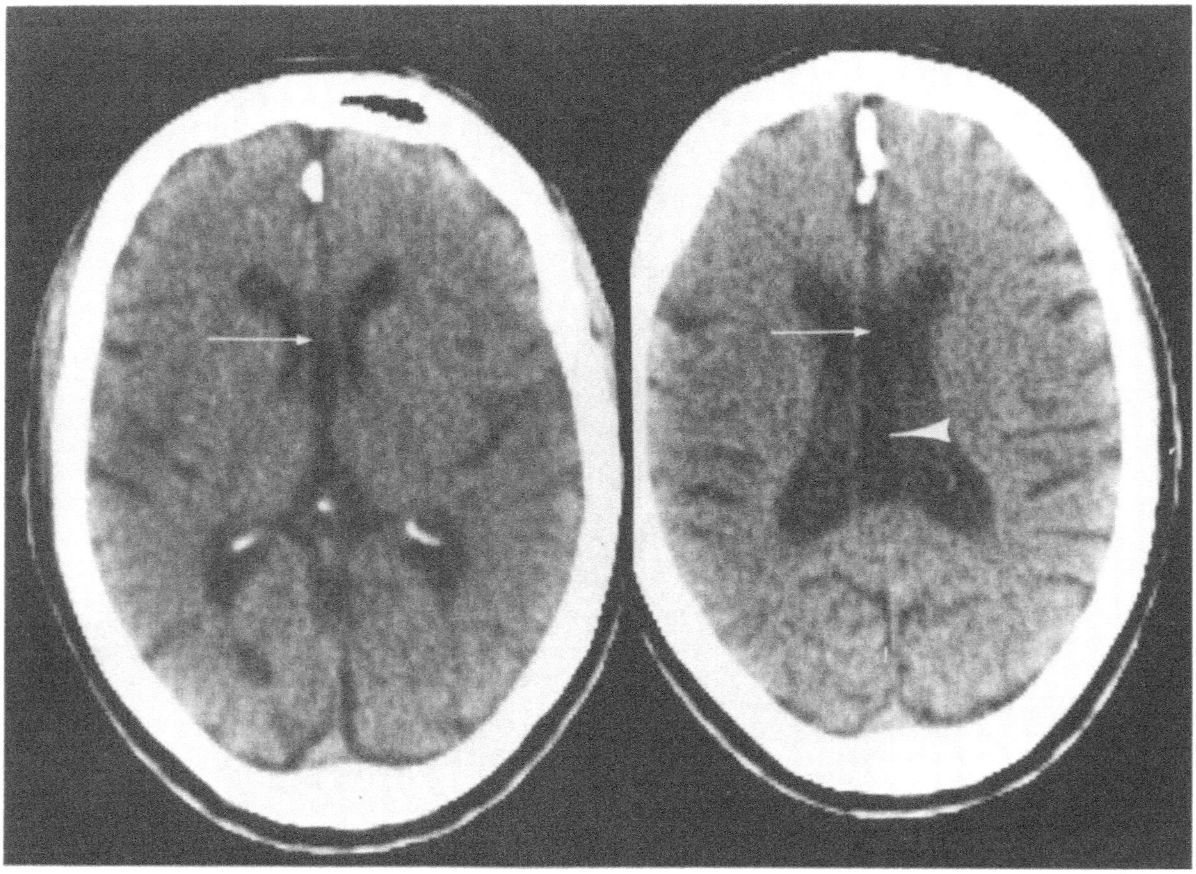

Figure 23. Cavum septum pellucidum **(arrows)** and cavum vergae **(large arrowhead).**

in children. It develops secondary to an unusual separation of crura of the fornix. It is located beneath the corpus callosum and fornices and above the tela chorioidea of the third ventricle. It is bounded anteriorly by the anterior pillars of the fornix. It may be termed a cyst when it is quite prominent. Such an enlargement may be isolated or concomitant with extraventricular obstruction of CSF passages. It is triangular dorsally and narrows anteriorly (Fig. 25). It is of no clinical consequence per se. Its appearance is different from cavum or cyst of the septum pellucidum and cavum vergae as the latter have parallel or laterally bulging borders.

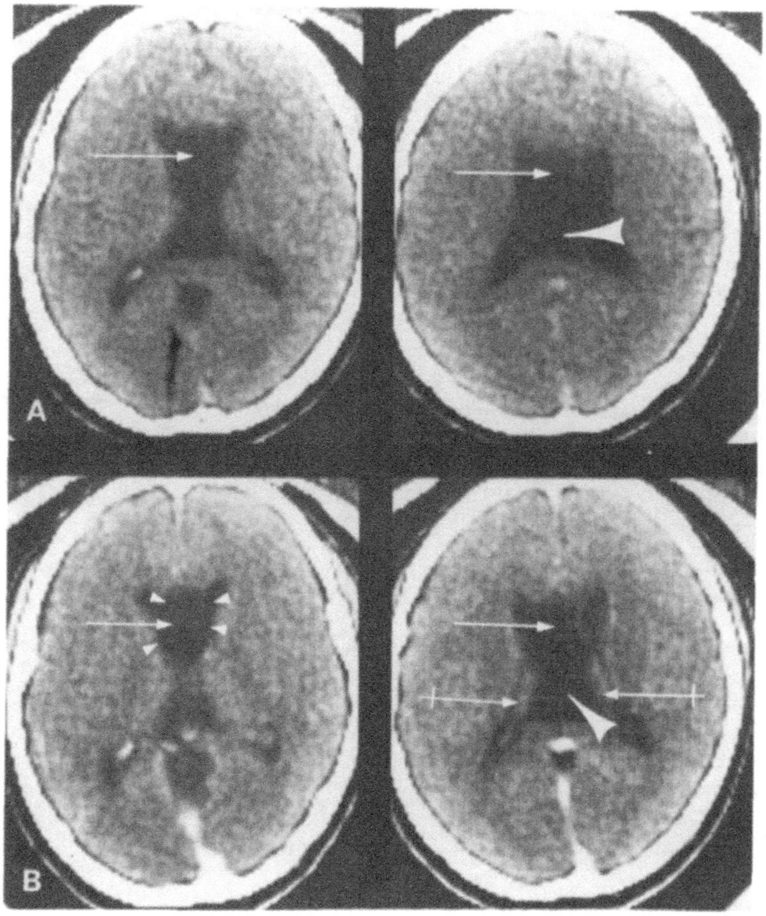

Figure 24. Cyst of the septum pellucidum (**arrows**) and large cavum vergae (**arrowheads**).

A) Non-contrast and B) contrast CT. Note laterally bulging walls of the cyst of the septum pellucidum (**small arrowheads**) and some separation of the choroid plexi (**crossed arrows**).

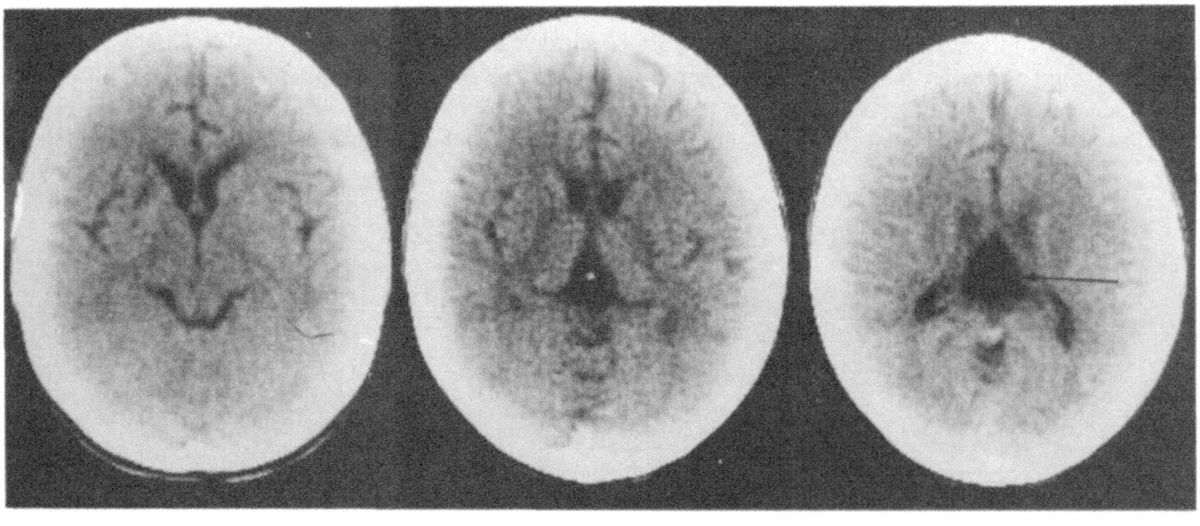

Figure 25. Cavum velum interpositum (**arrow**).

REFERENCES

Encephalocele and Meningoencephalocele

1. Byrd SE, Harwood-Nash DC, Fitz CR, Rogovita DM: Computed tomography in the evaluation of encephaloceles in infants and children. *J Comput Asst Tomogr, 2:*81-87, 1978.
2. Karch SB, Urich H: Occipital encephalocele: a morphological study. *J Neurol Sci, 15:*89, 1972.
3. Rahman N: Nasal encephalocele. *J Neural Sci, 42:*73-85, 1979.
4. Rapport RL, Dunn RC, Alhady F: Anterior encephalocele. *J Neurosurg, 54:*213-219, 1981.
5. Sakoda K, Ishikawa S, Uozumi T, *et al.*: Sphenoethmoidal meningocele associated with agenesis of corpus callosum and medium cleft lip and palate. Case report. *J Neurosurg, 51:*397-401, 1979.
6. Suwanwela C, Hongsprabhas C: Fronto-ethmoidal encephalomeningocele. *J Neurosurg, 25:*172, 1966.
7. Suwanwela C, Suwanwela N: A morphological classification of sincipital encephalomeningoceles. *J Neurosurg, 36:*201, 1972.
8. Van Nouhuys JM, Bruyn GW: Nasopharyngeal transsphenoidal encephalocele, crater like hole in the optic disc and agenesis of the corpus callosum: pneumoencephalographic visualization in a case. *J Psychiatr Neurol Neurochir, 67:*243-258, 1964.

Porencephaly

9. Yakovlev PI, Wadsworth RC: Schizencephalies; study of the congenital clefts in the cerebral mantle. I. Clefts with fused lips. II. Clefts with hydrocephalus and lips separated. *J Neuropathol Exp Neurol, 5:*116, 169, 1946.
10. Tardieu M, Eurad P, Lyon A: Progressive expanding congenital porencephalies: A treatable cause of progressive encephalopathy. *Pediatrics, 68:*198-202, 1981.
11. Ramsey RG, Huckman MS: Computed tomography of porencephaly and other cerebrospinal fluid-containing lesions. *Radiology, 123:*73-77, 1977.

Micrencephaly

12. Coffey VP, Jessop WJE: Study of 137 cases of anencephaly. *Br J Prevent and Soc Med, 11:*174-189, 1957.

Median Cleft Face Syndrome

13. DeMyer W: The median cleft face syndrome. Differential diagnosis of cranium bifidum ococultum, hypertelorism, and median cleft nose, lip, and palate. *Neurology, 17:*961-971, 1967.
14. Kurlander GJ, DeMyer W, Campbell JA: Roentgenology of the median cleft face syndrome. *Radiology, 88:*473-478, 1967.
15. Currarino G, Silverman FN: Orbital hypotelorism, arhinencephaly and trigonocephaly. *Radiology, 74:*206-217, 1960.

Lissencephaly

16. Chi JG, Dooling EC, Gilles FH: Gyral development of the human brain. *Ann Neurol, 1:*86-93, 1977.
17. Dieker H, Edwards RH, zu Rhein G, *et al.*: The lissencephaly syndrome. Birth defects: *Orig Art Ser, 5/2:*53-64, 1969.
18. Garcia CA, Dunn D, Trevor R: The lissencephaly (agyria) syndrome in siblings: Computerized tomographic and neuropathologic finds. *Arch Neurol, 35:*608-611, 1978.
19. Ohno K, Enomoto T, Imamoto J, *et al.*: Lissencephaly (agyria) on computed tomography. *J Comput Asst Tomogr, 3:*92-95, 1979.
20. Wesenberg RL, Juhl JH, Daube RJ: Radiological findings in lissencephaly (congenital agyria). *Radiology, 87:*437-445, 1966.

Colpocephaly

21. Benda CE: Microcephaly. *Am J Psychiat, 97:* 1135-1146, 1940.
22. Garg BP: Colpocephaly. An error of morphogenesis? *Arch Neurol, 39:*243-246, 1982.
23. Yakovlev PI, Wadsworth RC: Schizencephalies: A study of the congenital clefts in the cerebral mantle: 1. clefts with fused lips. *J Neuropathol Exp Neurol, 5:*116-130, 1946.

Fetal Alcohol Syndrome

24. Clarren SK: Recognition of fetal alcohol syndrome. *JAMA, 245:*2435-2439, 1981.
25. Clarren SK, Alvord EC, Sumi SM, *et al.*: Brain malformations related to prenatal exposure to ethanol. *J Pediatr, 90:* 630-633, 1978.
26. O'Shea KS, Kaufman MH: The teratogenic effect of acetaldehyde: Implications for the study of the fetal alcohol syndrome. *J Anat, 128:*65-76, 1979.

Arachnoid Cyst

27. Robinson RG: Congenital cysts of the brain: arachnoid malformations. *Prog Neurol Surg, 4:*133, 1971.
28. Galassi E, Tognetti F, Gaist G, *et al.*: CT scan and metrizamide CT cisternography in arachnoid cysts of the middle cranial fossa: Classification and pathophysiological aspects. *Surg Neurol, 17:* 363-769, 1982.

Megalencephaly

29. Fletcher HM: A case of megalencephaly. *Trans Pathol Soc London, 51:*230, 1900.
30. DeMyer W: Megalencephaly in children. Clinical syndromes, genetic patterns and differential diagnosis from other causes of megalocephaly. *Neurology, 22:*634, 1972.

Amniotic Band Disruption Complex Syndrome

31. Portal P: (1685) *LaPratique des accouchements.* Paris
32. Ossipoff V, Hall BD: Etiologic factors in amniotic band syndrome: a study of 24 patients. *Birth Defects, 13:*117, 1977.
33. Higginbottom MC, Jones KL, Hall BD, Smith DW: The amniotic band disruption complex: timing of amniotic rupture and variable spectra of consequent defects. *J Pediat, 95:*544, 1979.
34. Carter CO, Oxon DM: The risk of recurrence after two children with central-nervous-syndrome malformations. *Lancet, 1:*306, 1967.
35. Jones KL, Smith DW, Hall BD, Hall JG, Ebbin AJ, Massoud H, Golbus M: A pattern of craniofacial and limb defects secondary to aberrant tissue bands. *J Pediat, 84:*90, 1974.

Cavum and Cyst Septum Pellucidum and Cavum Velum Interposition

36. Larroche JC, Baudey J: Cavum septi lucidi, cavum vergea, cavum veli interpositi: cavites de la ligne mediane. *Biol Neonat, 3:*193-236, 1961.
37. Nakano S, Hojo H, Kataoka K, Yamasaki S: Age related incidence of cavum septi pellucidi and cavum vergae on CT scans of pediatric patients. *J Comput Asst Tomogr, 5:*348-349, 1981.
38. Aicardi J, Goutieresa F: The syndrome of absence of the septum pellucidum with porencephalies and other developmental defects. *Neuropediat, 12:* 319-329, 1981.
39. Cowley AR, Moody DM, Alexander E, Jr., Ball MR, Laster DW: Distinctive CT appearance of cyst of the cavum septi pellucidi. *AJR, 133:*548-550, 1979.

Index

GPSR Compliance

The European Union's (EU) General Product Safety Regulation (GPSR) is a set of rules that requires consumer products to be safe and our obligations to ensure this.

If you have any concerns about our products, you can contact us on ProductSafety@springernature.com

In case Publisher is established outside the EU, the EU authorized representative is:

Springer Nature Customer Service Center GmbH
Europaplatz 3
69115 Heidelberg, Germany

Batch number: 10816838

Printed by Printforce, the Netherlands